T0144755

Handbook of Regression and Modeling

Applications for the Clinical and Pharmaceutical Industries

Handbook of Regression and Modeling

Applications for the Clinical and Pharmaceutical Industries

Daryl S. Paulson

BioScience Laboratories, Inc.

Bozeman, Montana, U.S.A.

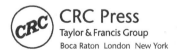

CRC Press
Taylor & Francis Group
Boca Raton London New York

CRC Press is an imprint of the
Taylor & Francis Group, an **informa** business

A CHAPMAN & HALL BOOK

CRC Press
Taylor & Francis Group
6000 Broken Sound Parkway NW, Suite 300
Boca Raton, FL 33487-2742

First issued in paperback 2022

© 2007 by Taylor & Francis Group, LLC
CRC is an imprint of Taylor & Francis Group, an Informa business

No claim to original U.S. Government works

ISBN 13: 978-1-03-247785-5 (pbk)
ISBN 13: 978-1-57444-610-4 (hbk)

DOI: 10.1201/9781420017380

Library of Congress Cataloging-in-Publication Data

Paulson, Daryl S., 1947-
    Handbook of regression and modeling : applications for the clinical and pharmaceutical industries / Daryl S. Paulson.
        p. ; cm. -- (Biostatistics ; 18)
    Includes index.
    ISBN-13: 978-1-57444-610-4 (hardcover : alk. paper)
    ISBN-10: 1-57444-610-X (hardcover : alk. paper)
    1. Medicine--Research--Statistical methods--Handbooks, manuals, etc. 2. Regression analysis--Handbooks, manuals, etc. 3. Drugs--Research--Statistical methods--Handbooks, manuals, etc. 4. Clinical trials--Statistical methods--Handbooks, manuals, etc. I. Title. II. Series: Biostatistics (New York, N.Y.) ; 18.
    [DNLM: 1. Clinical Medicine. 2. Regression Analysis. 3. Biometry--methods. 4. Drug Industry. 5. Models, Statistical. WA 950 P332h 2007]

R853.S7P35 2007
610.72'7--dc22   2006030225

Visit the Taylor & Francis Web site at
http://www.taylorandfrancis.com

and the CRC Press Web site at
http://www.crcpress.com

Preface

In 2003, I wrote a book, *Applied Statistical Designs for the Researcher* (Marcel Dekker, Inc.), in which I covered experimental designs commonly encountered in the pharmaceutical, applied microbiological, and healthcare-product-formulation industries. It included two sample evaluations, analysis of variance, factorial, nested, chi-square, exploratory data analysis, nonparametric statistics, and a chapter on linear regression. Many researchers need more than simple linear regression methods to meet their research needs. It is for those researchers that this regression analysis book is written.

Chapter 1 is an overview of statistical methods and elementary concepts for statistical model building.

Chapter 2 covers simple linear regression applications in detail.

Chapter 3 deals with a problem that many applied researchers face when collecting data of time–serial correlation (the actual response values of y are correlated with one another). This chapter lays the foundation for the discussion on multiple regression in Chapter 8.

Chapter 4 introduces multiple linear regression procedures and matrix algebra. The knowledge of matrix algebra is not a prerequisite, and Appendix II presents the basics in matrix manipulation. Matrix notation is used because those readers without specific statistical software that contains "canned" statistical programs can still perform the statistical analyses presented in this book. However, I assume that the reader will perform most of the computations using statistical software such as SPSS, SAS, or MiniTab. This chapter also covers strategies for checking the contribution of each x_i variable in a regression equation to assure that it is actually contributing. Partial F-tests are used in stepwise, forward selection, and backward elimination procedures.

Chapter 5 focuses on aspects of correlation analysis and those of determining the contribution of x_i variables using partial correlation analysis.

Chapter 6 discusses common problems encountered in multiple linear regression and the ways to deal with them. One problem is multiple collinearity, in which some of the x_i variables are correlated with other x_i variables and the regression equation becomes unstable in applied work. A number of procedures are explained to deal with such problems and a biasing method called ridge regression is also discussed.

Chapter 7 describes aspects of polynomial regression and its uses.

Chapter 8 aids the researcher in determining outlier values of the variables y and x. It also includes residual analysis schemas, such as standardized, Studentized, and jackknife residual analyses. Another important feature of this chapter is leverage value identification, or identifying values, ys and xs, that have undue influence.

Chapter 9 applies indicator or dummy variables to an assortment of analyses.

Chapter 10 presents forward and stepwise selections of x_i variables, as well as backward elimination, in terms of statistical software.

Chapter 11 introduces covariance analysis, which combines regression and analysis of variance into one model.

The concepts presented in this book have been used for the past 25 years, in the clinical trials and new product development and formulation areas at BioScience Laboratories, Inc. They have also been used in analyzing data supporting studies submitted to the Food and Drug Administration (FDA) and the Environmental Protection Agency (EPA), and in my work as a statistician for the Association of Analytical Chemists (AOAC) in projects related to EPA regulation and Homeland Security.

This book has been two years in the making, from my standpoint. Certainly, it has not been solely an individual process on my part. I thank my friend and colleague, John A. Mitchell, PhD, also known as doctor for his excellent and persistent editing of this book, in spite of his many other duties at BioScience Laboratories, Inc. I also thank Tammy Anderson, my assistant, for again managing the entire manuscript process of this book, which is her sixth one for me. I also want to thank Marsha Paulson, my wife, for stepping up to the plate and helping us with the grueling final edit.

Daryl S. Paulson, PhD

Author

Daryl S. Paulson is the president and chief executive officer of BioScience Laboratories, Inc., Bozeman, Montana. Previously, he was the manager of laboratory services at Skyland Scientific Services (1987–1991), Belgrade, Montana. A developer of statistical models for clinical trials of drugs and cosmetics, he is the author of more than 40 articles on clinical evaluations, software validations, solid dosage validations, and quantitative management science. In addition, he has also authored several books, including *Topical Antimicrobial Testing and Evaluation*, the *Handbook of Topical Antimicrobials, Applied Statistical Designs for the Researcher* (Marcel Dekker, Inc.), *Competitive Business, Caring Business: An Integral Business Perspective for the 21st Century* (Paraview Press), and *The Handbook of Regression Analysis* (Taylor & Francis Group). Currently, his books *Biostatistics and Microbiology: A Survival Manual* (Springer Group) and the *Handbook of Applied Biomedical Microbiology: A Biofilms Approach* (Taylor & Francis Group) are in progress. He is a member of the American Society for Microbiology, the American Society for Testing and Materials, the Association for Practitioners in Infection Control, the American Society for Quality Control, the American Psychological Association, the American College of Forensic Examiners, and the Association of Analytical Chemists.

Dr. Paulson received a BA (1972) in business administration and an MS (1981) in medical microbiology and biostatistics from the University of Montana, Missoula. He also received a PhD (1988) in psychology from Sierra University, Riverside, California; a PhD (1992) in psychoneuro-immunology from Saybrook Graduate School and Research Center, San Francisco, California; an MBA (2002) from the University of Montana, Missoula; and a PhD in art from Warnborough University, United Kingdom. He is currently working toward a PhD in both psychology and statistics and performs statistical services for the AOAC and the Department of Homeland Security.

Series Introduction

The primary objectives of the *Biostatistics Book Series* are to provide useful reference books for researchers and scientists in academia, industry, and government, and also to offer textbooks for undergraduate and graduate courses in the area of biostatistics. This book series will provide comprehensive and unified presentations of statistical designs and analyses of important applications in biostatistics, such as those in biopharmaceuticals. A well-balanced summary is given of current and recently developed statistical methods, and interpretations for both statisticians and researchers or scientists with minimal statistical knowledge and engaged in the field of applied biostatistics. The series is committed to providing easy-to-understand, state-of-the-art references and textbooks. In each volume, statistical concepts and methodologies are illustrated through real-world examples.

Regression and modeling are commonly employed in pharmaceutical research and development. The purpose is not only to provide a valid and fair assessment of the pharmaceutical entity under investigation before regulatory approval, but also to assure that the pharmaceutical entity possesses good characteristics with the desired accuracy and reliability. In addition, it is to establish a predictive model for identifying patients who are most likely to respond to the test treatment under investigation. This volume is a condensation of various useful statistical methods that are commonly employed in pharmaceutical research and development. It covers important topics in pharmaceutical research and development such as multiple linear regression, model building or model selection, and analysis of covariance. This handbook provides useful approaches to pharmaceutical research and development. It would be beneficial to biostatisticians, medical researchers, and pharmaceutical scientists who are engaged in the areas of pharmaceutical research and development.

Shein-Chung Chow

Table of Contents

1 Basic Statistical Concepts

The use of statistics in clinical and pharmaceutical settings is extremely common. Because the data are generally collected under experimental conditions that result in measurements containing a certain amount of error,* statistical analyses, though not perfect, are the most effective way of making sense of the data. The situation is often portrayed as

$$T = t + e.$$

Here, the true but unknown value of a measurement, T, consists of a sample measurement, t, and random error or variation, e. Statistical error is considered to be the random variability inherent in any system, not a mistake. For example, the incubation temperature of bacteria in an incubator might have a normal random fluctuation of $\pm 1°C$, which is considered a statistical error. A timer might have an inherent fluctuation of ± 0.01 sec for each minute of actual time. Statistical analysis enables the researcher to account for this random error.

Fundamental to statistical measurement are two basic parameters: the population mean, μ, and the population standard deviation, σ. The population parameters are generally unknown and are estimated by the sample mean, $\bar{x}$, and sample standard deviation, s. The sample mean is simply the central tendency of a sample set of data that is an unbiased estimate of the population mean, μ. The central tendency is the sum of values in a set, or population, of numbers divided by the number of values in that set or population. For example, for the sample set of values 10, 13, 19, 9, 11, and 17, the sum is 79. When 79 is divided by the number of values in the set, 6, the average is $79 \div 6 = 13.17$. The statistical formula for average is

$$\bar{x} = \frac{\sum_{i=1}^{n} x_i}{n},$$

---

*Statistical error is not a wrong measurement or a mistaken measurement. It is, instead, a representation of uncertainty concerning random fluctuations.

where the operator, $\sum_{i=1}^{n} x_i$, means to sum (add) the values beginning with $i = 1$ and ending with the value n; where n is the sample size.

The standard deviation for the population is written as σ, and for a sample as s.

$$\sigma = \sqrt{\frac{\sum\limits_{i=1}^{n} (x_i - \mu)^2}{N}},$$

where $\sum_{i=1}^{n} (x_i - \mu)^2$ is the sum of the actual x_i values minus the population mean, the quantities squared; and N the total population size.

The sample standard deviation is given by

$$s = \sqrt{\frac{\sum\limits_{i=1}^{n} (x_i - \bar{x})^2}{n - 1}},$$

where $\sum_{i=1}^{n} (x_i - \bar{x})^2$ is the sum of the actual sample values minus the sample mean, the quantities squared; and $n - 1$ is the sample size minus 1, to account for the loss of one degree of freedom from estimating μ by $\bar{x}$. Note that the standard deviation σ or s is the square root of the variance σ^2 or s^2.

MEANING OF STANDARD DEVIATION

The standard deviation provides a measure of variability about the mean or average value. If two data sets have the same mean, but their data range differ,* so will their standard deviations. The larger the range, the larger the standard deviation.

For instance, using our previous example, the six data points—10, 13, 19, 9, 11, and 17—have a range of $19 - 9 = 10$. The standard deviation is calculated as

$$\sqrt{\frac{(10-13.1667)^2+(13-13.1667)^2+(19-13.1667)^2+(9-13.1667)^2+(11-13.1667)^2+(17-13.1667)^2}{6-1}}$$

$$= 4.0208.$$

Suppose the values were 1, 7, 11, 3, 28, and 29,

$$\bar{x} = \frac{1 + 7 + 11 + 3 + 28 + 29}{6} = 13.1667.$$

---

*Range = maximum value − minimum value.

The range is $29 - 1 = 28$, and the standard deviation is

$$\sqrt{\frac{(1 - 13.1667)^2 + (7 - 13.1667)^2 + (11 - 13.1667)^2 + (3 - 13.1667)^2 + (28 - 13.1667)^2 + (29 - 13.1667)^2}{6 - 1}}$$

$= 12.3680.$

Given a sample set is normally distributed,* the standard deviation has a very useful property, in that one knows where the data points reside. The mean ± 1 standard deviation encompasses 68% of the data set. The mean ± 2 standard deviations encompass about 95% of the data. The mean ± 3 standard deviations encompass about 99.7% of the data. For a more in-depth discussion of this, see D.S. Paulson, *Applied Statistical Designs for the Researcher* (Marcel Dekker, 2003, pp. 21–34).

In this book, we restrict our analyses to data sets that approximate the normal distribution. Fortunately, as sample size increases, even nonnormal populations tend to become normal-like, at least in the distribution of their error terms, $e = (y_i - \bar{y})$, about the value 0. Formally, this was known as the central limit theorem, which states that in simulation and real-world conditions, the error terms e become more normally distributed as the sample size increases (Paulson, 2003). The error itself, random fluctuation about the predicted value (mean), is usually composed of multiple unknown influences, not just one.

HYPOTHESIS TESTING

In statistical analysis, often a central objective is to evaluate a claim made about a specific population. A statistical hypothesis consists of two mutually exclusive, dichotomous statements of which one will be accepted and the other rejected (Lapin, 1977; Salsburg, 1992).

The first of the dichotomous statements is the test hypothesis, also known as the alternative hypothesis (H_A). It always hypothesizes the results of a statistical test to be significant (greater than, less than, or not equal). For example, the test of the significance (alternative hypothesis) of a regression function may be that β_1 (the slope) is not equal to 0 ($\beta_1 \neq 0$). The null hypothesis (H_0, the hypothesis of no effect) would state the opposite that $\beta_1 = 0$. In significance testing, it is generally easier to state the alternative hypothesis first and then the null hypothesis. Restricting ourselves to two sample groups (e.g., test vs. control or group A vs. group B), any of the three basic conditions of hypothesis tests can be employed—an upper-tail, a lower-tail, or a two-tail condition.

---

*A normally distributed set of data are symmetrical about the mean, and the mean = mode = median at one central peak, a bell-shaped or Gaussian distribution.

Upper-Tail Test

The alternative or test hypothesis H_A asserts that one test group is larger in value than the other in terms of a parameter, such as the mean or the slope of a regression. For example, the slope (β_1) of one regression function is larger than that of another.* The null hypothesis H_0 states that the test group value is less than or equal to that of the other test group or the control. The upper-tail statements written for comparative slopes of regression, for example, would be as follows:

H_0: $\beta_1 \leq \beta_2$ (the slope β_1 is less than or equal to β_2 in rate value),
H_A: $\beta_1 > \beta_2$ (the slope β_1 is greater than β_2 in rate value).

Lower-Tail Test

For the lower-tail test, the researcher claims that a certain group's parameter of interest is less than that of the other. Hence, the alternative hypothesis states that $\beta_1 < \beta_2$. The null hypothesis is stated in the opposite direction with the equality symbol:

H_0: $\beta_1 \geq \beta_2$ (the slope β_1 is equal to or greater than β_2 in rate value),
H_A: $\beta_1 < \beta_2$ (the slope of β_1 is less than β_2 in rate value).

Two-Tail Test

A two-tail test is used to determine if a difference exists between the two groups in a parameter of interest, either larger or smaller. The null hypothesis states that there is no such difference.

H_0: $\beta_1 = \beta_2$ (the slope β_1 equals β_2),
H_A: $\beta_1 \neq \beta_2$ (the two slopes differ).

Hypothesis tests are never presented as absolute statements, but as probability statements, generally for alpha or type I error. Alpha (α) error is the probability of accepting an untrue alternative hypothesis; that is, rejecting the null hypothesis when it is, in fact, true. For example, concluding one drug is better than another when, in fact, it is not. The alpha error level is a researcher's set probability value, such as $\alpha = 0.05$, or 0.10, or 0.01. Setting alpha at 0.05 means that, over repeated testing, a type I error would be made 5 times out of 100 times. The probability is never in terms of a particular trial, but over the long run. Unwary researchers may try to protect themselves from committing

---

*The upper- and lower-tail tests can also be used to compare data from one sample group to a fixed number, such as 0 in the test: $\beta_1 \neq 0$.

this error by setting α at a smaller level, say 0.01; that is, the probability of committing a type I error is 1 time in 100 experiments, over the long run. However, reducing the probability of type I error generally creates another problem. When the probability of type I (α) error is reduced by setting α at a smaller value, the probability of type II or beta (β) error will increase, with all the other things equal. Type II or beta error is the probability of rejecting an alternative hypothesis when it is true—for example, stating that there is no difference in drugs or treatments when there really is.

Consider the case of antibiotics, in which a new drug and a standard drug are compared. If the new antibiotic is compared with the standard one for antimicrobial effectiveness, a type I (α) error is committed if the researcher concludes that the new antibiotic is more effective than the old one, when it is actually not. Type II (β) error occurs if the researcher concludes that the new antibiotic is not better than the standard one, when it really is.

For a given sample size n, alpha and beta errors are inversely related in that, as one reduces the α error rate, one increases the β error rate, and vice versa. If one wishes to reduce the possibility of both types of errors, one must increase n. In many medical and pharmaceutical experiments, the alpha level is set by convention at 0.05 and beta at 0.20 (Sokal and Rohlf, 1994; Riffenburg, 2006). The power of a statistic $(1 - \beta)$ is its ability to reject both false alternative and null hypotheses; that is, to make correct decisions.

True Condition	Accept H_0	Reject H_0
H_0 true	Correct decision	Type I error
H_0 false	Type II error	Correct decision

There are several ways to reduce both type I and type II errors available to researchers. First, one can select a more powerful statistical method that reduces the error term by blocking, for example. This is usually a major goal for researchers and a primary reason they plan the experimental phase of a study in great detail. Second, as mentioned earlier, a researcher can increase the sample size. An increase in the sample size tends to reduce type II error, when holding type I error constant; that is, if the alpha error is set at 0.05, increasing the sample size generally will reduce the rate of beta error.

Random variability of the experimental data plays a major role in the power and detection levels of a statistic. The smaller the variance s^2, the greater the power of any statistical test. The lesser the variability, the smaller the value s^2 and the greater the detection level of the statistic. An effective way to determine if the power of a specific statistic is adequate for the researcher is to compute the detection limit δ. The detection limit simply informs the researcher how sensitive the test is by stating what the difference needs to be between test groups to state that a significant difference exists.

To prevent undue frustration for a researcher, to perform a hypothesis test in this book, we use a six-step procedure to simplify the statistical testing process. If the readers desire a basic introduction to hypothesis testing, they can consult *Applied Statistical Designs for the Researcher* (Marcel Dekker, 2003, pp. 35–47). The six steps to hypothesis testing are as follows:

Step 1: Formulate the hypothesis statement, which consists of the null (H_0) and alternative (H_A) hypotheses. Begin with the alternative hypothesis. For example, the slope β_1 is greater in value than the slope β_2; that is, H_A: $\beta_1 > \beta_2$. On the other hand, the $\log_{10}$ microbial reductions for formula MP1 are less than those for MP2; that is, H_A: MP1 $<$ MP2. Alternatively, the absorption rate of antimicrobial product A is different from that of antimicrobial product B; that is, H_A: product A $\neq$ product B.

Once the alternative hypothesis is determined, the null hypothesis can be written, which is the opposite of the H_A hypothesis, with the addition of equality. Constructing the null hypothesis after the alternative is often easier for the researcher. If H_A is an upper-tail test, such as A is greater than B, then H_A: A $>$ B. The null hypothesis is written as A is equal to or less than B; that is, H_0: A $\leq$ B. If H_A is a lower-tail test, then H_0 is an upper-tail with an equality:

H_A: A $<$ B,
H_0: A $\geq$ B.

If H_A is a two-tail test, where two groups are considered to differ, the null hypothesis is that of equivalence:

H_A: A $\neq$ B,
H_0: A $=$ B.

By convention, the null hypothesis is the lead or first hypothesis presented in the hypothesis statement; so formally, the hypothesis tests are written as

Upper-Tail Test:
H_0: A $\leq$ B,
H_A: A $>$ B.

Lower-Tail Test:
H_0: A $\geq$ B,
H_A: A $<$ B.

Two-Tail Test:
H_0: A $=$ B,
H_A: A $\neq$ B.

Note that an upper-tail test can be written as a lower-tail test, and a lower-tail test can be written as an upper-tail test simply by reversing the order of the test groups.

Upper-Tail Test		Lower-Tail Test
H_0: A $\leq$ B		H_0: B $\geq$ A
	=	
H_A: A $>$ B		H_A: B $<$ A

Step 2: Establish the α level and the sample size n. The α level is generally set at $\alpha = 0.05$. This is by convention and really depends on the research goals. The sample size of the test groups is often a specific preset number. The sample size ideally should be determined based on the required detectable difference δ an established β level and an estimate of the sample variance s^2. For example, in a clinical setting, one may determine that a detection level is adequate if the statistic can detect a 10% change in serum blood levels; for a drug stability study, detection of a 20% change in drug potency may be acceptable; and in an antimicrobial time-kill study, a ± 0.5 $\log_{10}$ detection level may be adequate.

Beta error (β), the probability of rejecting a true H_A hypothesis, is often set at 0.20, again, by convention. The variance (s^2) is generally estimated based on prior experimentation. For example, the standard deviation in a surgical scrub evaluation for normal resident flora populations on human subjects is about 0.5 $\log_{10}$; thus, 0.5^2 is a reasonable variance estimate. If no prior variance levels have been collected, it must be estimated, ideally, by means of a pilot study.

Often, two sample groups are contrasted. In this case, the joint standard deviation must be computed. For example, assume that $s_1^2 = 0.70$ and $s_2^2 = 0.81$ $\log_{10}$, representing the variances of group 1 and group 2 data. An easy and conservative way of doing this is to compute $\hat{s} = \sqrt{s_1^2 + s_2^2}$ or $\sqrt{0.70 + 0.81} = 1.23$, the estimated joint standard deviation. If one wants, say a detection level (δ) of 0.5 $\log_{10}$ and sets $\alpha = 0.05$ and $\beta = 0.20$, a rough sample size computation is given by

$$n \geq \frac{ms^2(Z_{\alpha/2} + Z_\beta)^2}{\delta^2},$$

where n is the sample size for each of the sample groups; m is the number of groups to be compared, $m = 2$ in this example; s^2 is the estimate of the common variance. Suppose here $s^2 = (1.23)^2$; $Z_{\alpha/2}$ is the normal tabled value for α. Suppose $\alpha = 0.05$, then $\alpha/2 = 0.025$, so $Z_{\alpha/2} = 1.96$, from the standard normal distribution table (Table A); Z_β is the normal tabled value for β. Suppose $\beta = 0.20$, then $Z_\beta = 0.842$, from the standard normal distribution table; δ is the detection level, say ± 0.5 $\log_{10}$.

TABLE 1.1
Three Possible Hypothesis Test Conditions

Lower-Tail Test	**Upper-Tail Test**	**Two-Tail Test**
H_0: A $\geq$ B	H_0: A $\leq$ B	H_0: A $=$ B
H_A: A $<$ B	H_A: A $>$ B	H_A: A $\neq$ B
Visual	Visual	Visual

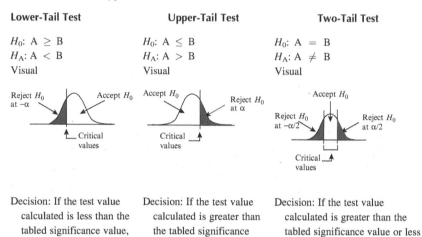

Decision: If the test value calculated is less than the tabled significance value, reject H_0.	Decision: If the test value calculated is greater than the tabled significance value, reject H_0.	Decision: If the test value calculated is greater than the tabled significance value or less than the tabled significance value, reject H_0.

The sample size estimation is

$$n \geq \frac{2(1.23)^2(1.96 + 0.842)^2}{0.5^2} = 95.02.$$

Hence, $n \geq 95$ subjects each of the two groups at $\alpha = 0.05$, $\beta = 0.20$, and $\hat{s} = 1.23$. The test can detect a 0.5 $\log_{10}$ difference between the two groups.

Step 3: Next, the researcher selects the statistic to be used. In this book, the statistics used are parametric ones.

Step 4: The decision rule is next determined. Recall the three possible hypothesis test conditions as shown in Table 1.1.

Step 5: Collect the sample data by running the experiment.

Step 6: Apply the decision rule (Step 4) to the null hypothesis, accepting or rejecting it at the specified α level.*

---

*Some researchers do not report the set α value, but instead use a p value so that the readers can make their own test significance conclusions. The p value is defined as the probability of observing the computed significance test value or a larger one, if the H_0 hypothesis is true. For example, $P[t \geq 2.1 \mid H_0 \; true] \leq 0.047$. The probability of observing a t-calculated value of 2.1, or a more extreme value, given the H_0 hypothesis is true is less than or equal to 0.047. Note that this value is less than 0.05, thus at $\alpha = 0.05$, it is statistically significant.

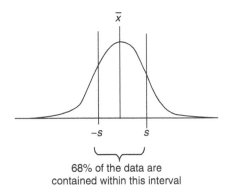

68% of the data are
contained within this interval

FIGURE 1.1 Normal distribution of data.

CONFIDENCE INTERVALS

Making interval predictions about a parameter, such as the mean value, is a very important and useful aspect of statistics. Recall that, for a normal distribution, the mean value $\pm$ the standard deviation provides a confidence interval in which about 68% of the data lie.

The $\bar{x} \pm s$ interval contains approximately 68% of the data in the entire sample set of data (Figure 1.1). If the mean value is 80 with a standard deviation of 10, then the 68% confidence interval is 80 ± 10; therefore, the interval 70–90 contains 68% of the data set.

The interval $\bar{x} \pm 2s$ contains 95% of the sample data set, and the interval $\bar{x} \pm 3s$ contains 99% of the data. In practice, knowing the spread of the data about the mean is valuable, but from a practical standpoint, the interval of the mean is a confidence interval of the mean, not of the data about the mean. Fortunately, the same basic principle holds when we are interested in the standard deviation of the mean, which is $s/\sqrt{n}$, and not the standard deviation of the data set, s. Many statisticians refer to the standard deviation of the mean as the standard error of the mean.

Roughly, then, $\bar{x} \pm s/\sqrt{n}$ is the interval in which the true population mean μ will be found 68 times out of 100. The 95% confidence interval for the population mean μ is $\bar{x} \pm 2.0s/\sqrt{n}$. However, because $s/\sqrt{n}$ slightly overestimates the interval, 95 out of 100 times, the true μ will be contained in the interval, $\bar{x} \pm 1.96s/\sqrt{n}$, given the sample size is large enough to assure a normal distribution. If not, the Student's t distribution (Table B) is used, instead of the Z distribution (Table A).

APPLIED RESEARCH AND STATISTICS

The vast majority of researchers are not professional statisticians but are, instead, experts in other areas, such as medicine, microbiology, chemistry, pharmacology, engineering, or epidemiology. Many professionals of these

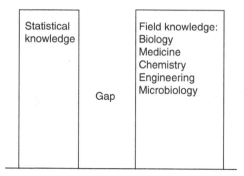

FIGURE 1.2 Knowledge gap between fields.

kinds, at times, work in collaboration with statisticians with varying success. A problem that repeatedly occurs between researchers and statisticians is a knowledge gap between fields (Figure 1.2). Try as they might, statisticians tend to be only partially literate in the sciences, and scientists only partially literate in statistics. When they attempt to communicate, neither of them can perceive fully the experimental situation from the other's point of view. Hence, statisticians interpret as best they can what the scientists are doing, and the scientists interpret as best they can what the statisticians are doing. How close they come to mutual understanding is variable and error-prone (Paulson, 2003).

In this author's view, the best researchers are trained primarily in the sciences, augmented by strong backgrounds in research design and applied statistics. When this is the case, they can effectively ground the statistical analyses into their primary field of scientific knowledge. If the statistical test and their scientific acumen are at variance, they will suspect the statistic and use their field knowledge to uncover an explanation.

EXPERIMENTAL VALIDITY

Experimental validity means that the conclusions drawn on inference are true, relative to the perspective of the research design. There are several threats to inference conclusions drawn from experimentation, and they include (1) internal validity, (2) external validity, (3) statistical conclusion validity, and (4) construct validity.

Internal validity is the validity of a particular study and its claims. It is a cause–effect phenomenon. To assure internal validity, researchers are strongly advised to include a reference or control arm when evaluating a test condition. A reference arm is a treatment or condition in which the researcher has *a priori* knowledge of the outcome. For example, if a bacterial strain of *Staphylococcus aureus*, when exposed to a 4% chlorhexidine gluconate (CHG) product, is generally observed to undergo a $2 \log_{10}$ reduction in population after 30 sec of exposure, it can be used as a reference or control, given that data from a sufficient number of historical studies confirm this. A control arm is another alternative to increase the internal validity of a study. A control is essentially a standard with which a test arm is compared in relative terms.

Researchers assume that, by exposing *S. aureus* to 4% CHG (cause), a 2 $\log_{10}$ reduction in population will result (effect). Hence, if investigators evaluated two products under the conditions of this test and reported a 3 $\log_{10}$ and 4 $\log_{10}$ reduction, respectively, they would have no way of assuring the internal validity of the study. However, if the reference or control product, 4% CHG, was also tested with the two products, and it demonstrated a 4 $\log_{10}$ reduction, researchers would suspect that a third, unknown variable had influenced the study. With that knowledge, they could no longer state that the products themselves produced the 3 $\log_{10}$ and 4 $\log_{10}$ reductions, because the reference or control product's results were greater than the 2 $\log_{10}$ expected.

External validity is the degree to which one can generalize from a specific study's findings based on a population sample to the general population. For example, if a presurgical skin preparation study of an antimicrobial product is conducted in Bozeman, Montana, using local residents as participants, can the results of the study be generalized across the country to all humans? To increase the external validity, the use of heterogeneous groups of persons (different ages, sexes, and races) drawn from different settings (sampling in various parts of the country), at different times of year (summer, spring, winter, and fall) is of immense value. Hence, to assure external validity, the FDA requires that similar studies be conducted at several different laboratories located in different geophysical settings using different subjects.

Statistical conclusion validity deals with the power of a statistic $(1-\beta)$, type I (α), and type II (β) errors (Box et al., 2005). Recall, type I (α) error is the probability of rejecting a true null hypothesis whereas type II (β) error is the probability of accepting a false null hypothesis. A type I error is generally considered more serious than a type II error. For example, if one concludes that a new surgical procedure is more effective than the standard one, and the conclusion is untrue (type I error), this mistake is viewed as a more serious error than stating that a new surgical procedure is not better than the standard one, when it really is (type II error). Hence, when α is set at 0.05, and β is set at 0.20, as previously stated, as one lessens the probability of committing one type of error, one increases the probability of committing the other, given the other conditions are held constant. Generally, the α error acceptance level is set by the experimenter, and the β error is influenced by its value. For example, if one decreases $\alpha = 0.05$ to $\alpha = 0.01$, the probability of a type I error decreases, but type II error increases, given the other parameters (detection level, sample size, and variance) are constant. Both error levels are reduced, however, when the sample size is increased.

Most people think of the power of a statistic as its ability to enable the researcher to make a correct decision—to reject the null hypotheses when it is incorrect, and accept the alternative hypotheses when it is correct. However, this is not the precise statistical definition. Statistical power is simply $1 - \beta$, or the probability of selecting the alternative hypothesis when it is true. Generally, employing the correct statistical method and assuring the method's validity and robustness provide the most powerful and valid statistic. In regression analysis, using a simple linear model to portray polynomial data is a less powerful, and, sometimes, even nonvalid model. A residual analysis is recommended in evaluating the regression model's fit to the actual data; that is, how closely the predicted values of $\hat{y}$ match the actual values of y. The residuals, $e = \hat{y} - y$, are of extreme value in regression, for they provide a firm answer to just how valid the regression model is.

For example (Figure 1.3), the predicted regression values, $\hat{y}_i$, are linear, but the actual, y_i, values are curvilinear. A residual analysis quickly would show this. The e_i values initially are negative, then are positive in the middle range of x_i values, and then negative again in the upper x_i values (Figure 1.4). If the model fits the data, there would be no discernable pattern about 0, just random e_i values.

Although researchers need not be statisticians to perform quality research, they do need to understand the basic principles of experimental design and apply them. In this way, the statistical model usually can be kept relatively low in complexity and provide straightforward, unambiguous answers. Underlying all research is the need to present the findings in a clear, concise manner. This is particularly important if one is defending those findings

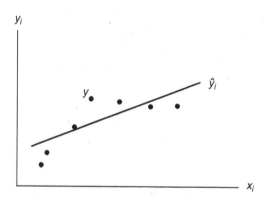

where x_i, the independent variable;
y_i, the dependent variable with respect to x_i;
$\hat{y}_i$, the predicted dependent variable with respect to x_i.

FIGURE 1.3 Predicted regression values.

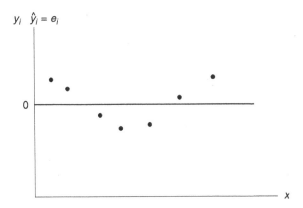

FIGURE 1.4 Residual δ graph.

before a regulatory agency, explaining them to management, or looking for funding from a particular group, such as marketing.

Research quality can be better assured through a thorough understanding of how to employ statistical methods properly, and in this book, they consist of regression methods. Research quality is often compromised when one conducts an experiment before designing the study statistically, and afterward, determining "what the numbers mean." In this situation, researchers often must consult a professional statistician to extract any useful information. An even more unacceptable situation can occur when a researcher evaluates the data using a battery of statistical methods and selects the one that provides the results most favorable to a preconceived conclusion. This should not be confused with fitting a regression model to explain the data, but rather, is fitting a model to a predetermined outcome (Box et al., 2005).

EMPIRICAL RESEARCH

Statistical regression methods, as described in this text, require objective observational data that result from measuring specific events or phenomena under controlled conditions in which as many extraneous influences as possible, other than the variable(s) under consideration, are eliminated. To be valid, regression methods employed in experimentation require at least four conditions to be satisfied:

1. Collection of sample response data in an unbiased manner
2. Accurate, objective observations and measurements
3. Unbiased interpretation of data-based results
4. Reproducibility of the observations and measurements

The controlled experiment is a fundamental tool for the researcher.* In controlled experiments, a researcher collects the dependent sample data (y) from the population or populations of interest at particular preestablished levels of a set of x values.

BIASES

Measurement error has two general components, a random error and a systematic error (Paulson, 2003). Random error is an unexplainable fluctuation in the data for which the researcher cannot identify a specific cause and, therefore, cannot be controlled. Systematic error, or bias, is an error that is not the consequence of chance alone. In addition, systematic error, unlike random fluctuation, has a direction and magnitude.

Researchers cannot will themselves to take a purely objective perspective toward research, even if they think they can. Researchers have personal desires, needs, wants, and fears that will unconsciously come into play by filtering, to some degree, the research, particularly when interpreting the data's meaning (Polkinghorne, 1983). In addition, shared, cultural values of the scientific research community bias researchers' interpretations with preset expectations (Searle, 1995). Therefore, the belief of researchers that they are without bias is particularly dangerous (Varela and Shear, 1999).

Knowing the human predisposition to bias, it is important to collect data using methods for randomization and blinding. It is also helpful for researchers continually to hone their minds toward strengthening three important characteristics:

Openness
Discernment
Understanding

Openness

The research problem, the research implementation, and the interpretation of the data must receive the full, *open* attention of the researcher. Open attention can be likened to the Taoist term, *wu wei*, or noninterfering awareness

---

*However, at least three data types can be treated in regression analysis: observational, experimental, and completely randomized. Observational data are those collected via non-experimental processes—for example, going through quality assurance records to determine if the age of media affects its bacterial growth-promoting ability. Perhaps over a period of months, the agar media dries and becomes less supportive of growth. Experimental data are collected when, say, five time points are set by the experimenter in a time-kill study, and the $\log_{10}$ microbial colony counts are allowed to vary, dependent on the exposure time. Completely randomized data require that the independent variable be assigned at random.

(Maslow, 1971); that is, the researcher does not try to interpret initially but is, instead, simply aware. In this respect, even though unconscious bias remains, the researcher must not consciously overlay data with theoretical constructs concerning how the results should appear (Polkinghorne, 1983); that is, the researcher should strive to avoid consciously bringing to the research process any preconceived values. This is difficult, because those of us who perform research have conscious biases. Probably the best way to remain consciously open for *what is* is to avoid becoming overly invested, *a priori*, in specific theories and explanations.

Discernment

Accompanying openness is discernment—the ability not only to be passively aware, but also to go a step further to see into the heart of the experiment and uncover information not immediately evident, but not adding information that is not present. Discernment can be thought of as one's internal nonsense detector. Unlike openness, discernment enables the researcher to draw on experience to differentiate fact from supposition, association from causation, and intuition from fantasy. Discernment is an accurate discrimination with respect to sources, relevance, pattern, and motives by grounding interpretation in the data and one's direct experience (Assagioli, 1973).

Understanding (*Verstehen*)

Interwoven with openness and discernment is understanding. Researchers cannot merely observe an experiment, but must understand—that is, correctly interpret—the data (Polkinghorne, 1983). Understanding what is, then, is knowing accurately and precisely what the phenomena mean. This type of understanding is attained when intimacy with the data and their meaning is achieved and integrated. In research, it is not possible to gain understanding by merely observing phenomena and analyzing them statistically. One must interpret the data correctly, a process enhanced by at least three conditions:

1. *Familiarity* with the mental processes by which understanding and, hence, meaning is obtained must exist. In addition, much of this meaning is shared. Researchers do not live in isolation, but within a culture—albeit scientific—which operates through shared meaning, shared values, shared beliefs, and shared goals (Sears et al., 1991). Additionally, one's language—both technical and conversant—is held together through both shared meaning and concepts. Because each researcher must communicate meaning to others, understanding the semiotics of communication is important. For example, the letters— marks—on this page are signifiers. They are symbols that refer to collectively defined (by language) objects or concepts known as refer- ents. However, each individual has a slightly unique concept of each

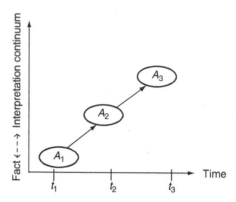

FIGURE 1.5 Fact interpretation gradient of experimental processes.

referent stored in their memory, termed the signified. For instance, when one says or writes tree, the utterance or letter markings of t-r-e-e, this is a signifier that represents a culturally shared referent, the symbol of a wooden object with branches and leaves. Yet, unavoidably, we have a slightly different concept of the referent, tree. This author's mental signified may be an oak tree; the reader's may be a pine tree.

2. *Realization* that an event and the perception of an event are not the same. Suppose a researcher observes event A_1 at time t_1 (Figure 1.5). The researcher describes what was witnessed at time t_1, which is now a description, A_2, of event A_1 at time t_2. Later, the researcher will distance even farther from event A_1 by reviewing laboratory notes on A_2, a process that produces A_3. Note that this process hardly represents a direct, unbiased view of A_1. The researcher will generally interpret data (A_3), which, themselves, are interpretations of data to some degree (A_2), based on the actual occurrence of the event, A_1 (Varela and Shear, 1999).

3. *Understanding* that a scientific system, itself (e.g., biology, geology), provides a definition of most observed events that transfer interpretation, which is again reinterpreted by researchers. This, in itself, is biasing, particularly in that it provides a preconception of what is.

EXPERIMENTAL PROCESS

In practice, the experimental process is usually iterative. The results of experiment A become the starting point for experiment B, the next experiment (Figure 1.6). The results of experiment B become the starting point for experiment C. Let us look more closely at the iterative process in an example.

Suppose one desires to evaluate a newly developed product at five incremental concentration levels (0.25%, 0.50%, 0.75%, 1.00%, and 1.25%)

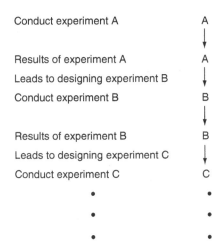

FIGURE 1.6 Iterative approach to research.

for its antimicrobial effects against two representative pathogenic bacterial species—*S. aureus*, a Gram-positive bacterium, and *Escherichia coli*, a Gram-negative one. The researcher designs a simple, straightforward test to observe the antimicrobial action of the five concentration levels when challenged for 1 min with specific inoculum levels of *S. aureus* and *E. coli*. Exposure to the five levels of the drug, relative to the kill produced in populations of the two bacterial species, demonstrates that the 0.75% and the 1.00% concentrations were equivalent in their antimicrobial effects, and that 0.25%, 0.50%, and 1.25% were much less antimicrobially effective.

Encouraged by these results, the researcher designs another study focusing on the comparison of the 0.75% and the 1.00% drug formulations, when challenged for 1 min with 13 different microbial species to identify the better (more antimicrobially active) product. However, the two products perform equally well against the 13 different microorganism species at 1 min exposures. The researcher then designs the next study to use the same 13 microorganism species, but at reduced exposure times, 15 and 30 sec, and adds a competitor product to use as a reference.

The two formulations again perform equally well and significantly better than the competitor. The researcher now believes that one of the products may truly be a candidate to market, but at which active concentration? Product cost studies, product stability studies, etc. are conducted, and still the two products are equivalent.

Finally, the researcher performs a clinical trial with human volunteer subjects to compare the two products' antibacterial efficacy, as well as their skin irritation potential. Although the antimicrobial portion of the study had revealed activity equivalence, the skin irritation evaluation demonstrates that the 1.00% product was significantly more irritating to users' hands. Hence, the candidate formulation is the 0.75% preparation.

This is the type of process commonly employed in new product development projects (Paulson, 2003). Because research and development efforts are generally subject to tight budgets, small pilot studies are preferred to larger, more costly ones. Moreover, usually this is fine, because the experimenter has intimate, first-hand knowledge of their research area, as well as an understanding of its theoretical aspects. With this knowledge and understanding, they can usually ground the meaning of the data in the observations, even when the number of observations is small.

Yet, researchers must be aware that there is a downside to this step-by-step approach. When experiments are conducted one factor at a time, if interaction between factors is present, it will not be discovered. Statistical interaction occurs when two or more products do not produce the same proportional response at different levels of measurement. Figure 1.7 depicts $\log_{10}$ microbial counts after three time exposures with product A (50% strength) and product B (full strength). No interaction is apparent because, over the three time intervals, the difference between the product responses is constant.

Figure 1.8 shows statistical interaction between factors. At time t_1, product A provides more microbial reduction (lower counts) than product B. At time t_2, product A demonstrates less reduction in microorganisms than does product B. At time t_3, products A and B are equivalent. When statistical

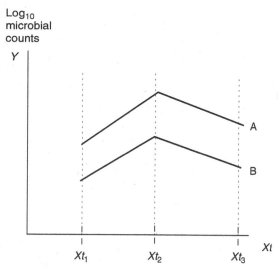

FIGURE 1.7 No interaction present.

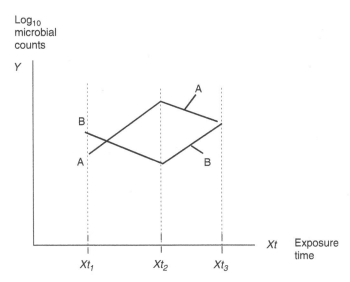

FIGURE 1.8 Interaction present.

interaction is present, it makes no sense to discuss the general effects of products A and B, individually. Instead, one must discuss product performance relative to a specific exposure time frame; that is, at times xt_1, xt_2, and xt_3.

Additionally, researchers must realize that reality cannot be broken into small increments to know it *in toto*. This book is devoted mainly to small study designs, and although much practical information can be gained from small studies, by themselves, they rarely provide a clear perspective on the whole situation.

We humans tend to think and describe reality in simple cause-and-effect relationships (e.g., A causes B). However, in reality, phenomena seldom share merely linear relationships, nor do they have simple, one-factor causes. For example, in medical practice, when a physician examines a patient infected with *S. aureus*, they will likely conclude that *S. aureus* caused the disease and proceed to eliminate the offending microorganism from the body. Yet, this is not the complete story. The person's immune system—composed of the reticuloendothelial system, immunocytes, phagocytes, etc.—acts to prevent infectious diseases from occurring, and to fight them, once the infection is established. The immune system is directly dependent on genetic predisposition, modified through one's nutritional state, psychological state (e.g., a sense of life's meaning and purpose), and stress level. In a simple case like this, where oral administration of an antibiotic cures the disease, knowledge of these other influences does not usually matter. However, in more complicated chronic diseases such as cancer, those other factors may play an important role in treatment efficacy and survival of the patient.

OTHER DIFFICULTIES IN RESEARCH

There are three other phenomena that may pose difficulties for the experimenter:

Experimental (random) error
Confusing correlation with causation
Employing a study design that is complex, when a simpler one would be as good

EXPERIMENTAL ERROR

Random variability—experimental error—is produced by a multitude of uncontrolled factors that tend to obscure the conclusions one can draw from an experiment based on a small sample size. This is a very critical consideration in research where small sample sizes are the rule, because it is more difficult to detect significant treatment effects when they truly exist, a type II error.

One or two wild data points (outliers) in a small sample can distort the mean and hugely inflate the variance, making it nearly impossible to make inferences—at least meaningful ones. Therefore, before experimenters become heavily invested in a research project, they should have an approximation of what the variability of the data is and establish the tolerable limits for both the alpha (α) and beta (β) errors, so that the appropriate sample size is tested.

Although, traditionally, type I (α) error is considered more serious than type II (β) error, this is not always the case. In research and development (R&D) studies, type II error can be very serious. For example, if one is evaluating several compounds, using a small sample size pilot study, there is a real problem of concluding statistically that the compounds are not different from each other, when actually they are. Here, type II (β) error can cause a researcher to reject a promising compound. One way around this is to increase the α level to reduce β error; that is, use an α of 0.10 or 0.15, instead of 0.05 or 0.01. In addition, using more powerful statistical procedures can immensely reduce the probability of committing β error.

CONFUSING CORRELATION WITH CAUSATION

Correlation is a measure of the degree to which two variables vary linearly with relation to each other. Thus, for example, in comparing the number of lightning storms in Kansas to the number of births in New York City, you discover a strong positive correlation: the more lightning storms in Kansas, the more children born in New York City (Figure 1.9).

Although the two variables appear to be correlated sufficiently to claim that the increased incidence of Kansas lightning storms caused increased childbirth in New York, correlation is not causation. Correlation between

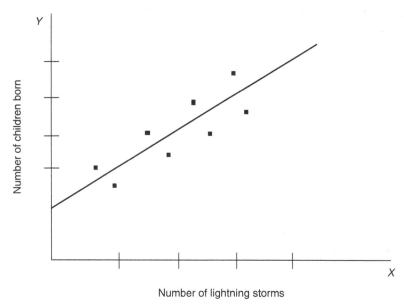

FIGURE 1.9 Correlation between unrelated variables.

two variables, X and Y, often occurs because they are both associated with a third factor, Z, which is unknown. There are a number of empirical ways to verify causation, and generally these do not rely on statistical inference. Therefore, until causation is truly demonstrated, it is preferred to state that correlated data are "associated," rather than causally related.

COMPLEX STUDY DESIGN

In many research situations, especially those involving human subjects in medical research clinical trials, such as blood level absorption rates of a drug, the study design must be complex to evaluate the dependent variable(s) better. However, whenever possible, it is wise to use the rule of parsimony; that is, use the simplest and most straightforward study design available. Even simple experiments can quickly become complex. Adding other questions, although interesting, will quickly increase complexity. This author finds it useful to state formally the study objectives, the choice of experimental factors and levels (i.e., independent variables), the dependent variable one intends to measure to fulfill the study objectives, and the study design selected. For example, suppose biochemists evaluate the $\log_{10}$ reduction in *S. aureus* bacteria after a 15 sec exposure to a new antimicrobial compound produced in several pilot batches. They want to determine the 95% confidence interval for the true $\log_{10}$ microbial average reduction. This is simple enough, but then the chemists ask:

1. Is there significant lot-to-lot variation in the pilot batches? If there is, perhaps one is significantly more antimicrobially active than another.
2. What about subculture-to-subculture variability in the antimicrobial resistance of the strain of S. *aureus* used in testing? If one is interested in knowing if the product is effective against S. *aureus*, how many strains must be evaluated?
3. What about lot-to-lot variability in the culture medium used to grow the bacteria? The chemists remember supplier A's medium routinely supporting larger microbial populations than that of supplier B. Should both be tested? Does the medium contribute significantly to $\log_{10}$ microbial reduction variability?
4. What about procedural error by technicians and variability between technicians? The training records show technician A to be more accurate in handling data than technicians B and C. How should this be addressed?

As one can see, even a simple study can—and often will—become complex.

BASIC TOOLS IN EXPERIMENTAL DESIGN

There are three basic tools in statistical experimental design (Paulson, 2003):

Replication
Randomization
Blocking

Replication means that the basic experimental measurement is repeated. For example, if one is measuring the CO_2 concentration of blood, those measurements would be repeated several times under controlled circumstances. Replication serves several important functions. First, it allows the investigator to estimate the variance of the experimental or random error through the sample standard deviation (s) or sample variance (s^2). This estimate becomes a basic unit of measurement for determining whether observed differences in the data are statistically significant. Second, because the sample mean ($\bar{x}$) is used to estimate the true population mean (μ), replication enables an investigator to obtain a more precise estimate of the treatment effect's value. If s^2 is the sample variance of the data for n replicates, then the variance of the sample mean is $s_{\bar{x}}^2 = s^2/n$.

The practical aspect of this is that if few or no replicates are made, then the investigator may be unable to make a useful inference about the true population mean, μ. However, if the sample mean is derived from replicated data, the population mean, μ, can be estimated more accurately and precisely.

Randomization of a sampling process is a mainstay of statistical analysis. No matter how careful an investigator is in eliminating bias, it can still creep into the study. Additionally, when a variable cannot be controlled, randomized sampling can modulate any biasing effect. Randomization schemes can be achieved by using a table of random digits or a computer-generated randomization subroutine. Through randomization, each experimental unit is as likely to be selected for a particular treatment or measurement as are any of the others.

Blocking is another common statistical technique used to increase the precision of an experimental design by reducing or even eliminating nuisance factors that influence the measured responses, but are not of interest to the study. Blocks consist of groups of the experimental unit, such that each group is more homogenous with respect to some variable than is the collection of experimental units as a whole. Blocking involves subjecting the block to all the experimental treatments and comparing the treatment effects within each block. For example, in a drug absorption study, an investigator may have four different drugs to compare. They may block according to similar weights of test subjects. The rationale is that the closer the subjects are to the same weight, the closer the baseline liver functions will be. The four individuals between 120 and 125 pounds in block 1 each randomly receive one of the four test drugs. Block 2 may contain the four individuals between 130 and 135 pounds.

STATISTICAL METHOD SELECTION: OVERVIEW

The statistical method, to be appropriate, must measure and reflect the data accurately and precisely. The test hypothesis should be formulated clearly and concisely. If, for example, the study is designed to test whether products A and B are different, statistical analysis should provide an answer.

Roger H. Green, in his book *Sampling Designs and Statistical Methods for Environmental Biologists*, describes 10 steps for effective statistical analysis (Green, 1979). These steps are applicable to any analysis:

1. State the test hypothesis concisely to be sure that what you are testing is what you want to test.
2. Always replicate the treatments. Without replication, measurements of variability may not be reliable.
3. As far as possible, keep the number of replicates equal throughout the study. This practice makes it much easier to analyze the data.
4. When determining whether a particular treatment has a significant effect, it is important to take measurements both where the test condition is present and where it is absent.

5. Perform a small-scale study to assess the effectiveness of the design and statistical method selection, before going to the effort and expense of a larger study.

6. Verify that the sampling scheme one devises actually results in a representative sample of the target population. Guard against systematic bias by using techniques of random sampling.

7. Break a large-scale sampling process into smaller components.

8. Verify that the collected data meet the statistical distribution assumptions. In the days before computers were commonly used and programs were readily available, some assumptions had to be made about distributions. Now it is easy to test these assumptions, to verify their validity.

9. Test the method thoroughly to make sure that it is valid and useful for the process under study. Moreover, even if the method is satisfactory for one set of data, be certain that it is adequate for other sets of data derived from the same process.

10. Once these nine steps have been carried out, one can accept the results of analysis with confidence. Much time, money, and effort can be saved by following these steps to statistical analysis.

Before assembling a large-scale study, the investigator should reexamine (a) the test hypothesis, (b) the choice of variables, (c) the number of replicates required to protect against type I and type II errors, (d) the order of experimentation process, (e) the randomization process, (f) the appropriateness of the design used to describe the data, and (g) the data collection and data-processing procedures to ensure that they continue to be relevant to the study. We have discussed aspects of statistical theory as applied to statistical practices. We study basic linear regression in the following chapters.

2 Simple Linear Regression

Simple linear regression analysis provides bivariate statistical tools essential to the applied researcher in many instances. Regression is a methodology that is grounded in the relationship between two quantitative variables (y, x) such that the value of y (dependent variable) can be predicted based on the value of x (independent variable). Determining the mathematical relationship between these two variables, such as exposure time and lethality or wash time and $\log_{10}$ microbial reductions, is very common in applied research. From a mathematical perspective, two types of relationships must be discussed: (1) a functional relationship and (2) a statistical relationship. Recall that, mathematically, a functional relationship has the form

$$y = f(x),$$

where y is the resultant value, on the function of x ($f(x)$), and $f(x)$ is any set of mathematical procedure or formula such as $x + 1$, $2x + 10$, or $4x^3 - 2x^2 + 5x - 10$, or $\log_{10} x^2 + 10$, and so on. Let us look at an example in which $y = 3x$. Hence,

y	x
3	1
6	2
9	3

Graphing the function y on x, we have a linear graph (Figure 2.1). Given a particular value of x, y is said to be determined by x.

A statistical relationship, unlike a mathematical one, does not provide an exact or perfect data fit in the way that a functional one does. Even in the best of conditions, y is composed of the estimate of x, as well as some amount of unexplained error or disturbance called statistical error, e. That is,

$$\hat{y} = f(x) + e.$$

So, using the previous example, $y = 3x$, now $\hat{y} = 3x + e$ ($\hat{y}$ indicates that $\hat{y}$ estimates y, but is not exact, as in a mathematical function). They differ by

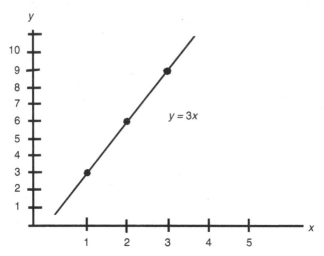

FIGURE 2.1 Linear graph.

some random amount termed e (Figure 2.2). Here, the estimates of y on x do not fit the data estimate precisely.

GENERAL PRINCIPLES OF REGRESSION ANALYSIS

REGRESSION AND CAUSALITY

A statistical relationship demonstrated between two variables, y (the response or dependent variable) and x (the independent variable), is not necessarily a

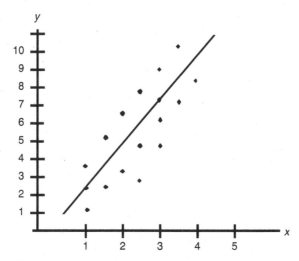

FIGURE 2.2 Linear graph.

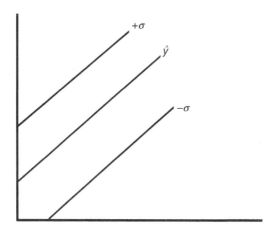

FIGURE 2.3 Constant, equidistant variability.

causal one, but can be. Ideally, it is, but unless one knows this for sure, y and x are said to be associated.

The fundamental model for a simple regression is

$$Y_i = \beta_0 + \beta_1 x_i + \varepsilon_i, \tag{2.1}$$

where Y is the response or dependent variable for the ith observation; β_0 is the population y intercept, when $x = 0$; β_1 is the population regression parameter (slope or (rise/run)); x_i is the independent variable; ε_i is the random error for the ith observation, where $\varepsilon = N(0, \sigma^2)$; that is, the errors are normally and independently distributed with a mean of zero and a variance of σ^2; ε_i and ε_{i-1} are assumed to be uncorrelated (an error term is not influenced by the magnitude of the previous or other error terms), so the covariance is equal to 0.

This model is linear in the parameters (β_0, β_1) and in the x_i values, and there is only one predictor value, x_i, in only a power of 1. In actually applying the regression function to sample data, we use the form $\hat{y}_i = b_0 + b_1 + e_i$. Often, this function is also written as $\hat{y}_i = a + bx + e_i$. This form is also known as a first-order model. As previously stated, the actual y value is composed of two components: (1) $b_0 + b_1 x$, the constant term and (2) e, the random variable term. The expected value of y is $E(Y) = \beta_0 + \beta_1 x$. The variability of σ is assumed to be constant and equidistant over the regression function's entirety (Figure 2.3). Examples of nonconstant, nonequidistant variabilities are presented in Figure 2.4.

MEANING OF REGRESSION PARAMETERS

A researcher is performing a steam–heat thermal–death curve calculation on a 10^6 microbial population of *Bacillus stearothermophilus*, where the steam

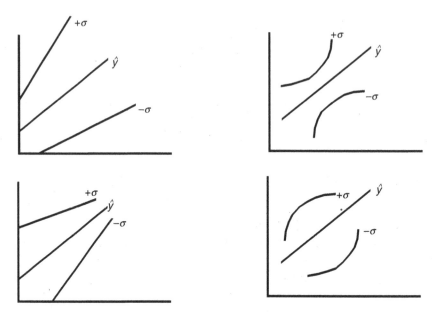

FIGURE 2.4 Nonconstant, nonequidistant variability.

sterilization temperature is 121°C. Generally, a $\log_{10}$ reexpression is used to linearize the microbial population. In $\log_{10}$ scale, 10^6 is 6. In this example, assume that the microbial population is reduced to 1 $\log_{10}$ for every 30 sec of exposure to steam (this example is presented graphically in Figure 2.5):

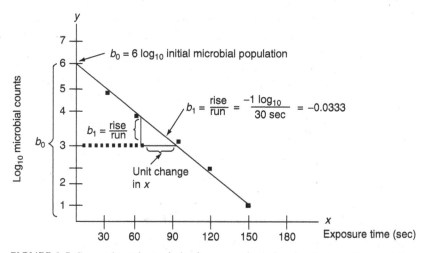

FIGURE 2.5 Steam–heat thermal–death curve calculation for *B. stearothermophilus*.

$$\hat{y} = b_0 + b_1 x,$$

$$\hat{y} = 6 - 0.0333(x),$$

where b_0 represents the value of $\hat{y}$ when $x = 0$, which is $\hat{y} = 6 - 0.0333(0) = 6$ in this example. It is also known as the y intercept value when $x = 0$. b_1 represents the slope of the regression line, which is the rise/run or tangent. This rise is negative in this example, meaning that the slope is decreasing over exposure time, so

$$b_1 = \frac{\text{rise}}{\text{run}} = \frac{-1}{30} = -0.0333.$$

For $x = 60$ sec, $\hat{y} = 6 - 0.0333(60) = 4$. For every second of exposure time, the reduction in microorganisms is $0.0333 \log_{10}$.

DATA FOR REGRESSION ANALYSIS

The researcher ordinarily will not know the population values of β_0 or β_1. They have to be estimated by a b_0 and b_1 computation, termed the method of least squares. In this design, two types of data are collected: the response or dependent variable (y_i) and the independent variable (x_i). The x_i values are usually preset and not random variables; hence, they are considered to be measured without error (Kutner et al., 2005; Neter et al., 1983).

Recall that observational data are obtained by nonexperimental methods. There are times a researcher may collect data (x and y) within the environment to perform a regression evaluation. For example, a quality assurance person may suspect that a relationship exists between warm weather (winter to spring to summer) and microbial contamination levels in a laboratory. The microbial counts (y) are then compared with the months, $x(1-6)$, to determine whether this theory holds (Figure 2.6).

In experimental designs, usually the values of x are preselected at specific levels, and the y values corresponding to these are dependent on the x levels set. This provides y or x values, and a controlled regimen or process is implemented. Generally, multiple observations of y at a specific x value are taken to increase the precision of the error term estimate.

On the other hand, in completely randomized regression design, the designated values of x are selected randomly, not specifically set. Hence, both x and y are random variables. Although this is a useful design, it is not as common as the other two.

REGRESSION PARAMETER CALCULATION

To find the estimates of both b_0 and b_1, we use the least-squares method. This method provides the best estimate (the one with the least error) by minimizing

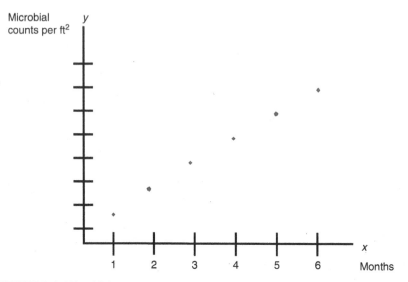

FIGURE 2.6 Microbial counts compared with months.

the difference between the actual and predicted values from the set of collected values:

$$y - \hat{y} \quad \text{or} \quad y - b_0 + b_1 x,$$

where y is the dependent variable and $\hat{y}$ is the predicted dependent variable. The computation utilizes all the observations in a set of data. The sum of the squares is denoted by Q; that is,

$$Q = \sum_{i=1}^{n} (y_i - b_0 - b_1 x_i)^2,$$

where Q is the smallest possible value, as determined by the least-squares method. The actual computational formulas are

$$b_1 = \text{slope} = \frac{\sum\limits_{i=1}^{n} (x_i - \bar{x})(y_i - \bar{y})}{\sum\limits_{i=1}^{n} (x_i - \bar{x})^2} \tag{2.2}$$

and

$$b_0 = y \text{ intercept} = \frac{\sum\limits_{i=1}^{n} y_i - b_1 \sum\limits_{i=1}^{n} x_i}{n}$$

or simply

$$b_0 = \bar{y} - b_1\bar{x}. \tag{2.3}$$

PROPERTIES OF THE LEAST-SQUARES ESTIMATION

The expected value of $b_0 = E[b_0] = \beta_0$. The expected value of $b_1 = E[b_1] = \beta_1$. The least-squares estimators of b_0 and b_1 are unbiased estimators and have the minimum variance of all other possible linear combinations.

Example 2.1: An experimenter challenges a benzalkonium chloride disinfectant with 1×10^6 *Staphylococcus aureus* bacteria in a series of timed exposures. As noted earlier, exponential microbial colony counts are customarily linearized via a $\log_{10}$ scale transformation, which has been performed in this example. The resultant data are presented in Table 2.1.

The researcher would like to perform regression analysis on the data to construct a chemical microbial inactivation curve, where x is the exposure time in seconds and y is the $\log_{10}$ colony-forming units recovered.

Note that the data are replicated in triplicate for each exposure time, x. First, we compute the slope of the data

$$b_1 = \frac{\sum_{i=1}^{n}(x_i - \bar{x})(y_i - \bar{y})}{\sum_{i=1}^{n}(x_i - \bar{x})^2},$$

TABLE 2.1
Resultant Data

n	x	y
1	0	6.09
2	0	6.10
3	0	6.08
4	15	5.48
5	15	5.39
6	15	5.51
7	30	5.01
8	30	4.88
9	30	4.93
10	45	4.53
11	45	4.62
12	45	4.49
13	60	3.57
14	60	3.42
15	60	3.44

where $\bar{x} = 30$ and $\bar{y} = 4.90$,

$$\sum_{i=1}^{15} (x_i - \bar{x})(y_i - \bar{y}) = (0 - 30)(6.09 - 4.90) + (0 - 30)(6.10 - 4.90)$$

$$+ \cdots + (60 - 30)(3.42 - 4.90) + (60 - 30)(3.44 - 4.90) = -276.60,$$

$$\sum_{i=1}^{15} (x_i - \bar{x})^2 = (0 - 30)^2 + (0 - 30)^2 + \cdots + (60 - 30)^2$$

$$+ (60 - 30)^2 + (60 - 30)^2 = 6750,$$

$$b_1 = \frac{-276.60}{6750} = -0.041.^*$$

The negative sign of b_1 means the regression line estimated by $\hat{y}$ is descending, from the y intercept:

$$b_0 = \bar{y} - b_1\bar{x} = 4.90 - (-0.041)(30),$$
$$b_0 = 6.13, \text{ the } y \text{ intercept point when } x = 0.$$

The complete regression equation is

$$\hat{y}_i = b_0 + b_1 x_i,$$
$$\hat{y}_i = 6.13 - 0.041 x_i. \tag{2.4}$$

This regression equation can then be used to predict each $\hat{y}$, a procedure known as point estimation.

For example, for $x = 0$, $\hat{y} = 6.13 - 0.041(0) = 6.130$

$$15, \hat{y} = 6.13 - 0.041(15) = 5.515,$$
$$30, \hat{y} = 6.13 - 0.041(30) = 4.900,$$

---

*There is a faster machine computational formula for b_1, useful with a hand-held calculator, although many scientific calculators provide b_1 as a standard routine. It is

$$b_1 = \frac{\sum_{i=1}^{n} x_i y_i - \dfrac{\left(\sum_{i=1}^{n} x\right)\left(\sum_{i=1}^{n} y_i\right)}{n}}{\sum_{i=1}^{n} x_i^2 - \dfrac{\left(\sum_{i=1}^{n} x_i\right)^2}{n}}.$$

$$45, \hat{y} = 6.13 - 0.041(45) = 4.285,$$
$$60, \hat{y} = 6.13 - 0.041(60) = 3.670.$$

From these data, we can now make a regression diagrammatic table to see how well the model fits the data. Regression functions are standard on most scientific calculators and computer software packages. One of the statistical software packages that is easiest to use, and has a considerable number of options, is MiniTab. We first learn to perform the computations by hand and then switch to this software package because of its simplicity and efficiency. Table 2.2 presents the data.

In regression, it is very useful to plot the predicted regression values, $\hat{y}$ with the actual observations, y, superimposed. In addition, exploratory data analysis (EDA) is useful, particularly when using regression methods with the residual values $(e = y - \hat{y})$ to ensure that no pattern or trending is seen that would suggest inaccuracy. Although regression analysis can be extremely valuable, it is particularly prone to certain problems, as follows:

1. The regression line computed on $\hat{y}$ will be a straight line or linear. Often experimental data are not linear and must be transformed to a linear scale, if possible, so that the regression analysis provides an

TABLE 2.2
Regression Data

n	x = Time	y = Actual $\log_{10}$ Values	$\hat{y}$ = Predicted $\log_{10}$ Values	$e = y - \hat{y}$ (e = Actual–Predicted y Values)
1	0.00	6.0900	6.1307	−0.0407
2	0.00	6.1000	6.1307	−0.0307
3	0.00	6.0800	6.1307	−0.0507
4	15.00	5.4800	5.5167	−0.0367
5	15.00	5.3900	5.5167	−0.1267
6	15.00	5.5100	5.5167	−0.0067
7	30.00	5.0100	4.9027	0.1073
8	30.00	4.8800	4.9027	−0.0227
9	30.00	4.9300	4.9027	0.0273
10	45.00	4.5300	4.2887	0.2413
11	45.00	4.6200	4.2887	0.3313
12	45.00	4.4900	4.2887	0.2013
13	60.00	3.5700	3.6747	−0.1047
14	60.00	3.4200	3.6747	−0.2547
15	60.00	3.4400	3.6747	−0.2347

accurate and reliable model of the data. The EDA methods described in Chapter 3 (Paulson, 2003) are particularly useful in this procedure. However, some data transformations may confuse the intended audience. For example, if the y values are transformed to a cube root ($\sqrt[3]{}$) scale, the audience receiving the data analysis may have trouble understanding the regression's meaning in real life because they cannot translate the original scale to a cube root scale in their heads. That is, they cannot make sense of the data. In this case, the researcher is in a dilemma. Although it would be useful to perform the cube root transformation to linearize the data, the researcher may then need to take the audience through the transformation process verbally and graphically in an attempt to enlighten them. As an alternative, however, a nonparametric method could be applied to analyze the nonlinear data. Unfortunately, this too is likely to require a detailed explanation.

2. Sometimes, a model must be expanded in the b_i parameters to better estimate the actual data. For example, the regression equation may expand to

$$\hat{y} = b_0 + b_1 x_1 + b_2 x_2 \tag{2.5}$$

or

$$\hat{y} = b_0 + b_1 x_1 + \cdots + b_k x_k, \tag{2.6}$$

where the b_i values will always be linear values.

However, we concentrate on simple linear regression procedures, that is, $\hat{y} = b_0 + b_1 x_i$ in this chapter. Before continuing, let us look at a regression model to understand better what $\hat{y}$, y, and ε represent (as in Figure 2.7). Note $e = y - \hat{y}$ or the error term, which is merely the actual y value minus the predicted $\hat{y}$ value.

DIAGNOSTICS

One of the most important steps in regression analysis is to plot the actual data values (y_i) and the fitted data ($\hat{y}_i$) on the same graph to visualize clearly how closely the predicted regression line ($\hat{y}_i$) fits or mirrors the actual data (y_i). Figure 2.8 presents a MiniTab graphic plot of this, as an example.

In the figure, R^2 (i.e., R-Sq) is the coefficient of determination, a value used to evaluate the adequacy of the model, which in this example indicates that the regression equation is about a 96.8% better predictor of y than using $\bar{x}$. An R^2 of 1.00 or 100% is a perfect fit (the $\hat{y} = y$). We discuss both R and R^2 later in this chapter.

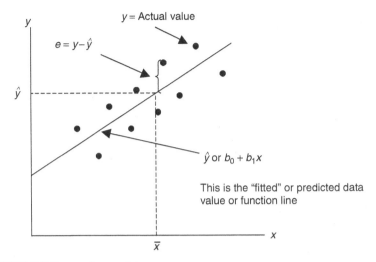

FIGURE 2.7 Regression model.

Note that on examining the regression plot (Figure 2.8), it appears that the data are adequately modeled by the linear regression equation used. To check this, the researcher should next perform a stem–leaf display, a letter–value display, and a boxplot display of the residuals, $y - \hat{y} = e$ values. Moreover, it is often useful to plot the y values and the residual values, e, and the $\hat{y}$ values

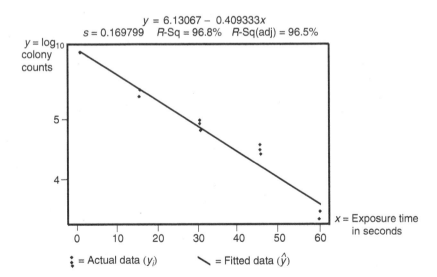

FIGURE 2.8 MiniTab regression plot.

Stem-and-leaf display of
residuals
$N = 15$
Leaf unit = 0.010

2	-2	53
4	-1	20
(6)	-0	543320
5	0	2
4	1	0
3	2	04
1	3	3

FIGURE 2.9 Stem-and-leaf display.

and the residual values, e. Figure 2.9 presents a stem–leaf display of the residual data $(e = y_i - \hat{y})$.

The stem–leaf display of the residual data $(e = y_i - \hat{y}_i)$ shows nothing of great concern, that is, no abnormal patterns. Residual value (e_i) plots should be patternless if the model is adequate. The residual median is not precisely 0 but very close to it.

Figure 2.10 presents the letter–value display of the residual data. Note that the letter–value display Mid column trends toward increased values, meaning that the residual values are skewed slightly to the right or to the values greater than the mean value. In regression analysis, this is a clue that the predicted regression line function may not adequately model the data.* The researcher then wants to examine a residual value (e_i) vs. actual (y_i) value graph (Figure 2.11), and a residual (e_i) vs. predicted $(\hat{y})$ value graph (Figure 2.12) and review the actual regression graph (Figure 2.8). Looking closely at these graphs, and the letter–value display, we see clearly that the regression model does not completely describe the data. The actual data appear not quite $\log_{10}$ linear. For example, note that beyond time $x_i = 0$, the regression model overestimates the actual $\log_{10}$ microbial kill by about 0.25 $\log_{10}$, underestimates the actual $\log_{10}$ kill at $x_i = 45$ sec by about 0.25 $\log_{10}$, and again overestimates at $x_i = 60$ sec. Is this significant or not?

	Depth	Lower	Upper	Mid	Spread
$N =$	15				
M	8.0	-0.031		-0.031	
H	4.5	-0.078	0.067	-0.005	0.145
E	2.5	-0.181	0.221	0.020	0.402
D	1.5	-0.245	0.286	0.021	0.531
	1	-0.255	0.331	0.038	0.586

FIGURE 2.10 Letter–value display.

*For an in-depth discussion of exploratory data analysis, see Paulson, 2003.

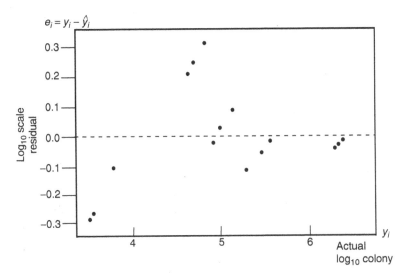

FIGURE 2.11 Residual (e_i) vs. actual (y_i) value graph.

Researchers can draw on their primary field knowledge to determine this, whereas a card-carrying statistician usually cannot. The statistician may decide to use a polynomial regression model and is sure that, with some manipulation, it can model the data better, particularly in that the error at each

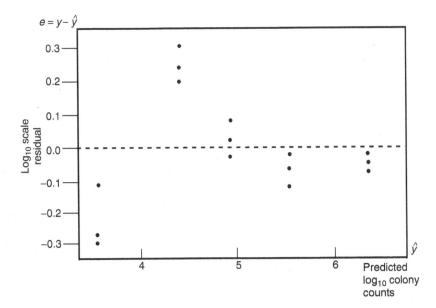

FIGURE 2.12 Residual (e_i) vs. predicted ($\hat{y}_i$) value graph.

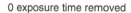

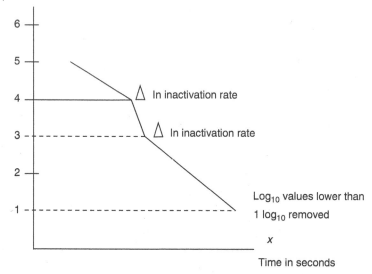

FIGURE 2.13 Piecewise regression model.

observation is considerably reduced (as supported by several indicators we have yet to discuss, the regression f-test and the coefficient of determination, r^2). However, the applied microbiology researcher has an advantage over the statistician, knowing that often the initial value at time 0 ($x = 0$) is not reliable in microbial death rate kinetics and, in practice, is often dropped from the analysis. Additionally, from experience, the applied microbiology researcher knows that, once the data drop below 4 $\log_{10}$, a different inactivation rate (i.e., slope of b_1) occurs with this microbial species until the population is reduced to about two logs, where the microbial inactivation rate slows because of survivors genetically resistant to the antimicrobial. Hence, the microbial researcher may decide to perform a piecewise regression (to be explained later) to better model the data and explain the inactivation properties at a level more basic than that resulting from a polynomial regression. The final regression, when carried out over sufficient time, could be modeled using a form such as that in Figure 2.13.

In conclusion, field microbiology researchers generally have a definite advantage over statisticians in understanding and modeling the data, given they ground their interpretation in basic knowledge of the field.

ESTIMATION OF THE ERROR TERM

To continue, the variance (σ^2) of the error term (written as ε^2 for a population estimate or e^2 for the sample variance) needs to be estimated. As a general principle of parametric statistics, the sample variance (s^2) is obtained by first measuring the squared deviation between each of the actual values (x_i) and the average value ($\bar{x}$), and summing these:

$$\sum_{i=1}^{n} (x_i - \bar{x})^2 = \text{sum of squares.}$$

The sample variance is then derived by dividing the sum of squares by the degrees of freedom ($n - 1$):

$$s^2 = \frac{\sum_{i=1}^{n} (x_i - \bar{x})^2}{n - 1}. \tag{2.7}$$

This formulaic process is also applicable in regression. Hence, the sum of squares for the error term in regression analysis is

$$SS_E = \sum_{i=1}^{n} (y_i - \hat{y})^2 = \sum_{i=1}^{n} e^2 = \text{sum-of-squares error term.} \tag{2.8}$$

The mean square error (MS_E) is used to predict the sample variance or s^2. Hence,

$$MS_E = s^2, \tag{2.9}$$

where

$$MS_E = \frac{SS_E}{n - 2}. \tag{2.10}$$

Two degrees of freedom are lost, because both b_0 and b_1 are estimated in the regression model ($b_0 + b_1 x_i$) to predict $\hat{y}$. The standard deviation is simply the square root of MS_E:

$$s = \sqrt{MS_E}, \tag{2.11}$$

where the value of s is considered to be constant for the x, y ranges of the regression analysis.

REGRESSION INFERENCES

Recall that the simple regression model equation is

$$Y_i = \beta_0 + \beta_1 x_i + \varepsilon_i,$$

where β_0 and β_1 are the regression parameters; x_i are the known (set) independent values; and $\varepsilon = (y - \hat{y})$, normally and independently distributed, $N(0, \sigma^2)$.

Frequently, the investigator wants to know whether the slope, β_1, is significant, that is, not equal to zero ($\beta_1 \neq 0$). If $\beta_1 = 0$, then regression analysis should not be used, for β_0 is a good estimate of y, that is, $\beta_0 = \bar{y}$. The significance test for β_1 is a hypothesis test:

H_0: $\beta_1 = 0$ (slope is not significantly different from 0),
H_A: $\beta_1 \neq 0$ (slope is significantly different from 0).

The conclusions that are made when $\beta_1 = 0$ are the following:

1. There is no linear association between y and x.
2. There is no relationship of any type between y and x.

Recall that β_1 is estimated by b_1, which is computed as

$$b_1 = \frac{\sum_{i=1}^{n}(x_i - \bar{x})(y_i - \bar{y})}{\sum_{i=1}^{n}(x_i - \bar{x})^2}$$

and b_1, the mean slope value, is an unbiased estimator of β_1.
The population variance of β_1 is

$$\sigma_{\beta_1}^2 = \frac{\sigma^2}{\sum_{i=1}^{n}(x_i - \bar{x})^2}. \qquad (2.12)$$

In practice, $\sigma_{\beta_1}^2$ will be estimated by

$$s_{b_1}^2 = \frac{MS_E}{\sum_{i=1}^{n}(x_i - \bar{x})^2}$$

and

$$\sqrt{s_{b_1}^2} = s_{b_1}, \text{ or the standard deviation value for } \beta_1. \qquad (2.13)$$

Returning to the β_1 test, to evaluate whether β_1 is significant ($\beta_1 \neq 0$), the researchers set up a two-tail hypothesis, using the six-step procedure.

Step 1: Determine the hypothesis.

$H_0: \beta_1 = 0,$

$H_A: \beta_1 \neq 0.$

Step 2: Set the α level.

Step 3: Select the test statistic, $t_{calculated}$

$$t_{calculated} = t_c = \frac{b_1}{s_{b_1}}, \text{ where}$$

$$b_1 = \frac{\sum_{i=1}^{n} (x_i - \bar{x})(y_i - \bar{y})}{\sum_{i=1}^{n} (x_i - \bar{x})^2} \text{ and}$$

$$s_{b_1} = \sqrt{\frac{MS_E}{\sum_{i=1}^{n} (x_i - \bar{x})^2}}.$$

Step 4: State the decision rule for $t_{tabled} = t_{(\alpha/2, \, n-2)}$ from Table B.

If $|t_c| > t_{(\alpha/2, n-2)}$, reject H_0; the slope (β_1) differs significantly from 0 at α.
If $|t_c| \leq t_{(\alpha/2, n-2)}$, the researcher cannot reject the null hypothesis at α.

Step 5: Compute the calculated test statistic (t_c).

Step 6: State the conclusion when comparing $t_{calculated}$ with t_{tabled}.

Let us now calculate whether the slope is 0 for data presented in Table 2.1 for Example 2.1.

Step 1: Establish the hypothesis.

$H_0: \beta_1 = 0,$

$H_A: \beta_1 \neq 0.$

Step 2: Set α. Let us set α at 0.05.

Step 3: Select the test statistic:

$$t_c = \frac{b_1}{s_{b_1}}.$$

Step 4: Decision rule.

If $|t_c| > t_{(\alpha/2, \, n-2)}$, reject the null hypothesis (H_0) at $\alpha = 0.05$. Using Student's t table (Table B) $t_{(0.05/2, 15-2)} = t_{0.025, 13} = 2.160$. So if $|t_{calculated}| > 2.160$, reject H_0 at $\alpha = 0.05$.

Step 5: Calculate the test statistic, $t_c = \frac{b_1}{s_{b_1}}$.

Recall from Example 2.1 that $b_1 = -0.041$. Also, recall from the initial computation of b_1 that $\sum_{i=1}^{n}(x_i - \bar{x})^2 = 6750$:

$$MS_E = \frac{\sum_{i=1}^{n}(y_i - \hat{y})^2}{n-2} = \frac{\sum_{i=1}^{n}e_i^2}{n-2},$$

$$= \frac{(0.0407)^2 + (-0.0307)^2 + \cdots + (-0.2547)^2 + (-0.2347)^2}{13},$$

$$= \frac{0.3750}{13} = 0.0288,$$

$$s_{b_1} = \sqrt{\frac{MS_E}{\sum_{i=1}^{n}(x_i - \bar{x})^2}} = \sqrt{\frac{0.0288}{6750}} = 0.0021,$$

$$t_c = \frac{b_1}{s_{b_1}} = \frac{-0.041}{0.0021} = -19.5238.$$

Step 6: Draw conclusion.

Because $|t_c| = |-19.5238| > 2.160$, the researcher rejects H_0, that the slope (rate of bacterial destruction per second) is 0 at $\alpha = 0.05$.

One-tail tests (upper or lower tail) for b_1 are also possible. If the researcher wants to conduct an upper-tail test (hypothesize that β_1 is significantly positive, that is, an ascending regression line), the hypothesis would be

$$H_0: \beta_1 \leq 0,$$

$$H_A: \beta_1 > 0,$$

with the same test statistic as that used in the two-tail test,

$$t_c = \frac{b_1}{s_{b_1}}.$$

The test is: if $t_c > t_{(\alpha, n-2)}$, reject H_0 at α.

Note: The upper-tail t_{tabled} value from Table B, which is a positive value, will be used.

For the lower-tail test, the test hypothesis for β_1 will be a negative t_{tabled} value (descending regression line):

$$H_0: \beta_1 \geq 0,$$

$$H_A: \beta_1 < 0,$$

with the test calculated value

$$t_c = \frac{b_1}{s_{b_1}}.$$

If $t_c < t_{(\alpha, n-2)}$, reject H_0 at α.

Note: The lower-tail value from Table B, which is negative, is used to find the $t_{(\alpha, n-2)}$ value.

Finally, if the researcher wants to compare β_1 with a specific value (k), that too can be accomplished using a two-tail or one-tail test. For the two-tail test, the hypothesis is

$$H_0: \beta_1 = k,$$

$$H_A: \beta_1 \neq k,$$

where k is a set value.

$$t_c = \frac{b_1 - k}{s_{b_1}}.$$

If $|t_c| > t_{(\alpha/2, n-2)}$, reject H_0. Both upper- and lower-tail tests can be evaluated for a k value, using the procedures just described. The only modification is that $t_c = (b_1 - k)/s_{b_1}$ is compared, respectively, with the positive or negative values of $t_{(\alpha, n-2)}$ tabled.

COMPUTER OUTPUT

Generally, it will be most efficient to use a computer for regression analyses. A regression analysis using MiniTab, a common software program, is presented in Table 2.3, using the data from Example 2.1.

CONFIDENCE INTERVAL FOR β_1

A $1 - \alpha$ confidence interval (CI) for β_1 is a straightforward computation:

$$\beta_1 = b_1 \pm t_{(\alpha/2, n-2)} s_{b_j}.$$

Example 2.2: To determine the 95% CI on β_1, using the data from Example 2.1 and our regression analysis data, we find $t_{(0.05/2, 15-2)}$ (from Table B, Student's t table) $= \pm 2.16$:

TABLE 2.3
Computer Printout of Regression Analysis

Predictor	Coef	SE Coef	T	P
[a]b_0	6.13067	0.07594	80.73	0.000
[b]b_1	−0.040933	0.002057	−19.81	0.000
[c]$s = 0.1698$	[d]$R\text{-}Sq = 96.8\%$			

The regression equation is $y = 6.13 - 0.041x$.

[a]b_0 value row = constant = y intercept when $x = 0$. The value beneath Coef is b_0 (6.13067); the value beneath SE Coef (0.07594) is the standard error of b_0. The value beneath T (80.73) is the t-test calculated value for b_0, hypothesizing it as 0, from H_0. The value (0.00) beneath P is the probability, when H_0 is true, of seeing a value of t greater than or the same as 80.73, and this is essentially 0.

[b]b_1 value row = slope. The value beneath Coef (−0.040933) is b_1; the value beneath SE Coef (0.002057) is the standard error of b_1; the value beneath T (−19.81) is the t-test calculated value for the null hypothesis that $b_1 = 0$. The value beneath P (0.00) is the probability of computing a value of −19.81, or more extreme, given the b_1 value is actually 0.

[c]$s = \sqrt{\text{MS}_E}$.

[d]r^2 or coefficient of determination.

$$b_1 = -0.0409,$$

$$s_{b_1} = \sqrt{\frac{\text{MS}_E}{\sum (x - \bar{x})^2}} = \sqrt{\frac{0.0288}{6750}} = 0.0021,$$

$$b_1 + t_{\alpha/2}s_{b_1} = -0.0409 + (2.16)(0.0021) = -0.0364,$$

$$b_1 - t_{\alpha/2}s_{b_1} = -0.0409 - (2.16)(0.0021) = -0.0454,$$

$$-0.0454 \le \beta_1 \le -0.0364.$$

The researcher is confident at the 95% level that the true slope (β_1) lies within this CI. In addition, the researcher can determine whether $\beta_1 = 0$ is from the CI. If the CI includes 0 (which it does not), the H_0 hypothesis, $\beta_1 = 0$, cannot be rejected at α.

INFERENCES WITH β_0

The point estimator of β_0, the y intercept, is

$$b_0 = \bar{y} - b_1\bar{x}. \tag{2.14}$$

The expected value of b_0 is

$$E(b_0) = \beta_0. \tag{2.15}$$

The expected variance of β_0 is

$$\sigma_{b_0}^2 = \sigma^2 \left[\frac{1}{n} + \frac{\bar{x}^2}{\sum\limits_{i=1}^{n}(x_i - \bar{x})^2} \right], \tag{2.16}$$

which is estimated by $s_{b_0}^2$:

$$s_{b_0}^2 = \text{MS}_E \left[\frac{1}{n} + \frac{\bar{x}^2}{\sum\limits_{i=1}^{n}(x_i - \bar{x})^2} \right], \tag{2.17}$$

where

$$\text{MS}_E = \frac{\sum\limits_{i=1}^{n}(y_i - \hat{y})^2}{n-2} = \frac{\sum e^2}{n-2}.$$

Probably the most useful procedure for evaluating β_0 is to determine a $1-\alpha$ CI for its true value. The procedure is straightforward. Using our previous Example 2.1,

$$\beta_0 = b_0 \pm t_{(\alpha/2, n-2)} s_{b_0},$$

$$b_0 = 6.1307.$$

$t_{(0.05/2, 15-2)} = \pm 2.16$ from Table B (Student's t table).

$$s_{b_0} = \sqrt{\text{MS}_E \left[\frac{1}{n} + \frac{\bar{x}^2}{\sum\limits_{i=1}^{n}(x_i - \bar{x})^2} \right]},$$

$$s_{b_0} = \sqrt{0.0288 \left[\frac{1}{15} + \frac{30^2}{6750} \right]} = 0.0759,$$

$$b_0 + t_{(\alpha/2, n-2)} s_{b_0} = 6.1307 + 2.16(0.0759) = 6.2946,$$
$$b_0 - t_{(\alpha/2, n-2)} s_{b_0} = 6.1307 - 2.16(0.0759) = 5.9668,$$
$$5.9668 \le \beta_0 \le 6.2946 \quad \text{at} \quad \alpha = 0.05.$$

The researcher is $1 - \alpha$ (or 95%) confident that the true β_0 value lies within the CI of 5.9668 to 6.2946.

Notes:

1. In making inferences about β_0 and/or β_1, the distribution of the y_i values, as with our previous work with the x_i values using Student's t-test or the analysis of variance (ANOVA), does not have to be perfectly normal. It can approximate normality. Even if the distribution is rather far from normal, the estimators b_0 and b_1 are said to be asymptotically normal. That is, as the sample size increases, the y distribution used to estimate both b_0 and b_1 approaches normality. In cases where the y_i data are clearly not normal, however, the researcher can use nonparametric regression approaches.

2. The regression procedure we use assumes that the x_i values are fixed and have not been collected at random. The CIs and tests concerning β_0 and β_1 are interpreted with respect to the range the x values cover. They do not purport to estimate β_0 and β_1 outside of that range.

3. As with the t-test, the $1 - \alpha$ confidence level should not be interpreted that one is 95% confident that the true β_0 or β_1 lie within the $1 - \alpha$ CI. Instead, over 100 runs, one observes the b_0 or b_1 contained within the interval $(1 - \alpha)$ times. At $\alpha = 0.05$, for example, if one performed the experiment 100 times, 95 times out of 100, the calculated b_0 or b_1 would be contained within that calculated interval.

4. It is important that the researcher knows that the greater the range covered by the x_i values selected, the more generally useful will be the regression equation. In addition, the greatest weight in the regression computation lies with the outer values (Figure 2.14).

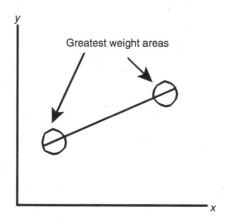

FIGURE 2.14 Greatest weight in regression computation.

The researcher will generally benefit by taking great pains to assure that those outer data regions are representative of the true condition. Recall that in our discussion of the example data set, when we noted the importance in the $\log_{10}$ linear equation of death curve kinetics, that the first value (time zero) and the last value are known to have disproportionate influence on the data, we dropped them. This sort of insight, afforded only by experience, must be drawn on constantly by the researcher. In research, it is often, but not always, wise to take the worst-case approach to make decisions. Hence, the researcher should constantly intersperse statistical theory with field knowledge and experience.

5. The greater the spread of the x values, the greater the value $\sum_{i=1}^{n} (x_i - \bar{x})^2$, which is the denominator of b_1 and s_{b_1} and a major portion of the denominator for b_0. Hence, the greater the spread, the smaller the variance of values for b_1 and b_0 will be. This is particularly important for statistical inferences concerning β_1.

POWER OF THE TESTS FOR β_0 AND β_1

To compute the power of the tests concerning β_0 and β_1, the approach is relatively simple:

$$H_0: \beta = \beta_x,$$

$$H_A: \beta \neq \beta_x,$$

where $\beta = \beta_1$ or β_0, and β_x = any constant value. If the test is to evaluate the power relative to 0 (e.g., $\beta_1 \neq 0$), the β_x value should be set at 0. As always, the actual sample testing uses lower case b_i values:

$$t_c = \frac{b_i - \beta_x}{s_{b_i}} \qquad (2.18)$$

is the test statistic to be employed, where b_i is the ith regression parameter; $i = 0$, if b_0; and 1, if b_1; β_x is the constant value or 0; and s_{b_i} is the standard error of β_i, where $i = 0$, if b_0 and 1, if b_1.

The power computation of the statistic is $1 - \beta$. It is found by computing δ, which is essentially a t-test (2.20). Using δ, at a specific α level corresponding to the degrees of freedom, one finds the corresponding $(1 - \beta)$ value:

$$\delta = \frac{|\beta_i - \beta_x|}{\sigma_{b_i}}, \qquad (2.19)$$

where σ_{b_i} is the standard error of β_i:

$$\beta_i = \beta_0, \quad \sigma_{(\beta_0)} = \sqrt{\sigma^2 \left[\frac{1}{n} + \frac{\bar{x}^2}{\sum_{i=1}^{n}(x_i - \bar{x})^2} \right]}, \quad \text{which in practice is}$$

$$s_{b_0} = \sqrt{MS_E \left[\frac{1}{n} + \frac{\bar{x}^2}{\sum_{i=1}^{n}(x_i - \bar{x})^2} \right]}.$$

Note: Generally, the power of the test is calculated before the evaluation to ensure that the sample size is adequate, and σ^2 is estimated from previous experiments, because MS_E cannot be known if the power is computed before performing the experiment. The value of σ^2 is estimated using MS_E when the power is computed after the sample data have been collected:

$$\beta_i = \beta_1, \quad \sigma_{(\beta_1)} = \sqrt{\frac{\sigma^2}{\sum_{i=1}^{n}(x_i - \bar{x})^2}},$$

which is estimated by $s_{\beta_1} = \sqrt{\dfrac{MS_E}{\sum_{i=1}^{n}(x_i - \bar{x})^2}}.$

Let us work an example. The researcher wants to compute the power of the statistic for β_1:

$H_0: \beta_1 = \beta_x,$

$H_A: \beta_1 \neq \beta_x.$

Let $\beta_x = 0$, in this example. Recall that $b_1 = -0.0409$. Let us estimate σ^2 with MS_E and, as an exercise, evaluate the power after the study has been conducted, instead of before:

$$s_{b_1}^2 = \frac{MS_E}{\sum_{i=1}^{n}(x_i - \bar{x})^2},$$

$$s_{b_1}^2 = \frac{0.0288}{6750},$$

$$s_{(b_1)} = \sqrt{\frac{0.0288}{6750}} = 0.0021,$$

$$\delta = \frac{|0.0409 - 0|}{0.0021} = \frac{0.0409}{0.0021} = 19.4762.$$

Using Table D (Power table for two-tail t-test), $df = n-2 = 15-2 = 13$, $\alpha = 0.05$, $\delta = 19.4762$, and the power $= 1-\beta \approx 1.00$ or 100% at $\delta = 9$, which is the largest value of δ available in the table. Hence, the researcher is assured that the power of the test is adequate to determine that the slope (β_1) is not 0, given it is not 0, at a σ of 0.0021 and $n = 15$.

ESTIMATING $\hat{y}$ VIA CONFIDENCE INTERVALS

A very common aspect of interval estimation involves estimating the regression line value, $\hat{y}$, with simultaneous CIs, for a specific value of x. That value $\hat{y}$ can be further subcategorized as an average predicted $\hat{y}$ value, or a specific $\hat{y}$. Figure 2.15 shows which regions on the regression plot can and cannot be estimated reliably via point and interval measurements.

The region—interpolation range—based on actual x, y values can be predicted confidently by regression methods. If intervals between the y values are small, the prediction is usually more reliable than if they are extended. The determining factor is the background—field—experience. If one, for example, has worked with lethality curves and has an understanding of a particular microorganism's death rate, the reliability of the model is greatly enhanced by the grounding in this knowledge. Any region not represented by both smaller and larger actual values of x, y is a region of extrapolation. It is usually very dangerous to assume accuracy and reliability of an estimate

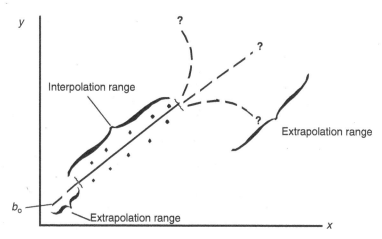

FIGURE 2.15 Regions on the regression plot.

made in an extrapolation region because this assumes that the data respond identically to the regression function computed from the observed x, y data. This usually cannot be safely assumed, so it is better not to attempt extrapolation. Such prediction is better dealt with using forecasting and time-series procedures. The researcher should focus exclusively on the region of the regression, the interpolation region, where actual x, y data have been collected, and so we shall, in this text.

Up to this point, we have considered the sampling regions of both b_0 and b_1, but not $\hat{y}$. Recall that the expected value of a predicted $\hat{y}$ at a given x is

$$E(\hat{y}) = b_0 + b_1 x. \tag{2.20}$$

The variance of $E(\hat{y})$ is

$$\sigma_{\hat{y}}^2 = \sigma^2 \left[\frac{1}{n} + \frac{(x_i - \bar{x})^2}{\sum_{i=1}^{n}(x_i - \bar{x})^2} \right].$$

In addition, as stated earlier, the greater the numerical range of the x_i values, the smaller the corresponding $\sigma_{\hat{y}}^2$ value is. However, note that the $\sigma_{\hat{y}}^2$ value is the variance for a specific x_i point. The farther the individual x_i is from the mean ($\bar{x}$), the larger $\sigma_{\hat{y}}^2$ will be. The $\sigma_{\hat{y}}^2$ value is smallest at $x_i = \bar{x}$. This phenomenon is important from a practical and a theoretical point of view. In the regression equation $b_0 + b_1 x_i$, there will always be some error in b_0 and b_1 estimates. In addition, the regression line will always go through ($\bar{x}$, $\bar{y}$), the pivot point. The more the variability in $\sigma_{\hat{y}}^2$, the greater the swing on the pivot point, as illustrated in Figure 2.16.

The true regression equation ($\hat{y}_P$) is somewhere between $\hat{y}_L$ and $\hat{y}_U$ (estimate of y lower and upper). The regression line pivots on the $\bar{y}$, $\bar{x}$ axis to a certain degree, with both b_0 and b_1 varying.

Because the researcher does not know exactly what the true regression linear function is, it must be estimated. Any of the $\hat{y}$ (y-predicted) values on particular x_i values will be wider, the farther away from the mean ($\bar{x}$) one estimates in either direction. This means that the $\hat{y}$ CI is not parallel to the regression line, but curvilinear (see Figure 2.17).

CONFIDENCE INTERVAL OF $\hat{y}$

A $1 - \alpha$ CI for the expected value—average value—of $\hat{y}$ for a specific x is calculated using the following equation:

$$\hat{y} \pm t_{(\alpha/2;\, n-2)} s_{\bar{y}}, \tag{2.21}$$

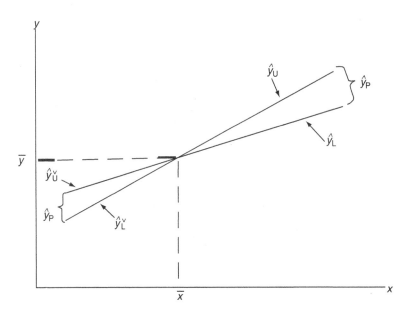

FIGURE 2.16 Regression line pivots.

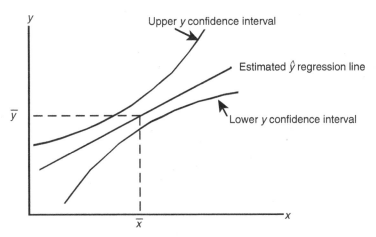

FIGURE 2.17 Confidence intervals.

where

$$\hat{y} = b_0 + b_1 x$$

and

$$s_{\bar{y}} = \sqrt{MS_E \left[\frac{1}{n} + \frac{(x_i - \bar{x})^2}{\sum_{i=1}^{n}(x_i - \bar{x})^2} \right]} \qquad (2.22)$$

and where x_i is the x value of interest used to predict $\hat{y}_i$:

$$MS_E = \frac{\sum_{i=1}^{n}(y_i - \hat{y}_i)^2}{n-2} = \frac{\sum_{i=1}^{n} e_i^2}{n-2}.$$

Example 2.3: Using the data in Table 2.1 and from Equation 2.1, we note that the regression equation is $\hat{y} = 6.13 - 0.041x$. Suppose the researcher would like to know the expected (average) value of y, as predicted by x_i, when $x_i = 15$ sec. What is the 95% confidence interval for the expected $\hat{y}$ average value?

$$\hat{y}_{15} = 6.13 - 0.041(15) = 5.515,$$

$$n = 15,$$

$$\bar{x} = 30,$$

$$\sum_{i=1}^{n}(x_i - \bar{x})^2 = 6750,$$

$$MS_E = \frac{\sum(y_i - \hat{y})^2}{n-2} = 0.0288,$$

$$s_{\bar{y}}^2 = MS_E \left[\frac{1}{n} + \frac{(x_i - \bar{x})^2}{\sum_{i=1}^{n}(x_i - \bar{x})^2} \right] = 0.0288 \left[\frac{1}{15} + \frac{(15 - 30)^2}{6750} \right],$$

$$s_{\bar{y}_{15}}^2 = 0.0029,$$

$$s_{\bar{y}_{15}} = 0.0537.$$

$t_{(\alpha/2; n-2)} = t_{(0.025; 15-2)} = 2.16$ (from Table B, Student's t table).
    The 95% CI $= \hat{y} \pm t_{(\alpha/2, n-2)} s_{\bar{y}} = 5.515 \pm 2.16(0.0537) = 5.515 \pm 0.1160$ or $5.40 \le \hat{y}_{15} \le 5.63$, at $\alpha = 0.05$.

Hence, the expected or average $\log_{10}$ population of microorganisms remaining after exposure to a 15 sec treatment with an antimicrobial is between 5.40 and 5.63 $\log_{10}$ at the 95% confidence level. This CI is a prediction for one value, not multiple ones. Multiple estimation will be discussed later.

PREDICTION OF A SPECIFIC OBSERVATION

Many times researchers are not interested in an expected (mean) value or mean value CI. They instead want an interval for a specific y_i value corresponding to a specific x_i. The process for this is very similar to that for the expected (mean) value procedure, but the CI for a single, new y_i value results in a wider CI than does predicting for an average y_i value. The formula for a specific y_i value is

$$\hat{y} \pm t_{(\alpha/2, n-2)}(s_{\hat{y}}), \tag{2.23}$$

where

$$\hat{y} = b_0 + b_1 x,$$

$$s_{\hat{y}}^2 = \text{MS}_E \left[1 + \frac{1}{n} + \frac{(x_i - \bar{x})^2}{\displaystyle\sum_{i=1}^{n} (x_i - \bar{x})^2} \right] \tag{2.24}$$

and

$$\text{MS}_E = \frac{\displaystyle\sum_{i=1}^{n} (y_i - \hat{y}_i)^2}{n - 2} = \frac{\displaystyle\sum_{i=1}^{n} e^2}{n - 2}.$$

Example 2.4: Again, using data from Table 2.1 and Equation 2.1, suppose the researcher wants to construct a 95% CI for an individual value, y_i, at a specific x_i, say 15 sec, $\hat{y} = b_0 + b_1 x$ and $\hat{y}_{15} = 6.13 - 0.041(15) = 5.515$, as mentioned earlier:

$$n = 15,$$

$$\bar{x} = 30,$$

$$\sum (x_i - \bar{x})^2 = 6750,$$

$$MS_E = \frac{\sum (y - \hat{y})^2}{n - 2} = 0.0288.$$

$s_{\hat{y}}^2$ is the standard error of a specific y on x,

$$s_{\hat{y}}^2 = MS_E \left[1 + \frac{1}{n} + \frac{(x_i - \bar{x})^2}{\sum (x_i - \bar{x})^2} \right] = 0.0288 \left[1 + \frac{1}{15} + \frac{(15 - 30)^2}{6750} \right],$$

$$s_{\hat{y}}^2 = 0.0317,$$

$$s_{\hat{y}} = 0.1780.$$

$t_{(\alpha/2; n-2)} = t_{(0.025; 15-2)} = 2.16$ (from Table B, Student's t table).

The 95% CI $= \hat{y} \pm t_{(\alpha/2, n-2)} s_{\hat{y}} = 5.515 \pm 2.16(0.1780) = 5.515 \pm 0.3845$ or $5.13 \leq \hat{y}_{15} \leq 5.90$ at $\alpha = 0.05$.

Hence, the researcher can expect the value $\hat{y}_i$ ($\log_{10}$ microorganisms) to be contained within the 5.13 to 5.90 $\log_{10}$ interval at a 15 sec exposure at a 95% confidence level. This does not mean that there is a 95% chance of the value being within the CI. It means that, if the experimental procedure was conducted 100 times, approximately 95 times out of 100, the value would lie within this interval. Again, this is a prediction interval of one y_i value on one x_i value.

CONFIDENCE INTERVAL FOR THE ENTIRE REGRESSION MODEL

There are many cases in which a researcher would like to map out the entire regression model (including both b_0 and b_1) with a $1 - \alpha$ CI. If the data have excess variability, the CI will be wide. In fact, it may be too wide to be useful. If this occurs, the experimenter may want to rethink the entire experiment or conduct it in a more controlled manner. Perhaps more observations—particularly replicate observations—will be needed. In addition, if the error $(y - \hat{y}) = e$ values are not patternless, then the experimenter might transform the data to better fit the regression model to the data.

Given that these problems are insignificant, one straightforward way to compute the entire regression model is the Working–Hotelling Method, which enables the researcher not only to plot the entire regression function, but also, to find the upper and lower CI limits for $\hat{y}$ on any or all x_i values using the formula,

$$\hat{y} \pm W s_{\bar{y}}. \tag{2.25}$$

The F distribution (Table C) is used in this procedure, instead of the t table, where

$$W^2 = 2F_{\alpha;(2,n-2)}.$$

As given earlier,

$$\hat{y}_i = b_0 + b_1 x_i$$

and

$$s_{\bar{y}} = \sqrt{MS_E \left[\frac{1}{n} + \frac{(x_i - \bar{x})^2}{\sum_{i=1}^{n}(x_i - \bar{x})^2} \right]}. \qquad (2.26)$$

Note that the latter is the same formula (2.22) used previously to perform a $1-\alpha$ CI for the expected (mean) value of a specific y_i on a specific x_i. However, the CI in this procedure is wider than the previous CI calculations, because it accounts for all x_i values simultaneously.

Example 2.5: Suppose the experimenter wants to determine the 95% CI for the data in Example 2.1, using the x_i values, $x_i = 0$, 15, 30, 45, and 60 sec, termed $x_{predicted}$ or x_p. The $\hat{y}_i$ values predicted, in this case, are to predict the average value of the $\hat{y}_i$s. The linear regression formula is

$$\hat{y} = 6.13 - 0.041(x_i)$$

when

$$x_p = 0; \quad \hat{y} = 6.13 - 0.041(0) = 6.13,$$

$$x_p = 15; \quad \hat{y} = 6.13 - 0.041(15) = 5.52,$$

$$x_p = 30; \quad \hat{y} = 6.13 - 0.041(30) = 4.90,$$

$$x_p = 45; \quad \hat{y} = 6.13 - 0.041(45) = 4.29,$$

$$x_p = 60; \quad \hat{y} = 6.13 - 0.041(60) = 3.67,$$

$$W^2 = 2F_{(0.05;2,15-2)}.$$

The F tabled value (Table C) $= 3.81$:

$$W^2 = 2(3.81) = 7.62 \quad \text{and} \quad W = \sqrt{7.62} = 2.76,$$

$$S_{(\bar{y})} = \sqrt{MS_E \left[\frac{1}{n} + \frac{(x_i - \bar{x})^2}{\sum\limits_{i=1}^{n} (x_i - \bar{x})} \right]} \quad \text{for } x_{p_i} = 0, 15, 30, 45, 60,$$

$$S_{(\bar{y}_0)} = \sqrt{0.0288 \left[\frac{1}{15} + \frac{(0 - 30)^2}{6750} \right]} = 0.0759, \quad x_p = 0,$$

$$S_{(\bar{y}_{15})} = \sqrt{0.0288 \left[\frac{1}{15} + \frac{(15 - 30)^2}{6750} \right]} = 0.0537, \quad x_p = 15,$$

$$S_{(\bar{y}_{30})} = \sqrt{0.0288 \left[\frac{1}{15} + \frac{(30 - 30)^2}{6750} \right]} = 0.0438, \quad x_p = 30,$$

$$S_{(\bar{y}_{45})} = \sqrt{0.0288 \left[\frac{1}{15} + \frac{(45 - 30)^2}{6750} \right]} = 0.0537, \quad x_p = 45,$$

$$S_{(\bar{y}_{60})} = \sqrt{0.0288 \left[\frac{1}{15} + \frac{(60 - 30)^2}{6750} \right]} = 0.0759, \quad x_p = 60.$$

Putting these together, one can construct a simultaneous $1 - \alpha$ CI for each x_p:

$$\hat{y} \pm W s_{\bar{y}} \text{ for each } x_p.$$

For $x_p = 0$, $6.13 \pm 2.76 (0.0759) = 6.13 \pm 0.2095$
$5.92 \leq \hat{y}_0 \leq 6.34$ when $x_p = 0$ at $\alpha = 0.05$ for the expected (mean) value of $\hat{y}$.
For $x_p = 15$, $5.52 \pm 2.76 (0.0537) = 5.52 \pm 0.1482$
$5.37 \leq \hat{y}_{15} \leq 5.67$ when $x_p = 15$ at $\alpha = 0.05$ for the expected (mean) value of $\hat{y}$.
For $x_p = 30$, $4.90 \pm 2.76 (0.0438) = 4.90 \pm 0.1209$
$4.78 \leq \hat{y}_{30} \leq 5.02$ when $x_p = 30$ at $\alpha = 0.05$ for the expected (mean) value of $\hat{y}$.
For $x_p = 45$, $4.29 \pm 2.76 (0.0537) = 4.29 \pm 0.1482$
$4.14 \leq \hat{y}_{45} \leq 4.44$ when $x_p = 45$ at $\alpha = 0.05$ for the expected (mean) value of $\hat{y}$.
For $x_p = 60$, $3.67 \pm 2.76 (0.0759) = 3.67 \pm 0.2095$
$3.46 \leq \hat{y}_{60} \leq 3.88$ when $x_p = 60$ at $\alpha = 0.05$ for the expected (mean) value of $\hat{y}$.

Another way to do this, and more easily, is by means of a computer software program. Figure 2.18 provides a MiniTab computer graph of the 95% CI (outer two lines) and the predicted $\hat{y}_i$ values (inner line).

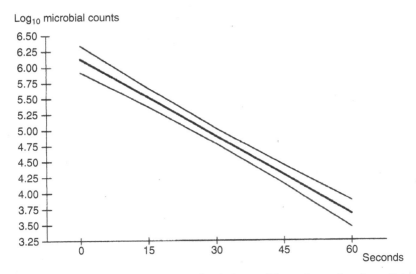

FIGURE 2.18 MiniTab computer graph of the confidence interval and predicted values.

Note that, though not dramatic, the CIs widen for the $\hat{y}_i$ regression line, as the data points move away from the mean ($\bar{x}$) value of 30. That is, the CI is the most narrow where $x_i = \bar{x}$ and increases in size as the values of x_i get further from $\bar{x}$, in either direction. In addition, one is not restricted to the values of x for which one has corresponding y data. One can interpolate for any value of x between and including 0 to 60 sec. The assumption, however, is that the actual y_i values for $x = (0, 60)$ follow the $\hat{y} = b_0 + b_1 x$ equation. Given that one has field experience, is familiar with the phenomena under investigation (here, antimicrobial death kinetics), and is sure the death curve remains $\log_{10}$ linear, there is no problem. If not, the researcher could make a huge mistake in thinking that the interpolated data follow the computed regression line, when they actually oscillate around the predicted regression line. Figure 2.19 illustrates this point graphically.

ANOVA AND REGRESSION

ANOVA is a statistical method very commonly used in checking the significance and adequacy of the calculated linear regression model. In simple linear—straight line—regression models, such as the one under discussion now, ANOVA can be used for evaluating whether β_1 (slope) is 0 or not. However, it is particularly useful for evaluating models involving two or more β_is; for example, determining if extra β_is (e.g., β_2, β_3, β_k) are of statistical value. We discuss this in detail in later chapters of this book.

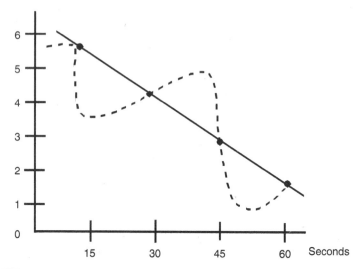

FIGURE 2.19 Antimicrobial death kinetics curve. (•) Actual collected data points; (—) predicted data points (regression analysis) that should be confirmed by the researcher's field experience; (- - - -) actual data trends known to the researcher but not measured. This example is exaggerated, but emphasizes that statistics must be grounded in field science.

For ANOVA employed in regression, three primary sum-of-squares values are needed: the total sum of squares, SS_T, the sum of squares explained by the regression SS_R, and the sum of squares due to the random error, SS_E. The total sum of squares is merely the sum of squares of the differences between actual y_i observations and the $\bar{y}$ mean:

$$SS_{total} = \sum_{i=1}^{n} (y_i - \bar{y})^2. \qquad (2.27)$$

Graphically, the total sum of squares $(y_i - \bar{y})^2$ includes both the regression and error effects in that it does not distinguish between them (Figure 2.20).

The total sum of squares, to be useful, is partitioned into the sum of squares due to regression (SS_R) and the sum of squares due to error (SS_E) or unexplained variability. The sum of squares, due to regression (SS_R), is the sum-of-squares value of the predicted values ($\hat{y}_i$) minus the $\bar{y}$ mean value:

$$SS_R = \sum_{i=1}^{n} (\hat{y}_i - \bar{y})^2. \qquad (2.28)$$

Figure 2.21 shows this graphically. If the slope is 0, the SS_R value is 0, because the regression parameters $\hat{y}$ and $\bar{y}$ are the same values.

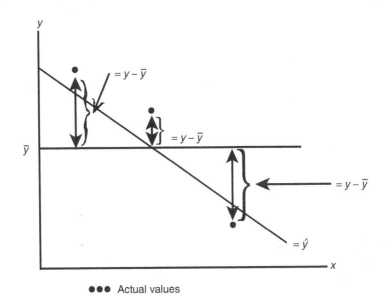

FIGURE 2.20 What the total sum-of-squares measures.

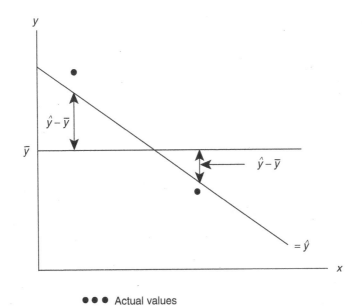

FIGURE 2.21 Sum-of-squares regression.

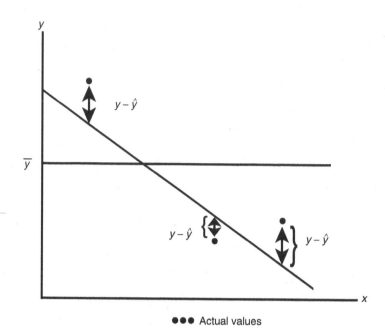

●●● Actual values

FIGURE 2.22 Sum-of-squares error term.

Finally, the sum-of-squares error term (SS_E) is the sum of the squares of the actual y_i values minus the predicted $\hat{y}_i$ value:

$$SS_E = \sum_{i=1}^{n} (y_i - \hat{y}_i)^2. \qquad (2.29)$$

Figure 2.22 shows this graphically.

As is obvious, the sums of SS_E and SS_R equal SS_{total}:

$$SS_R + SS_E = SS_{total}. \qquad (2.30)$$

The degrees of freedom for these three parameters, as well as the mean square error, are presented in Table 2.4. The entire ANOVA table is presented in Table 2.5.

The six-step procedure can be easily applied to the regression ANOVA for determining if $\beta_1 = 0$. Let us now use the data in Example 2.1 to construct an ANOVA table.

Step 1: Establish the hypothesis:

$H_0: \beta_1 = 0,$

$H_A: \beta_1 \neq 0.$

TABLE 2.4
Degrees of Freedom and Mean-Square Error

Sum of Squares (SS)	Degrees of Freedom (DF)	Mean-Square Error (MS$_E$)
SS$_R$	1	$\dfrac{SS_R}{1}$
SS$_E$	$n-2$	$\dfrac{SS_E}{n-2}$
SS$_{total}$	$n-1$	Not calculated

Step 2: Select the α significance level.
   Let us set α at 0.10.

Step 3: Specify the test statistic. The test statistic used to determine if $\beta_1 = 0$ is found in Table 2.5:

$$F_C = \frac{MS_R}{MS_E}.$$

Step 4: Decision rule: if $F_c > F_T$, reject H_0 at α.
   $F_T = F_{(\alpha;\, 1,\, n-a)} = F_{0.10\,(1,\,13)} = 3.14$ (from Table C, the F Distribution).
   If $F_c > 3.14$, reject H_0 at $\alpha = 0.10$.

Step 5: Compute ANOVA model.
   Recall from our calculations earlier, $\bar{y} = 4.90$:

$$SS_{total} = \sum_{i=1}^{n} (y_i - \bar{y})^2$$
$$= (6.09 - 4.90)^2 + (6.10 - 4.90)^2 + \cdots + (3.42 - 4.90)^2 + (3.44 - 4.90)^2$$
$$= 11.685$$

TABLE 2.5
ANOVA Table

Source	SS	DF	MS	F_c	F_T	Significant/ Non-Significant
Regression	$SS_R = \sum_{i=1}^{n} (\hat{y}_i - \bar{y})^2$	1	$\dfrac{SS_R}{1} = MS_R$ [a]	$\dfrac{MS_R}{MS_E} = F_c$	$F_{T(\alpha;\,1,n-2)}$	If $F_c > F_T$, reject H_0
Error	$SS_E = \sum_{i=1}^{n} (y_i - \hat{y}_i)^2$	$n-2$	$\dfrac{SS_E}{n-2} = MS_E$			
Total	$SS_{total} = \sum_{i=1}^{n} (y_i - \bar{y})^2$	$n-1$				

[a] An alternative that is often useful for calculating MS_R is $b_1^2 \sum_{i=1}^{n} (x_i - \bar{x})^2$.

TABLE 2.6
ANOVA Table

Source	SS	DF	MS	F_c	F_T	Significant/Nonsignificant
Regression	$SS_R = 11.310$	1	11.310	392.71	3.14	Significant
Error	$SS_E = 0.375$	13	0.0288			
Total	11.685	14				

SS_R (using the alternate formula):
Recall $\sum (x - \bar{x})^2 = 6750$, and $b_1 = -0.040933$

$$SS_R = b_1^2 \sum_{i=1}^{n} (x_i - \bar{x})^2 = -0.040933^2(6750) = 11.3097,$$

$$SS_E = SS_{total} - SS_R = 11.685 - 11.310 = 0.375.$$

Step 6: The researcher sees clearly that the regression slope b_1 is not equal to 0; that is, $F_c = 392.70 > F_T = 3.14$. Hence, the null hypothesis is rejected. Table 2.6 provides the completed ANOVA model of this evaluation. Table 2.7 provides a MiniTab version of this table.

LINEAR MODEL EVALUATION OF FIT OF THE MODEL

The ANOVA F test to determine the significance of the slope ($\beta_1 \neq 0$) is useful, but can it be expanded to evaluate the fit of the statistical model? That is, how well does the model predict the actual data? This procedure is often very important in multiple linear regression in determining whether increasing the number of variables (β_i) is statistically efficient and effective.

A lack-of-fit procedure, which is straightforward, can be used in this situation. However, it requires repeated measurements (i.e., replication) for

TABLE 2.7
MiniTab Printout ANOVA Table

Analysis of Variance

Source	DF	SS	MS	F	P
Regression	1	11.310	11.310	390.0	0.000
Residual error	13	0.375	0.029		
Total	14	11.685			

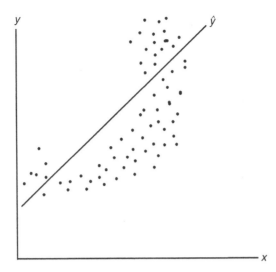

FIGURE 2.23 Inappropriate linear model.

at least some of the x_i values. The F test for lack of fit is used to determine if the regression model used (in our case, $\hat{y} = b_0 + b_1 x_i$) adequately predicts and models the data. If it does not, the researcher can (1) increase the beta variables, $\beta_2, \ldots, \beta_n$, by collecting additional experimental information or (2) transform the scale of the data to linearize them.

For example, in Figure 2.23, if the linear model is represented by a line and the data by dots, one can easily see that the model does not fit the data. In this case, a simple $\log_{10}$ transformation, without increasing the number of β_i values, may be the answer. Hence, a $\log_{10}$ transformation of the y values makes the simple regression model appropriate (Figure 2.24).

In computing the lack-of-fit F test, several assumptions about the data must be made:

1. The y_i values corresponding to each x_i are independent of each other.
2. The y_i values are normally distributed and share the same variance.

In practice, assumption 1 is often difficult to ensure. For example, in a time–kill study, the exposure values y at 1 min are related to the exposure values y at 30 sec. This author has found that, even if the y values are correlated, the regression is still very useful and appropriate. However, it may be more useful to use a different statistical model (Box–Jenkins, weighted average, etc.). This is particularly so if values beyond the data range collected are predicted.

It is important to realize that the F test for regression fit relies on the replication of various x_i levels. Note that this means the actual replication of

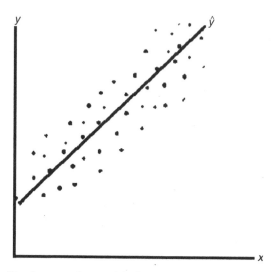

FIGURE 2.24 Simple regression model after $\log_{10}$ transformation.

these levels, not just repeated measurements. For example, if a researcher is evaluating the antimicrobial efficacy of a surgical scrub formulation by exposing a known number of microorganisms for 30 sec to the formulation, then neutralizing the antimicrobial activity and plating each dilution level three times, this would not constitute a triplicate replication. The entire procedure must be replicated or repeated three times, to include initial population, exposure to the antimicrobial, neutralization, dilutions, and plating.

The model the F test for lack of fit evaluates is $E[y] = b_0 + b_1 x_i$:

$$H_0 : E[y] = b_0 + b_1 x_i,$$
$$H_A : E[y] \neq b_0 + b_1 x_i,$$

where $E(y) = b_0 + b_1 x_i$ the expected value of y_i is adequately represented by $b_0 + b_1 x_i$.

The statistical process uses a full model and a reduced model. The full model is evaluated first, using the following formula:

$$y_{ij} = \mu_j + \varepsilon_{ij}, \tag{2.31}$$

where μ_j are the parameters $j = 1, \ldots, k$. The full model states that the y_{ij} values are made up of two components.

1. The expected mean response for the μ_j at a specific x_j value ($\mu_j = \bar{y}_j$).
2. The random error (ε_{ij}).

The sum-of-squares error for the full model is considered pure error, which will be used to determine the fit of the model. The pure error is any variation from $\bar{y}_j$ at a specific x_j level:

$$SSE_{full} = SS_{pure\ error} = \sum_{j=1}^{k} \sum_{i=1}^{n} (y_{ij} - \bar{y}_j)^2. \tag{2.32}$$

The $SS_{pure\ error}$ is the variation of the replicate y_j values from the $\bar{y}_j$ value at each replicated x_j level.

REDUCED ERROR MODEL

The reduced model determines if the actual regression model under the null hypothesis $(b_0 + b_1 x)$ is adequate to explain the data. The reduced model is

$$y_{ij} = b_0 + b_1 x_j + e_{ij}. \tag{2.33}$$

That is, the amount that error is reduced due to the regression equation $b_0 + b_1 x$ in terms of $e = y - \hat{y}$, or the actual value minus the predicted value, is determined.

More formally, the sum of squares reduced model is

$$SS_{(reduced)} = \sum_{i=1}^{k} \sum_{j=1}^{n} (y_{ij} - \hat{y}_{ij})^2 = \sum_{i=1}^{k} \sum_{j=1}^{n} [y_{ij} - (b_0 + b_1 x_j)]^2. \tag{2.34}$$

Note that

$$SS_{(reduced)} = SS_E. \tag{2.35}$$

The difference between SS_E and $SS_{pure\ error} = SS_{lack-of-fit}$:

$$SS_E = SS_{pure\ error} + SS_{lack-of-fit}, \tag{2.36}$$

$$\underbrace{(y_{ij} - \hat{y}_{ij})^2}_{total\ error} = \underbrace{(y_{ij} - \hat{y}_{\cdot j})^2}_{pure\ error} + \underbrace{(\bar{y}_{\cdot j} - \hat{y}_{ij})^2}_{lack-of-fit}. \tag{2.37}$$

Let us look at this diagrammatically (Figure 2.25). Pure error is the difference of actual y values from $\bar{y}$ at a specific x (in this case, $x = 4$):

$$y_i - \bar{y} = 23 - 21.33 = 1.67,$$

$$21 - 21.33 = -0.33,$$

$$20 - 21.33 = -1.33.$$

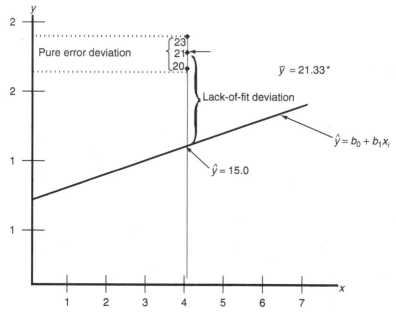

$$(y_{ij} - \hat{y}_{ij}) \quad = \quad (y_{ij} - \hat{y}_j) \quad + \quad (\bar{y}_j - \hat{y}_{ij})$$

Total deviation   Pure error deviation   Lack-of-fit deviation

*21.33 is the average of 23, 21, and 20.

FIGURE 2.25 Deviation decomposition using.

Lack of fit is the difference between the $\bar{y}$ value at a specific x and the predicted $\hat{y}$ at that specific x value or $\bar{y} - \hat{y}_4 = 21.33 - 15.00 = 6.33$.

The entire ANOVA procedure can be completed in conjunction with the previous F test ANOVA, by expanding the SS_E term to include both $SS_{\text{pure error}}$ and $SS_{\text{lack-of-fit}}$. This procedure can only be carried out with the replication of the x values (Table 2.8).

The test hypothesis for the lack-of-fit component is $H_0: E[y] = b_0 + b_1 x$ (the linear regression model adequately describes data).

$H_A: E[y] \neq b_0 + b_1 x$ (the linear regression model does not adequately describe data).

If

$$F_c = \left(\frac{MS_{LF}}{MS_{PE}}\right) > F_T, (F_{T\alpha(c-2; n-c)}), \text{ reject } H_0 \text{ at } \alpha,$$

TABLE 2.8
ANOVA Table

Source	Sum of Squares	Degrees of Freedom	MS	F_c	F_T
Regression	$SS_R = \sum_{i=1}^{n} \sum_{j=1}^{k} (\hat{y}_{ij} - \bar{y})^2$	1	$\dfrac{SS_R}{1} = MS_R$	$\dfrac{MS_R}{MS_E}$	$F_{\alpha(1, n-2)}$
Error	$SS_E = \sum_{i=1}^{n} \sum_{j=1}^{k} (y_{ij} - \hat{y}_{ij})^2$	$n - 2$	$\dfrac{SS_E}{n - 2} = MS_E$		
Lack-of-fit error	$SS_{\text{lack-of-fit}} = \sum_{i=1}^{n} \sum_{j=1}^{k} (\bar{y}_{\cdot j} - \hat{y}_{ij})^2$	$c - 2$	$\dfrac{SS_{\text{lack-of-fit}}}{c - 2} = MS_{LF}$	$\dfrac{MS_{LF}}{MS_{PE}}$	$F_{\alpha(c-2, n-c)}$
Pure error	$SS_{\text{pure error}} = \sum_{i=1}^{n} \sum_{j=1}^{k} (y_{ij} - \bar{y}_{\cdot j})^2$	$n - c$	$\dfrac{SS_{\text{pure error}}}{n - c} = MS_{PE}$		
Total	$SS_{\text{total}} = \sum_{i=1}^{k} \sum_{j=1}^{c} (y_{ij} - \bar{y})^2$	$n - 1$			

Note: c is the number of specific x observations (replicated x_i count as one value).

where c is the number of groups of data (replicated and nonreplicated), which is the number of different x_j levels. n is the number of observations.

Let us now work the data in Example 2.1.

The F test for lack of fit of the simple linear regression model is easily expressed in the six-step procedure.

Step 1: Determine the hypothesis:

$$H_0: E[y] = b_0 + b_1 x,$$

$$H_A: E[y] \neq b_0 + b_1 x.$$

Note: The null hypothesis for the lack of fit is that the simple linear regression model cannot be rejected at the specific α level.

Step 2: State the significance level (α).

In this example, let us set α at 0.10.

Step 3: Write the test statistic to be used

$$F_c = \frac{MS_{\text{lack-of-fit}}}{MS_{\text{pure error}}}.$$

Step 4: Specify the decision rule.

If $F_c > F_T$, reject H_0 at α. In this example, the value for F_T is

$$F_{\alpha(c-2; n-c)} = F_{0.10; (5-2; 15-5)} = F_{0.10 (3, 10)} = 2.73.$$

Therefore, if $F_c > 2.73$, reject H_0 at $\alpha = 0.10$.

Step 5: Perform the ANOVA. $N = 15$; $c = 5$

Level $= j = x_j$		1	2	3	4	5
		0	15	30	45	60
Replicate						
	1	6.09	5.48	5.01	4.53	3.57
	2	6.10	5.39	4.88	4.62	3.42
$y_{ij} =$	3	6.08	5.51	4.93	4.49	3.44
$\bar{y}_{\cdot j} =$		6.09	5.46	4.94	4.55	3.48

$$SS_{\text{pure error}} = \sum_{j=1}^{n} \sum_{j=1}^{k} (y_{ij} - \bar{y}_{\cdot j})^2 \text{ over the five levels of } x_j, \ c = 5.$$

$$SS_{PE} = (6.09 - 6.09)^2 + (6.10 - 6.09)^2 + (6.08 - 6.09)^2 + (5.48 - 5.46)^2$$
$$+ \cdots (3.57 - 3.48)^2 + (3.42 - 3.48)^2 + (3.44 - 3.48)^2$$
$$= 0.0388.$$

$SS_{\text{lack-of-fit}} = SS_E - SS_{PE}$, and SS_E (from Table 2.6) $= 0.375$.

$SS_{\text{lack-of-fit}} = 0.375 - 0.0388 = 0.3362$.

In anticipation of this kind of analysis, it is often useful to include the lack-of-fit and pure error within the basic ANOVA Table (Table 2.9). Note that the computation of lack-of-fit and pure error are a decomposition of SS_E.

Step 6: Decision.
Because F_c (28.74) $> F_T$ (2.73), we reject H_0 at the $\alpha = 0.10$ level. The rejection, i.e., the model is portrayed to lack fit, is primarily because there is too little variability within each of the j replicates used to obtain pure error. Therefore, even though the actual data are reasonably well represented by the regression model, the model could be better.

TABLE 2.9
New ANOVA Table

Source	SS	DF	MS	F_c	F_T	Significant/Nonsignificant
Regression	11.3100	1	11.3100	392.71	3.14	Significant
Error	0.375	13	0.0288			
Lack-of-fit error	0.3362	3	0.1121	28.74	2.73	Significant
Pure error	0.0388	10	0.0039			
Total	11.6850	14				

The researcher must now weigh the pros and cons of using the simple linear regression model. From a practical perspective, the model may very well be useful enough, even though the lack-of-fit error is significant. In many situations experienced by this author, this model would be good enough. However, to a purist, perhaps a third variable (β_2) could be useful. However, will a third variable hold up in different studies? It may be better to collect more data to determine if the simple linear regression model holds up in other cases. It is quite frustrating for the end user to have to compare different reports using different models to make decisions, apart from understanding the underlying data. For example, if, when a decision maker reviews several death-rate kinetic studies of a specific product and specific microorganisms, the statistical model is different for each study, the decision maker probably will not use the statistical analyst's services much longer. So, when possible, use general, but robust models.

This author would elect to use the simple linear regression model to approximate the antimicrobial activity, but would collect more data sets not only to see if the H_0 hypothesis would continue to be rejected, but also if the extra variable (β_2) model would be adequate for the new data. In statistics, data-pattern chasing can be an endless pursuit with no conclusion ever reached.

If the simple linear regression model, in the researcher's opinion, does not model the data properly, then there are several options:

1. Transform the data using EDA methods.
2. Abandon the simple linear regression approach for a more complex one, such as multiple regression.
3. Use a nonparametric statistic analog.

When possible, transform the data, because the simple linear regression model can still be used. However, there certainly is value in multiple regression procedures, in which the computations are done using matrix algebra. The only practical approach to performing multiple regression is via a computer using a statistical software package. Note that the replicate x_j values do not need to be consistent in number, as in our previous work in ANOVA. For example, if the data collected were as presented in Table 2.10, the computation would be performed the same way:

$$SS_{\text{pure error}} = (6.09 - 6.09)^2 + (6.10 - 6.09)^2 + (6.08 - 6.09)^2 + (5.48 - 5.46)^2$$
$$+ \cdots + (3.42 - 3.48)^2 + (3.44 - 3.48)^2 = 0.0388.$$

Degrees of freedom $= n - c = 15 - 5 = 10$.

Given SS_E as 0.375, $SS_{\text{lack-of-fit}}$ would equal

$$SS_{LF} = SS_E - SS_{\text{pure error}} = SS_{LF} = 0.375 - 0.0388 = 0.3362.$$

TABLE 2.10
Lack-of-Fit Computation (ns Are Not Equal)

Level j	1	2	3	4	5
x value	0	15	30	45	60
Corresponding y_{ij} values	6.09	5.48	5.01	4.53	3.57
		5.39	4.88	4.62	3.42
		5.51			3.44
Mean $\bar{y}_{\cdot j} =$	6.09	5.46	4.95	4.58	3.48
$n =$	1	3	2	2	3

Note: $n = 11, c = 5$.

Source	SS	DF	MS	F_c
SS_E	0.375	—	—	—
Error lack-of-fit	0.3362	3	0.1121	28.74
Pure error	0.0388	10	0.0039	

Let us now perform the lack-of-fit test with MiniTab using the original data as shown in Table 2.11.

As one can see, the ANOVA consists of the regression and residual error (SS_E) term. The regression is highly significant, with an F_c of 390.00. The residual error (SS_E) is broken into lack-of-fit and pure error. Moreover, the researcher sees that the lack-of-fit component is significant. That is, the linear model is not a precise fit, even though, from a practical perspective, the linear regression model may be adequate.

For many decision makers, as well as applied researchers, it is one thing to generate a complex regression model, but another entirely to explain its

TABLE 2.11
MiniTab Lack-of-Fit Test

Analysis of Variance

Source	DF	SS	MS	F	P
Regression	1	11.310	11.310	390.00	0.000
Residual error	13	0.375	0.029		
Lack-of-fit	3	0.336	0.112	28.00	0.000
Pure error	10	0.039	0.004		
Total	14	11.685			

meaning in terms of variables grounded in one's field of expertise. For those who are interested in regression in much more depth, see *Applied Regression Analysis* by Kleinbaum et al., *Applied Regression Analysis* by Draper and Smith, or *Applied Linear Statistical Models* by Kutner et al. Let us now focus on EDA, as it applies to regression.

EXPLORATORY DATA ANALYSIS AND REGRESSION

The vast majority of data can be linearized by merely performing a transformation. In addition, for those data that have nonconstant error variances, sigmoidal shapes, and other anomalies, the use of nonparametric regression is an option. In simple (linear) regression of the form $\hat{y} = b_0 + b_1 x$, the data must approximate a straight line. In practice, this often does not occur; so, to use the regression equation, the data must be straightened. Four common nonlinear data patterns can be straightened very simply. Figure 2.26 shows these patterns.

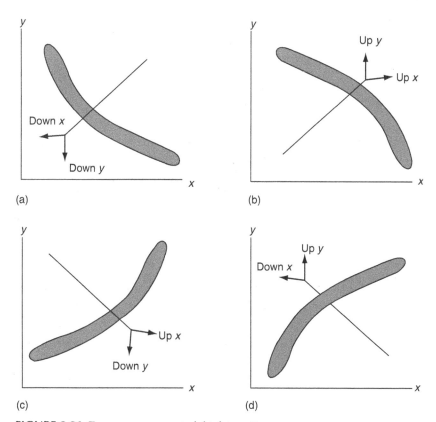

FIGURE 2.26 Four common nonstraight data patterns.

Pattern A

For Pattern A, the researcher will "go down" in the reexpression power of either x or y, or both. Often, nonstatistical audiences grasp the data more easily if the transformation is done on the y scale ($\sqrt{y}$, $\log_{10} y$, etc.) rather than on the x scale. The x scale is left at power 1, that is, it is not reexpressed. The regression is then refit, using the transformed data scale and checked to assure that the data have been straightened. If the plotted data do not appear straight line, the data are reexpressed again, say, from $\sqrt{y}$ to $\log y$ or even $-1\sqrt{y}$ (see Paulson, D.S., *Applied Statistical Designs for the Researcher*, Chapter 3). This process is done iteratively. In cases where one transformation almost straightens the data, but the next power transformation overstraightens the data slightly, the researcher may opt to choose the reexpression that has the smallest F_c value for lack of fit.

Pattern B

Data appearing like Pattern B may be linearized by increasing the power of the y values (e.g., y^2, y^3), increasing the power of the x values (e.g., x^2, x^3), or by increasing the power of both (y^2, x^2). Again, it is often easier for the intended audience—decision makers, business directors, or clients—to understand the data when y is reexpressed, and x is left in the original scale. As discussed earlier, the reexpression procedure is done sequentially (y^2 to y^3, etc.), computing the F_c value for lack of fit each time. The smaller the F_c value, the better. This author finds it most helpful to plot the data after each reexpression procedure, to select the best fit visually. The more linear the data are, the better.

Pattern C

For data that resemble Pattern C, the researcher needs to "up" the power scale of x (x^2, x^3, etc.) or "down" the power scale of y ($\sqrt{y}$, $\log y$, etc.) to linearize the data. For reasons previously discussed, it is recommended to transform the y values only, leaving the x values in the original form. In addition, once the data have been reexpressed, plot them to help determine visually if the reexpression adequately linearized them. If not, the next lower power transformation should be used, on the y value in this case. Once the data are reasonably linear, as determined visually, the F_c test for lack of fit can be used. Again, the smaller the F_c value, the better. If, say, the data are not quite linearized by $\sqrt{y}$ but are slightly curved in the opposite direction with the $\log y$ transformation, pick the reexpression with the smaller F_c value in the lack-of-fit test.

Pattern D

For data that resemble Pattern D, the researcher can go up the power scale in reexpressing y or down the power scale in reexpressing x, or do both. Again, it

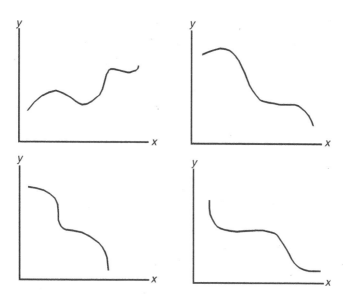

FIGURE 2.27 Polynomial regressions.

is recommended to reexpress the y values (y^2, y^3, etc.) only. The same strategy previously discussed should be used in determining the most appropriate reexpression, based on the F_c value.

DATA THAT CANNOT BE LINEARIZED BY REEXPRESSION

Data that are sigmoidal, or open up and down, or down and up, cannot be easily transformed. A change to one area (making it linear) makes the other areas even worse. Polynomial regression, a form of multiple regression, can be used for modeling these types of data and will be discussed in later chapters of this text (see Figure 2.27).

EXPLORATORY DATA ANALYSIS TO DETERMINE THE LINEARITY OF A REGRESSION LINE WITHOUT USING THE F_c TEST FOR LACK OF FIT

A relatively simple and effective way to determine if a selected reexpression procedure linearizes the data can be completed with EDA pencil–paper techniques (Figure 2.28). It is known as the "method of half-slopes" in EDA parlance. In practice, it is suggested, when reexpressing a data set to approximate a straight line, that this EDA procedure be used rather than the F_c test for lack of fit.

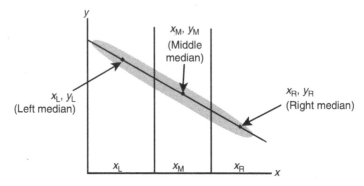

FIGURE 2.28 Half-slopes in EDA.

Step 1: Divide the data into thirds, finding the median (x, y) value of each group. Note that there is no need to be ultraaccurate, when partitioning the data into the three groups.

To find the left x, y medians (denoted x_L, y_L), use the left one-third of the data. To find the middle x, y medians, use the middle one-third of the data and label these as x_M, y_M. To find the right x, y medians, denoted by x_R, y_R, use the right one-third of the data.

Step 2: Estimate the slope (b_1) for both the left and right thirds of the data set:

$$b_L = \frac{y_M - y_L}{x_M - x_L}, \tag{2.38}$$

$$b_R = \frac{y_R - y_M}{x_R - x_M}, \tag{2.39}$$

where y_M is the median of the y values in the middle $1/3$ of the data set, y_L the median of the y values in the left $1/3$ of the data set, y_R the median of the y values in the right $1/3$ of the data set, x_M the median of the x values in the middle $1/3$ of the data set, x_L the median of the x values in the left $1/3$ of the data set, and x_R is the median of the x values in the right $1/3$ of the data set.

Step 3: Determine the slope coefficient:

$$\frac{b_R}{b_L}. \tag{2.40}$$

Step 4: If the b_R/b_L ratio is close to 1, the data are considered linear and good enough. If not, reexpress the data and repeat step 1 through step 3. Also, note that approximations of β_1 (slope) and β_0 (y intercept) can be computed using the median values of any data set:

$$b_1 = \frac{y_R - y_L}{x_R - x_L},$$ (2.41)

$$b_0 = y_M - b_1(x_M).$$ (2.42)

Let us use the data in Example 2.1 to perform the EDA procedures just discussed. Because these data cannot be partitioned into equal thirds, the data will be approximately separated into thirds. Because the left and right thirds have more influence on this EDA procedure than does the middle group, we use $x = 0$ and 15 in the left group, only $x = 30$ in the middle group, and $x = 45$ and 60 in the right group.

Step 1: Separate the data into thirds at the x levels.

Left Group	Middle Group	Right Group
$x = 0$ and 15	$x = 30$	$x = 45$ and 60
$x_L = 7.5$	$x_M = 30$	$x_R = 52.50$
$y_L = 5.80$	$y_M = 4.93$	$y_R = 4.03$

Step 2: Compute the slopes (β_1) for the left and right groups:

$$b_L = \frac{y_M - y_L}{x_M - x_L} = \frac{4.93 - 5.80}{30 - 7.5} = -0.0387,$$

$$b_R = \frac{y_R - y_M}{x_R - x_M} = \frac{4.03 - 4.93}{52.5 - 30} = -0.0400.$$

Step 3: Compute the slope coefficient, checking it to see if it equals 1:

$$\text{Slope coefficient} = \frac{b_R}{b_L} = \frac{-0.0400}{-0.0387} = 1.0336.$$

Note, in this procedure, that it is just as easy to see if $b_R = b_L$. If they are not exactly equal, it is the same as the slope coefficient not equaling 1. Because the slope coefficient ratio in our example is very close to 1 (and the values b_R and b_L are nearly equal), we can say that the data set is approximately linear.

If the researcher wants a rough idea as to what the slope (b_1) and y intercept (b_0) are, they can be computed using formula 2.42 and formula 2.43:

$$b_1 = \frac{y_R - y_L}{x_R - x_L} = \frac{4.03 - 5.80}{52.5 - 7.5} = -0.0393,$$

$$b_0 = y_M - b_1(x_M) = 4.93 - (-0.0393)30 = 6.109.$$

$\hat{y} = b_0 + b_1 x_1$ or $\hat{y} = 6.109 - 0.0393x$, which is very close to the parametric result, $\hat{y} = 6.13 - 0.041x$, computed by means of the least-squares regression procedure.

CORRELATION COEFFICIENT

The correlation coefficient, r, is a statistic frequently used to measure the strength of association between x and y. A correlation coefficient of 1.00 or 100% is a perfect fit (all the predicted $\hat{y}$ values equal the actual y values), and a 0 value is a completely random array of data (Figure 2.29). Theoretically, the range of r is -1 to 1, where -1 describes a perfect fit, descending slope (Figure 2.30).

The correlation coefficient (r) is a dimensionless value independent of x and y. Note that, in practice, the value for r^2 (coefficient of determination) is generally more directly useful. That is, knowing that $r = 0.80$ is not directly useful, but $r^2 = 0.80$ is, because the r^2 means that the regression equation is 80% better in predicting y than is the use of $\bar{y}$.

The more positive the r (closer to 1), the stronger the statistical association. That is, the accuracy and precision of predicting a y value from a value of x increases. It also means that, as the values of x increase, so do the y values. Likewise, the more negative the r value (closer to -1), the stronger the statistical association. In this case, as the x values increase, the y values decrease. The

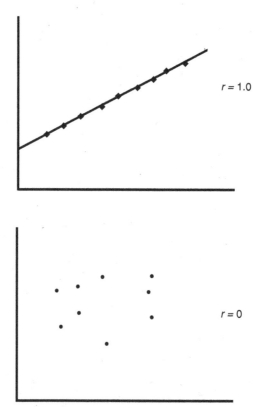

FIGURE 2.29 Correlation coefficients.

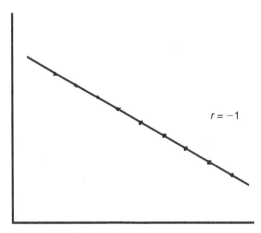

$r = -1$

FIGURE 2.30 Perfect descending slope.

closer the r value is to 0, the less linear association there is between x and y, meaning the accuracy in predictions of a y value from an x value decreases. By association, the author means dependence of y and x. That is, one can predict y by knowing x. The correlation coefficient value, r, is computed as

$$r = \frac{\sum_{i=1}^{n} (x_i - \bar{x})(y_i - \bar{y})}{\sqrt{\sum_{i=1}^{n} (x_i - \bar{x})^2 \sum_{i=1}^{n} (y_i - \bar{y})^2}}. \tag{2.43}$$

A simpler formula often is used for hand calculator computation:

$$r = \frac{\sum_{i=1}^{n} x_i y_i - \dfrac{\left(\sum_{i=1}^{n} x_i\right)\left(\sum_{i=1}^{n} y_i\right)}{n}}{\sqrt{\left[\sum_{i=1}^{n} x_i^2 - \dfrac{\left(\sum_{i=1}^{n} x_i\right)^2}{n}\right]\left[\sum_{i=1}^{n} y_i^2 - \dfrac{\left(\sum_{i=1}^{n} y_i\right)^2}{n}\right]}}. \tag{2.44}$$

Fortunately, even the relatively inexpensive scientific calculators usually have an internal program for calculating r. Let us compute r from the data in Example 2.1:

$$\sum_{i=1}^{n} x_i y_i = \sum_{i=1}^{15} (0 \times 6.09) + (0 \times 6.10) + \cdots + (60 \times 3.57) + (60 \times 3.42)$$

$$+ (60 \times 3.44) = 1929.90,$$

$$\sum_{i=1}^{15} x_i = 450,$$

$$\sum_{i=1}^{15} y_i = 73.54,$$

$$\sum_{i=1}^{15} x_i^2 = 20250.00,$$

$$\sum_{i=1}^{15} y_i^2 = 372.23,$$

$$n = 15,$$

$$r = \frac{1929.90 - \dfrac{(450)(73.54)}{15}}{\sqrt{\left[20250.00 - \dfrac{(450)^2}{15}\right]\left[372.23 - \dfrac{(73.54)^2}{15}\right]}} = -0.9837.$$

The correlation coefficient is −0.9837 or, as a percent, 98.37%. This value represents strong negative correlation. However, the more useful value to use, in this author's view, is the coefficient of determination, r^2. In this example, $r^2 = (-0.9837)^2 = 0.9677$. This r^2 value translates directly to the strength of association; that is, 96.77% of the variability of the (x, y) data can be explained through the linear regression function. Note in Table 2.3 that r^2 is given as 96.8% (or 0.968) from the MiniTab computer software regression routine. Also, note that

$$r^2 = \frac{SS_T - SS_E}{SS_T} = \frac{SS_R}{SS_T},$$

where

$$SS_T = \sum_{i=1}^{n} (y_i - \bar{y})^2$$

r^2 ranges between 0 and 1 or $0 \le r^2 \le 1$.

SS_R, as the reader will recall, is the amount of total variability directly due to the regression model. SS_E is the error not accounted for by the regression equation, which is generally called random error. Recall that $SS_T = SS_R + SS_E$. Therefore, the larger SS_R is relative to error, SS_E, the greater the r^2 value. Likewise, the larger SS_E is relative to SS_R, the smaller (closer to 0) the r^2 value will be.

Again, r^2 is, in this author's opinion, the better of the two (r^2 vs. r) to use, because r^2 can be applied directly to the outcome of the regression. If $r^2 = 0.50$, then the researcher can conclude that 50% of the total variability

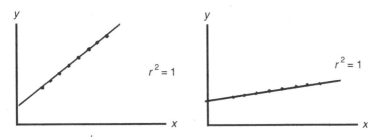

FIGURE 2.31 Correlation of slope rates.

is explained by the regression equation. This is no better than using the average $\bar{y}$ as predictor, and dropping the need for the $\bar{x}$ dimension entirely. Note that when $r^2 = 0.50$, $r = 0.71$. The correlation coefficient can be deceptive in cases like this, for it can lead a researcher to conclude that a higher degree of statistical association exists than actually does. Neither r^2 nor r is a measure of the magnitude of b_1, the slope. Hence, it cannot be said that the greater the slope value b_1, the larger will be r^2 or r (Figure 2.31).

If all the predicted values and actual values are the same, $r^2 = 1$, no matter what the slope, and as long as there is a slope. If there is no slope, b_1 drops out and b_0 becomes the best estimate of y, which turns out to be $\bar{y}$. Instead, r^2 is a measure of how close the actual y values are to the $\hat{y}$ values (Figure 2.32). Finally, r^2 is not a measure of the appropriateness of the linear model (see Figure 2.33) ($r^2 = 0.82$) for this model is high, but that a linear model is not appropriate is obvious. $r^2 = 0.12$ (Figure 2.34). Clearly, these data are not linear and not evaluated well by linear regression.

CORRELATION COEFFICIENT HYPOTHESIS TESTING

Because the researcher undoubtedly will be faced with describing regression functions via the correlation coefficient, r, which is such a popular statistic, we develop its use further. (Note: The correlation coefficient can be used to determine if $r = 0$, and if $r = 0$, then b_1 also equals 0.)

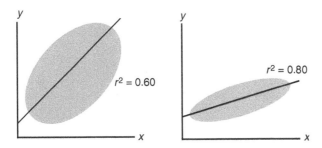

FIGURE 2.32 Degree of closeness of y to $\hat{y}$.

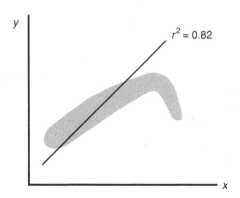

FIGURE 2.33 Inappropriate linear model.

This hypothesis test of $r = 0$ can be performed applying the six-step procedure.

Step 1: Determine the hypothesis.
   H_0: $R = 0$ (x and y are not associated, not correlational),
   H_A: $R \neq 0$ (x and y are associated, are correlational).

Step 2: Set the α level.

Step 3: Write out the test statistic, which is a t-test (Equation 2.45):

$$t_c = \frac{r\sqrt{n-2}}{\sqrt{1-r^2}} \text{ with } n-2 \text{ degrees of freedom.} \qquad (2.45)$$

Step 4: Decision rule:

$$\text{If } |t_c| > t_{(\alpha/2, n-2)}, \text{ reject } H_0 \text{ at } \alpha.$$

Step 5: Perform the computation (step 3).

Step 6: Make the decision based on step 5.

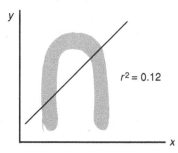

FIGURE 2.34 Nonlinear model.

Example 2.6: Using Example 2.1, the problem can be done as follows.

Step 1:
H_0: $R = 0$,
H_A: $R \neq 0$.

Step 2: Let us set $\alpha = 0.05$. Because this is a two-tail test, the t tabled (t_t) value uses $\alpha/2$ from Table B.

Step 3: The test statistic is

$$t_c = \frac{r\sqrt{n-2}}{\sqrt{1-r^2}}.$$

Step 4: If $|t_c| > t_{(0.05/2, 15-2)} = 2.16$, reject H_0 at $\alpha = 0.05$.

Step 5: Perform computation:

$$t_c = \frac{-0.9837\sqrt{15-2}}{\sqrt{1-0.9677}} = \frac{-3.5468}{0.1797} = -19.7348$$

Step 6: Decision.
Because $|t_c| = 19.7348 > t_{(\alpha/2, 13)} = 2.16$, the H_0 hypothesis is rejected at $\alpha = 0.05$. The correlation coefficient is not 0, nor does the slope $b_1 = 0$.

CONFIDENCE INTERVAL FOR THE CORRELATION COEFFICIENT

A $1 - \alpha$ CI on r can be derived using a modification of Fisher's Z transformation. The transformation has the form

$$\frac{1}{2}\ln\frac{1+r}{1-r}.$$

The researcher also uses the normal Z table (Table A) instead of Student's t table. The test is reasonably powerful, so long as $n \geq 20$.
    The complete CI is

$$\frac{1}{2}\ln\frac{1+r}{1-r} \pm Z_{\alpha/2}/\sqrt{n-3}. \qquad (2.46)$$

The quantity

$$\frac{1}{2}\ln\frac{1+r}{1-r}$$

approximates the mean and $Z_{\alpha/2}/\sqrt{n-3}$ the variance.

$$\text{Lower limit} = \frac{1}{2}\ln\frac{1+L_r}{1-L_r}. \tag{2.47}$$

The lower limit value is then found in Table O (Fisher's Z Transformation Table) for the corresponding r value.

$$\text{Upper limit} = \frac{1}{2}\ln\frac{1+U_r}{1-U_r}. \tag{2.48}$$

The upper limit is also found in Table O for the corresponding r value. The $(1-\alpha)$ 100% CI is of the form $L_r < R < U_r$. Let us use Example 2.1. Four steps are required for the calculator:

$$\frac{1}{2}\ln\frac{1+0.9837}{1-0.9837} \pm \frac{1.96}{\sqrt{15-3}}$$
$$2.4008 \pm 0.5658.$$

Step 1: Compute the basic interval, letting $\alpha = 0.05$ and $Z_{.05/2} = 1.96$ (from Table A).

Step 2: Compute lower or upper limits:

$$L_r = 2.4008 - 0.5658 = 1.8350,$$
$$U_r = 2.4008 + 0.5658 = 2.9660.$$

Step 3: Find L_r (1.8350) in Table O (Fisher's Z Transformation Table), and then find the corresponding value of r:

$$r \approx 0.95.$$

Find U_r (2.9660) in Table O (Fisher's Z Transformation Table), and again, find the corresponding value of r:

$$r \approx 0.994.$$

Step 4: Display $1 - \alpha$ confidence interval.

$$0.950 < r < 0.994,$$

$$\text{at } \alpha = 0.05 \quad \text{or} \quad 1 - \alpha = 0.95.$$

Note: This researcher has adapted the Fisher test to a t-tabled test, which is useful for smaller sample sizes. It is a more conservative test than the Z test, so the confidence intervals will be wider until the sample size of the t tabled r is large enough to equal the Z tabled value.

1. The basic formula

Basic modified interval:

$$\frac{1}{2}\ln\frac{1+r}{1-r} \pm \frac{t_{\alpha/2(n-2)}}{\sqrt{n-3}}.$$

Everything else is the same as for the Z-based confidence interval example.

Example 2.7: Let $\alpha = 0.05$; $t_{(\alpha/2;\,n-2)} = t_{(0.05/2,\,13)} = 2.16$, as found in the Student's t table (Table B).

Step 1: Compute the basic interval:

$$\frac{1}{2}\ln\frac{1+0.9837}{1-0.9837} \pm \frac{2.16}{\sqrt{15-3}} = 2.4008 \pm 0.6235.$$

Step 2: Compute the lower and upper limits, as done earlier:

$$L_r = 2.4008 - 0.6235 = 1.7773,$$
$$L_u = 2.4008 + 0.6235 = 3.0243.$$

Step 3: Find L_r (1.7773) in Table O (Fisher's Z table), and find the corresponding value of r:

$$r \approx 0.95r = 0.944.$$

Find U_r (3.0243) in Table O (Fisher's Z table), and find the corresponding value of r:

$$r = 0.995.$$

Step 4: Display the $1-\alpha$ confidence interval:

$$0.944 < R < 0.995 \text{ at } \alpha = 0.05, \text{ or } 1 - \alpha = 0.95.$$

PREDICTION OF A SPECIFIC x VALUE FROM A y VALUE

There are times when a researcher wants to predict a specific x value from a y value as well as generate confidence intervals for that estimated x value. For example, in microbial death kinetic studies (D values), a researcher often wants to know how much exposure time (x) is required to reduce a microbial population, say, three logs from the baseline value. Alternatively, a researcher may want to know how long an exposure time (x) is required for an antimicrobial sterilant to reduce the population to zero. In these situations, the researcher will predict x from y. Many microbial death kinetic studies, including those using dry heat, steam, ethylene oxide, and gamma radiation, can be computed in this way. The most common procedure uses the D value, which is the time (generally in minutes) in which the initial microbial population is reduced by 1 $\log_{10}$ value.

The procedure is quite straightforward, requiring just basic algebraic manipulation of the linear regression equation, $\hat{y} = b_0 + b_1 x$. As rearranged, then, the regression equation used to predict the x value is

$$\hat{x}_i = \frac{y_i - b_0}{b_1}.\qquad(2.49)$$

The process requires that a standard regression $\hat{y} = b_0 + b_1 x$ be computed to estimate β_0 and β_1. It is then necessary to ensure that the regression fit is adequate for the data described. At that point, the b_0 and b_1 values can be inserted into Equation 2.49. Equation 2.53 works from the results of Equation 2.49 to provide a confidence interval for $\hat{x}$. The $1 - \alpha$ confidence interval equation for $\hat{x}$ is

$$\hat{x} \pm t_{\alpha/2, n-2} s_x, \qquad(2.50)$$

where

$$s_x^2 = \frac{MS_E}{b_1^2}\left[1 + \frac{1}{n} + \frac{(\hat{x} - \bar{x})^2}{\sum\limits_{i=1}^{n}(x_i - \bar{x})^2}\right].\qquad(2.51)$$

Let us perform the computation using the data in Example 2.1 to demonstrate this procedure. The researcher's question is how long an exposure to the test antimicrobial product is required to achieve a 2 $\log_{10}$ reduction from the baseline?

Recall that the regression for this example has already been completed. It is $\hat{y} = 6.13067 - 0.040933x$, where $b_0 = 6.13067$ and $b_1 = -0.040933$. First, the researcher calculates the theoretical baseline or beginning value of y when $x = 0$ time: $\hat{y} = b_0 + b_1 x = 6.13067 - 0.040933(0) = 6.13$. The 2 $\log_{10}$ reduction time is found by using Equation 2.52, $\hat{x} = (y - b_0)/b_1$, where y is a 2 $\log_{10}$ reduction from $\hat{y}$ at time 0. We calculate this value as $6.13 - 2.0 = 4.13$. Then, using Equation 2.49, we can determine $\hat{x}$ or the time in seconds for the example:

$$\hat{x} = \frac{4.13 - 6.13}{-0.041} = 48.78 \text{ sec.}$$

The confidence interval for this $\hat{x}$ estimate is computed as follows, where $\hat{x} = 30$, $n = 15$, $\sum_{i=1}^{n}(x_i - \bar{x})^2 = 6750$, and $MS_E = 0.0288$. Using Equation 2.50, $\hat{x} \pm t_{\alpha/2, n-2} s_x$, and $t_{(0.0512, 15-2)} = 2.16$ from Table B:

$$s_x^2 = \frac{MS_E}{b_1^2}\left[1 + \frac{1}{n} + \frac{(\hat{x} - \bar{x})^2}{\sum\limits_{i=1}^{n}(x_i - \bar{x})^2}\right],$$

$$s_x^2 = \frac{0.0288}{(-0.041)^2}\left[1 + \frac{1}{15} + \frac{(48.78 - 30)^2}{6750}\right] = 19.170,$$

$$s_x = 4.378,$$

$$\hat{x} \pm t_{0.05/2, 13} s_x,$$

$$48.78 \pm 2.16(4.378),$$

$$48.78 \pm 9.46,$$

$$39.32 \le \hat{x} \le 58.24.$$

Therefore, the actual new value $\hat{x}$ on $y = 4.13$ is contained in the interval $39.32 \le \hat{x} \le 58.24$, when $\alpha = 0.05$. This is an 18.92 sec spread, which may not be very useful to the researcher. The main reasons for the wide confidence interval are variability in the data and that one is predicting a specific, not an average, value. The researcher may want to increase the sample size to reduce the variability or may settle for the average expected value of x because the confidence interval will be narrower.

PREDICTING AN AVERAGE $\hat{x}$

Often, a researcher is more interested in the average value of $\hat{x}$. In this case, the formula for determining x is the same as Equation 2.49:

$$\hat{x} \pm t_{\alpha/2, n-2} s_{\bar{x}}, \tag{2.52}$$

where

$$s_{\bar{x}} = \frac{MS_E}{b_1^2}\left[\frac{1}{n} + \frac{(\hat{x} - \bar{x})^2}{\sum\limits_{i=1}^{n}(x_i - \bar{x})^2}\right]. \tag{2.53}$$

Let us use Example 2.1 again. Here, the researcher wants to know, on an average, what the 95% confidence interval is for $\hat{x}$ when y is 4.13 (a 2 $\log_{10}$ reduction). $\hat{x} = 48.78$ sec, as discussed in the previous section:

$$s_x^2 = \frac{0.0288}{(-0.041)^2}\left[\frac{1}{15} + \frac{(48.78-30)^2}{6750}\right] = 2.037,$$

$$s_x = 1.427,$$

$$\hat{x} \pm t_{(\alpha/2, n-2)}s_{\bar{x}} = \hat{x} \pm t_{0.025, 13}s_{\bar{x}},$$

$$48.78 \pm 2.16(1.427),$$

$$48.78 \pm 3.08,$$

$$45.70 \le \hat{x} \le 51.86.$$

Therefore, on an average, the time required to reduce the initial population is between 45.70 and 51.86 sec. For practical purposes, the researcher may round up to a 1 min exposure.

D VALUE COMPUTATION

The D value is the time of exposure, usually in minutes, to steam, dry heat, or ethylene oxide that it takes to reduce the initial microbial population by 1 $\log_{10}$:

$$\hat{y} = b_0 + b_1 x,$$

$$\hat{x}_D = \frac{y - b_0}{b_1}. \tag{2.54}$$

Note that, when we look at a 1 $\log_{10}$ reduction, $y - b_0$ will always be 1. Hence, the D value, $\hat{x}_D$, will always equal $|1/b_1|$. The D value can also be computed for a new specific value. The complete formula is

$$\hat{x}_D \pm t_{(\alpha/2, n-2)}s_x,$$

where

$$s_x^2 = \frac{\text{MS}_E}{b_1^2}\left[1 + \frac{1}{n} + \frac{(\hat{x}_D - \bar{x})^2}{\sum_{i=1}^{n}(x_i - \bar{x})^2}\right]. \tag{2.55}$$

Alternatively, the D value can be computed for the average or expected value $E(x)$:

$$\hat{x}_D \pm t_{(\alpha/2,\, n-2)} s_x,$$

where

$$s_{\bar{x}}^2 = \frac{\text{MS}_E}{b_1^2} \left[\frac{1}{n} + \frac{(\hat{x}_D - \bar{x})^2}{\sum\limits_{i=1}^{n} (x_i - \bar{x})^2} \right].$$

Example 2.8: Suppose the researcher wants to compute the average D value or the time it takes to reduce the initial population 1 $\log_{10}$:

$$\hat{x}_D = \left| \frac{1}{b_1} \right| = \left| \frac{1}{-0.041} \right| = 24.39,$$

$$s_{\bar{x}}^2 = \frac{\text{MS}_E}{b_1^2} \left[\frac{1}{n} - \frac{(\hat{x}_D - \bar{x})^2}{\sum\limits_{i=1}^{n} (x_i - \bar{x})^2} \right] = \frac{0.0288}{(-0.041)^2} \left[\frac{1}{15} + \frac{(24.39 - 30)^2}{6750} \right] = 1.222,$$

$$s_{\bar{x}} = 1.11,$$

$$\hat{x}_D \pm t_{\alpha/2,\, n-2} s_{\bar{x}},$$

$$24.39 \pm 2.16(1.11),$$

$$24.39 \pm 2.40,$$

$$21.99 \le \hat{x}_D \le 26.79.$$

Hence, the D value, on an average, is contained within the interval $21.99 \le \hat{x}_D \le 26.79$ at the 95% level of confidence.

SIMULTANEOUS MEAN INFERENCES OF β_0 AND β_1

In certain situations, such as antimicrobial time–kill studies, an investigator may be interested in confidence intervals for both b_0 (initial population) and b_1 (rate of inactivation). In previous examples, confidence intervals were calculated for b_0 and b_1 separately. Now we discuss how confidence intervals for both b_0 and b_1 can be achieved simultaneously. We use the Bonferroni method for this procedure.

Recall

$$\beta_0 = b_0 \pm t_{(\alpha/2,\, n-2)} s_{b_0},$$
$$\beta_1 = b_1 \pm t_{(\alpha/2,\, n-2)} s_{b_1}.$$

Because we are estimating two parameters, b_0 and b_1, we use $\alpha/2 + \alpha/2 = \alpha/4$. Thus, the revised formulas for b_0 and b_1 are

$$\beta_0 = b_0 \pm t_{(\alpha/4, n-2)} s_{b_0} \text{ and}$$

$$\beta_1 = b_1 \pm t_{(\alpha/4, n-2)} s_{b_1}, \text{ where}$$

$$b_0 = y \text{ intercept},$$

$$b_1 = \text{slope},$$

$$s_{b_0}^2 = \text{MS}_\text{E} \left[\frac{1}{n} + \frac{\bar{x}^2}{\sum\limits_{i=1}^{n} (x_i - \bar{x})^2} \right],$$

$$s_{b_1}^2 = \frac{\text{MS}_\text{E}}{\sum\limits_{i=1}^{n} (x_i - \bar{x})^2}.$$

Let us now perform the computation using the data in Example 2.1. Recall that

$$b_0 = 6.13,$$

$$b_1 = -0.041,$$

$$\text{MS}_\text{E} = 0.0288,$$

$$\sum_{i=1}^{n} (x_i - \bar{x})^2 = 6750,$$

$$\bar{x} = 30,$$

$$n = 15, \text{ and}$$

$$\alpha = 0.05.$$

From Table B, the Student's t table, $t_{\alpha/4,\, n-2} = t_{0.05/4,\, 15-2} = t_{0.0125,\, 13} \approx 2.5$:

$$S_{b_1} = 0.0021,$$

$$S_{b_0} = 0.0759,$$

$$\beta_0 = b_0 \pm t_{(\alpha/4, n-2)}(s_{b_0})$$
$$= 6.13 + 0.1898 = 6.32$$
$$= 6.13 - 0.1898 = 5.94,$$

$$5.94 \leq \beta_0 \leq 6.32,$$

$$\beta_1 = b_1 \pm t_{(\alpha/4, n-2)}(s_{b_1})$$
$$= -0.041 + 0.0053 = -0.036$$
$$= -0.041 - 0.0053 = -0.046,$$

$$-0.046 \leq \beta_1 \leq -0.036.$$

Hence, the combined 95% confidence intervals for β_0 and β_1 are

$$5.94 \leq \beta_0 \leq 6.32,$$
$$-0.046 \leq \beta_1 \leq -0.036.$$

Therefore, the researcher can conclude, at the 95% confidence level, that the initial microbial population (β_0) is between 5.94 and 6.32 logs, and the rate of inactivation (β_1) is between 0.046 and 0.036 $\log_{10}$ per second of exposure.

SIMULTANEOUS MULTIPLE MEAN ESTIMATES OF y

There are times when a researcher wants to estimate the mean y values for multiple x values simultaneously. For example, suppose a researcher wants to predict the $\log_{10}$ microbial counts (y) at times 1, 10, 30, and 40 sec after the exposures and wants to be sure of their overall confidence at $\alpha = 0.10$. The Bonferroni procedure can again be used for $x_1, x_2, \ldots, x_r$ simultaneous estimates. $\hat{y} \pm t_{(\alpha/2r, n-2)} s_{\bar{y}}$ (mean response), where r is the number of x_i values estimated; $\hat{y} = b_0 + b_1 x$, for $i = 1, 2, \ldots, r$ simultaneous estimates

$$s_{\bar{y}}^2 = \text{MS}_E \left[\frac{1}{n} + \frac{(x_i - \bar{x})^2}{\sum\limits_{i=1}^{n} (x_i - \bar{x})^2} \right].$$

Example 2.9: Using the data from Example 2.1, a researcher wants a 0.90 confidence interval ($\alpha = 0.10$) for a series of estimates ($x_i = 0, 10, 30, 40$, so $r = 4$). What are they? Recall that $\hat{y}_i = 6.13 - 0.41 x_i$, $n = 15$, $\text{MS}_E = 0.0288$, and $\sum_{i=1}^{n} (x_i - \bar{x})^2 = 6750$:

$$s_{\bar{y}}^2 = \mathrm{MS_E} \left[\frac{1}{n} + \frac{(x_i - \bar{x})^2}{\sum\limits_{i=1}^{n}(x_i - \bar{x})^2} \right] = 0.0288 \left[\frac{1}{15} + \frac{(x_i - 30)^2}{6750} \right].$$

$t_{(0.10/2; 4, 13)} \approx 2.5$ from Table B, the Student's t table.

For $x = 0$

$$\hat{y}_0 = 6.13 - 0.041(0) = 6.13,$$

$$s_{\bar{y}}^2 = 0.0288 \left[\frac{1}{15} + \frac{(0 - 30)^2}{6750} \right] = 0.0058,$$

$$s_{\bar{y}} = 0.076,$$

$$\hat{y}_0 \pm t_{(0.10/2; 4, 13)}(s_{\bar{y}}),$$

$$6.13 \pm 2.5(0.076),$$

$$6.13 \pm 0.190,$$

$$5.94 \le \bar{y}_0 \le 6.32 \text{ for } x = 0, \text{ or no exposure, at } \alpha = 0.10.$$

For $x = 10$,

$$\hat{y}_{10} = 6.13 - 0.041(10) = 5.72,$$

$$s_{\bar{y}}^2 = 0.0288 \left[\frac{1}{15} + \frac{(10 - 30)^2}{6750} \right] = 0.0036,$$

$$s_{\bar{y}} = 0.060,$$

$$\hat{y}_{10} \pm t_{(0.10/2; 4, 13)}(s_{\bar{y}}),$$

$$5.72 \pm 2.5(0.060),$$

$$5.72 \pm 0.150,$$

$$5.57 \le \bar{y}_{10} \le 5.87 \text{ for } x = 10 \text{ sec, at } \alpha = 0.10.$$

For $x = 30$,

$$\hat{y}_{30} = 6.13 - 0.041(30) = 4.90,$$

$$s_{\bar{y}}^2 = 0.0288 \left[\frac{1}{15} + \frac{(30 - 30)^2}{6750} \right] = 0.0019,$$

$$s_{\bar{y}} = 0.044,$$

$$\hat{y}_{30} \pm t_{(0.10/2;\, 4,\, 13)}(S_{\bar{y}}),$$

$$4.90 \pm 2.5(0.044),$$

$$4.90 \pm 0.11,$$

$$4.79 \le \bar{y}_{30} \le 5.01 \quad \text{for } x = 30 \text{ sec, at } \alpha = 0.10.$$

For $x = 40$,

$$\hat{y}_{40} = 6.13 - 0.041(40) = 4.49,$$

$$s_{\bar{y}}^2 = 0.0288 \left[\frac{1}{15} + \frac{(40 - 30)^2}{6750} \right] = 0.0023,$$

$$s_{\bar{y}} = 0.0023,$$

$$\hat{y}_{40} \pm t_{(0.10/2;\, 4,\, 13)}(s_{\bar{y}}),$$

$$4.49 \pm 2.5(0.048),$$

$$4.49 \pm 0.12,$$

$$4.37 \le \bar{y}_{40} \le 4.61 \text{ for } x = 40 \text{ sec, at } \alpha = 0.10.$$

Note: Individual simultaneous confidence intervals can be made on not only the mean values, but on the individual values as well. The procedure is identical to the earlier one, except $s_{\bar{y}}$, is replaced by $s_{\hat{y}}$, where

$$s_{\hat{y}} = \text{MS}_{\text{E}} \left[1 + \frac{1}{n} + \frac{(x_i - \bar{x})^2}{\sum\limits_{i=1}^{n} (x_i - \bar{x})^2} \right]. \tag{2.56}$$

SPECIAL PROBLEMS IN SIMPLE LINEAR REGRESSION

PIECEWISE REGRESSION

There are times when it makes no sense to perform a transformation on a regression function. This is true, for example, when the audience will not make sense of the transformation or when the data are too complex. The data displayed in Figure 2.35 exemplify the latter circumstance. Figure 2.35 is a complicated data display that can easily be handled using multiple regression procedures, with dummy variables, which we will discuss later. Yet, data such as these can also be approximated by simple linear regression techniques, using three separate regression functions (see Figure 2.36).

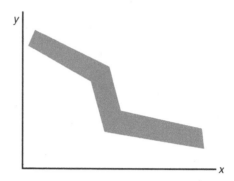

FIGURE 2.35 Regression functions.

Here,

$\hat{y}_a$ covers the range x_a; $b_0 =$ initial a value, when $x = 0$; $b_1 =$ slope of $\hat{y}_a$ over the x_a range,

$\hat{y}_b$ covers the range x_b; $b_0 =$ initial b value, when $x = 0$; $b_1 =$ slope of $\hat{y}_b$ over the x_b range,

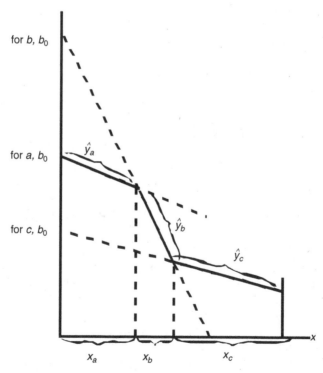

FIGURE 2.36 Complex data.

$\hat{y}_c$ covers the range x_c; $b_0 =$ initial c value, when $x = 0$; $b_1 =$ slope of $\hat{y}_c$ over the x_c range.

A regression of this kind, although rather simple to perform, is time-consuming. The process is greatly facilitated by using a computer.

The researcher can always take each x point and perform a t-test confidence interval, and this is often the course chosen. Although from a probability perspective, this is not correct; from a practical perspective, it is easy, useful, and more readily understood by audiences. We discuss this issue in greater detail using indicator or dummy variables in the multiple linear regression section of this book.

COMPARISON OF MULTIPLE SIMPLE LINEAR REGRESSION FUNCTIONS

There are times when a researcher would like to compare multiple regression function lines. One approach is to construct a series of 95% confidence intervals for each of the $\hat{y}$ values at specific x_i values. If the confidence intervals overlap, from regression line A to regression line B, the researcher simply states that no difference exists, and if the confidence intervals do not overlap, the researcher states that the y points are significantly different from each other at α (see Figure 2.37).

Furthermore, if any confidence intervals of $\hat{y}_a$ and $\hat{y}_b$ overlap, the $\hat{y}$ values on that specific x value are considered equivalent at α. Note that the

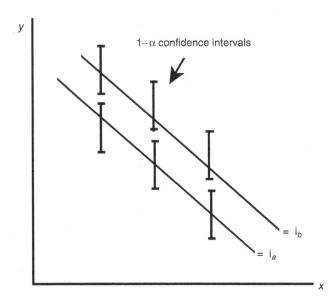

FIGURE 2.37 Nonoverlapping confidence levels.

confidence intervals in this figure do not overlap, so the two regression functions, in their entirety, are considered to differ at α. When using the $1-\alpha$ confidence interval (CI) approach, keep in mind that this is not $1-\alpha$ in probability. Moreover, the CI approach does not compare rates (b_1) or intercepts (b_0), but merely indicates whether the y values are the same or different. Hence, though the confidence interval procedure certainly has a place in describing regression functions, it is finite. There are other possibilities (see Figure 2.38). When a researcher must be more accurate and precise in deriving conclusions, more sophisticated procedures are necessary.

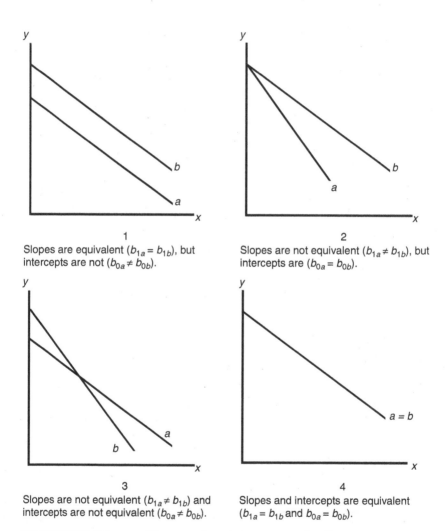

1

Slopes are equivalent ($b_{1a} = b_{1b}$), but intercepts are not ($b_{0a} \neq b_{0b}$).

2

Slopes are not equivalent ($b_{1a} \neq b_{1b}$), but intercepts are ($b_{0a} = b_{0b}$).

3

Slopes are not equivalent ($b_{1a} \neq b_{1b}$) and intercepts are not equivalent ($b_{0a} \neq b_{0b}$).

4

Slopes and intercepts are equivalent ($b_{1a} = b_{1b}$ and $b_{0a} = b_{0b}$).

FIGURE 2.38 Other possible comparisons between regression lines.

EVALUATING TWO SLOPES (b_{1a} AND b_{1b}) FOR EQUIVALENCE IN SLOPE VALUES

At the beginning of this chapter, we learned to evaluate b_1 to assure that the slope was not 0. Now we expand this process slightly to compare two slopes, b_{1a} and b_{1b}. The test hypothesis for a two-tail test will be

$$H_0: \beta_{1a} = \beta_{1b},$$

$$H_A: \beta_{1a} \neq \beta_{1b}.$$

However, the test can be adapted to perform one-tail tests, too.

Lower Tail	Upper Tail
$H_0: \beta_{1a} \geq \beta_{1b}$	$H_0: \beta_{1a} \leq \beta_{1b}$
$H_A: \beta_{1a} < \beta_{1b}$	$H_A: \beta_{1a} > \beta_{1b}$

The statistical procedure is an adaptation of the Student's t-test:

$$t_c = \frac{b_{1a} - b_{1b}}{s_{b_{a-b}}}, \tag{2.57}$$

where b_{1a} is the slope of regression function $a(\hat{y}_a)$ and b_{1b} is the slope of regression function $b(\hat{y}_b)$:

$$s_{b_{a-b}}^2 = s_{pooled}^2 \left[\frac{1}{(n_a - 1)s_{x_a}^2} + \frac{1}{(n_b - 1)s_{x_b}^2} \right],$$

where

$$s_{x_i}^2 = \frac{\sum_{i=1}^{n} x_i^2 - \frac{\left(\sum_{i=1}^{n} x_i \right)^2}{n}}{n - 1},$$

$$s_{pooled}^2 = \frac{(n_a - 2)\text{MS}_{E_a} + (n_b - 2)\text{MS}_{E_b}}{n_a + n_b - 4},$$

$$\text{MS}_{E_a} = \frac{\sum_{i=1}^{n} (y_{ia} - \hat{y}_a)^2}{n - 2} = \frac{\text{SS}_{E_a}}{n - 2},$$

$$\text{MS}_{E_b} = \frac{\sum_{i=1}^{n} (y_{ib} - \hat{y}_b)^2}{n - 2} = \frac{\text{SS}_{E_b}}{n - 2}.$$

This procedure can be easily performed applying the standard six-step procedure.

Step 1: Formulate hypothesis.

Two Tail	Lower Tail	Upper Tail
$H_0: \beta_{1a} = \beta_{1b}$	$H_0: \beta_{1a} \geq \beta_{1b}$	$H_0: \beta_{1a} \leq \beta_{1b}$
$H_A: \beta_{1a} \neq \beta_{1b}$	$H_A: \beta_{1a} < \beta_{1b}$	$H_A: \beta_{1a} > \beta_{1b}$

Step 2: State the α level.

Step 3: Write out the test statistic, which is

$$t_c = \frac{b_{1a} - b_{1b}}{s_{b_{a-b}}},$$

where b_{1a} is the slope estimate of the ath regression line and b_{1b} is that of the bth regression line.

Step 4: Determine hypothesis rejection criteria.

Two Tail	Lower Tail	Upper Tail
$H_0: \beta_{1a} = \beta_{1b}$	$H_0: \beta_{1a} \geq \beta_{1b}$	$H_0: \beta_{1a} \leq \beta_{1b}$
$H_A: \beta_{1a} \neq \beta_{1b}$	$H_A: \beta_{1a} < \beta_{1b}$	$H_A: \beta_{1a} > \beta_{1b}$

For a two-tail test (Figure 2.39),
    Decision rule: If $|t_c| > |t_t| = t_{\alpha/2,[(n_a-2)+(n_b-2)]}$, reject H_0 at α.
For a lower-tail test (Figure 2.40),
    Decision rule: If $t_c < t_t = t_{-\alpha,[(n_a-2)+(n_b-2)]}$, reject H_0 at α.
For upper-tail test (Figure 2.41),
    Decision rule: If $t_c > t_t = t_{-\alpha,[(n_a-2)+(n_b-2)]}$, reject H_0 at α.

Step 5: Perform statistical evaluation to determine t_c.

Step 6: Make decision based on comparing t_c and t_t.

    Let us look at an example.

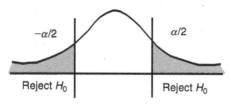

FIGURE 2.39 Step 4, decision rule for two-tail test.

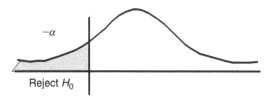

FIGURE 2.40 Step 4, decision rule for lower-tail test.

Example 2.10: Suppose the researcher exposed agar plates inoculated with *Escherichia coli* to forearms of human subjects that are treated with an anti-microbial formulation, as in an agar-patch test. In the study, four plates were attached to each of the treated forearms of each subject. In addition, one inoculated plate was attached to untreated skin on each forearm to provide baseline determinations of the initial microbial population exposure. A random selection schema was used to determine the order in which the plates would be removed from the treated forearms. Two plates were removed and incubated after a 15 min exposure to the antimicrobially treated forearms, two were removed and incubated after a 30 min exposure, two were removed and incubated after a 45 min exposure, and the remaining two after a 60 min exposure. Two test groups of five subjects each were used, one for antimicro-bial product A and the other for antimicrobial product B, for a total of 10 subjects. The agar plates were removed from 24 h of incubation at 35°C $\pm$ 2°C, and the colonies were counted. The duplicate plates at each time point for each subject were averaged to provide one value for each subject at each time.

The final average raw data provided the following results (Table 2.12). Hence, using the methods previously discussed throughout this chapter, the following data have been collected.

	Product A	**Product B**
Regression equation:	$\hat{y}_a = 5.28 - 0.060x$	$\hat{y}_b = 5.56 - 0.051x$
	$r^2 = 0.974$	$r^2 = 0.984$
	$MS_E = \dfrac{SS_E}{n-2} = 0.046$	$MS_E = \dfrac{SS_E}{n-2} = 0.021$
	$n_a = 25$	$n_b = 25$
	$SS_{E_a} = \displaystyle\sum_{i=1}^{n}(y_i - \hat{y})^2 = 1.069$	$SS_{E_b} = \displaystyle\sum_{i=1}^{n}(y_i - \hat{y})^2 = 0.483.$

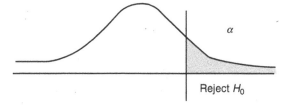

FIGURE 2.41 Step 4, decision rule for upper-tail test.

TABLE 2.12
Final Average Raw Data

Exposure Time in Minutes (x)	Log₁₀ Average Microbial Counts (y) Product A					Log₁₀ Average Microbial Counts (y) Product B				
Subject	5	1	3	4	2	1	3	2	5	4
0 (baseline counts)	5.32	5.15	5.92	4.99	5.23	5.74	5.63	5.52	5.61	5.43
15	4.23	4.44	4.18	4.33	4.27	4.75	4.63	4.82	4.98	4.62
30	3.72	3.25	3.65	3.41	3.37	3.91	4.11	4.05	4.00	3.98
45	3.01	2.75	2.68	2.39	2.49	3.24	3.16	3.33	3.72	3.27
60	1.55	1.63	1.52	1.75	1.67	2.47	2.40	2.31	2.69	2.53

The experimenter, we assume, has completed the model selection procedures, as previously discussed, and has found the linear regression models to be adequate. Figure 2.42 shows $\hat{y}$ (regression line) and the actual data at a 95% confidence interval for product A. Figure 2.43, likewise, shows the data for product B.

Experimenters want to compare the regression models of products A and B. They would like to know not only the $\log_{10}$ reduction values at specific times, as provided by each regression equation, but also if the death kinetic

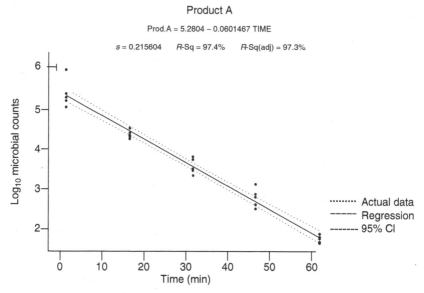

Product A

Prod.A = 5.2804 − 0.0601467 TIME

$s = 0.215604$ $R\text{-Sq} = 97.4\%$ $R\text{-Sq(adj)} = 97.3\%$

.... Actual data
– – – Regression
------- 95% CI

FIGURE 2.42 Linear regression model (product A).

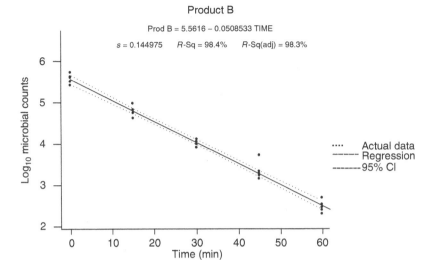

FIGURE 2.43 Linear regression model (product B).

rates (b_{1a} and b_{1b})—the slopes—are equivalent. The six-step procedure is used in this determination.

Step 1: Formulate the hypothesis.

Because the researchers want to know if the rates of inactivation are different, they want to perform a two-tail test.

H_0: $\beta_{1A} = \beta_{1B}$ (inactivation rates of products A and B are the same),

H_A: $\beta_{1A} \neq \beta_{1B}$ (inactivation rates of products A and B are different).

Step 2: Select α level. The researcher selects an α level of 0.05.

Step 3: Write out the test statistic:

$$s^2_{b_{a-b}} = s^2_{pooled}\left[\frac{1}{(n_a - 1)s^2_{x_a}} + \frac{1}{(n_b - 1)s^2_{x_b}}\right],$$

$$s^2_x = \sqrt{\frac{\sum\limits_{i=1}^{n}x_i^2 - \left(\sum\limits_{i=1}^{n}x_i\right)^2}{n-1}},$$

$$s^2_{pooled} = \frac{(n_a - 2)MS_{E_a} + (n_b - 2)MS_{E_b}}{n_a - n_b - 4},$$

$$MS_E = s^2_y = \frac{SS_E}{n-2} = \frac{\sum\limits_{i=1}^{n}(y_i - \hat{y})^2}{n-2} = \frac{\sum\limits_{i=1}^{n}\varepsilon^2}{n-2}.$$

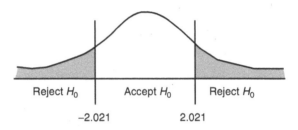

Reject H_0 Accept H_0 Reject H_0

−2.021   2.021

FIGURE 2.44 Step 4, decision rule.

Step 4: Decision rule.

$t_{\text{tabled}} = t_{(\alpha/2;\ n_a+n_b-4)}$, using Table B, the Student's t table,

$$= t_{(0.05/2;\ 25+25-4)} = t_{(0.025;\ 46)} = -2.021 \text{ and } 2.021 \text{ or } |2.021|.$$

If $|t_{\text{calculated}}| > |2.021|$, reject H_0 (Figure 2.44).

Step 5: Calculate t_c:

$$s^2_{\beta_{a-b}} = s^2_{\text{pooled}} \left[\frac{1}{(n_a-1)s^2_{x_a}} + \frac{1}{(n_b-1)s^2_{x_b}} \right],$$

$$s^2_{\text{pooled}} = \frac{(n_a-2)\text{MS}_{E_a} + (n_b-2)\text{MS}_{E_b}}{n_a+n_b-4} = \frac{(25-2)0.046 + (25-2)0.021}{25+25-4} = 0.0335,$$

$$s^2_{x_a} = \frac{\sum\limits_{i=1}^{n} x_i^2 - \left(\sum x_i\right)^2}{n}{n-1},$$

where

$$\sum_{i=1}^{n} x_i^2 = 33{,}750 \quad \text{and} \quad \left(\sum_{i=1}^{n} x_i\right)^2 = (750)^2 = 562{,}500,$$

$$s^2_{x_a} = \frac{33{,}750 - \left(\dfrac{562{,}500}{25}\right)}{25-1} = 468.75 \quad \text{and} \quad s_{x_a} = 21.65,$$

$$s^2_{x_b} = \frac{\sum\limits_{i=1}^{n} x_i^2 - \left(\sum x_i\right)^2}{n}{n-1},$$

where

$$\sum_{i=1}^{n} x_i^2 = 33,750 \text{ and } \left(\sum_{i=1}^{n} x_i\right)^2 = (750)^2 = 562,500,$$

$$s_{x_b}^2 = 468.75 \text{ and } s_{x_b} = 21.65,$$

$$s_{b_{a-b}}^2 = s_{pooled}^2 \left[\frac{1}{(n_a - 1)s_{x_a}^2} + \frac{1}{(n_b - 1)s_{x_b}^2}\right]$$

$$= 0.0335 \left[\frac{1}{(25 - 1)(468.75)} + \frac{1}{(25 - 1)(468.75)}\right],$$

$$s_{b_{a-b}}^2 = 0.0000060 \text{ and } s_{b_{a-b}} = 0.0024.$$

For $b_{1_a} = -0.060$ and $b_{1_b} = -0.051$,

$$t_c = \frac{b_{1a} - b_{1b}}{s_{b_{a-b}}} = \frac{-0.060 - (-0.051)}{0.0024} = -3.75.$$

Step 6: Because $t_c = -3.75 < F_{tabled}$ (-2.021) or $|t_c| > |t_t|$, one can reject the null hypothesis (H_0) at $\alpha = 0.05$. We can conclude that the slopes (b_1) are significantly different from each other.

EVALUATING THE TWO y INTERCEPTS (β_0) FOR EQUIVALENCE

There are times in regression evaluations when a researcher wants to be assured that the y intercepts of the two regression models are equivalent. For example, in microbial inactivation studies, in the comparison of $\log_{10}$ reductions attributable directly to antimicrobials, it must be assured that the test exposures begin at the same y intercept and have the same baseline for number of microorganisms.

Using a t-test procedure, this can be done with a slight modification to what we have already done in determining a $1 - \alpha$ confidence interval for β_0. The two separate β_0 values can be evaluated as a two-tail test, a lower-tail test, or an upper-tail test.

The test statistic used is

$$t_{calculated} = t_c = \frac{\beta_{0_a} - \beta_{0_b}}{s_{0_{a-b}}},$$

$$s_{0_{a-b}}^2 = s_{pooled}^2 \left[\frac{1}{n_a} + \frac{1}{n_b} + \frac{\bar{x}_a^2}{(n_a - 1)s_{x_a}^2} + \frac{\bar{x}_b^2}{(n_b - 1)s_{x_b}^2}\right],$$

$$s_x^2 = \frac{\displaystyle\sum_{i=1}^{n} x_i^2 - \frac{\left(\displaystyle\sum_{i=1}^{n} x_i\right)^2}{n}}{n-1},$$

$$s_{\text{pooled}}^2 = \frac{(n_a - 2)\text{MS}_{E_a} + (n_b - 2)\text{MS}_{E_b}}{n_a + n_b - 4}.$$

This test can also be framed into the six-step procedure.

Step 1: Formulate test hypothesis.

Two Tail	Lower Tail	Upper Tail
$H_0: \beta_{0a} = \beta_{0b}$	$H_0: \beta_{0a} \geq \beta_{0b}$	$H_0: \beta_{0a} \leq \beta_{0b}$
$H_A: \beta_{0a} \neq \beta_{0b}$	$H_A: \beta_{0a} < \beta_{0b}$	$H_A: \beta_{0a} > \beta_{0b}$

Note: The order of a or b makes no difference; the three hypotheses could be written in reverse order.

Two Tail	Lower Tail	Upper Tail
$H_0: \beta_{0b} = \beta_{0a}$	$H_0: \beta_{0b} \geq \beta_{0a}$	$H_0: \beta_{0b} \leq \beta_{0a}$

Step 2: State the α.

Step 3: Write the test statistic:

$$t_c = \frac{b_{0_a} - b_{0_b}}{s_{0_{a-b}}}.$$

Step 4: Determine the decision rule.
For two-tail test (Figure 2.45),

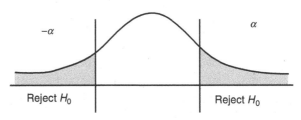

FIGURE 2.45 Step 4, decision rule for two-tail test.

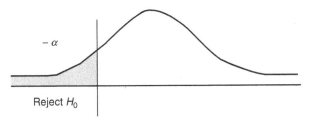

FIGURE 2.46 Step 4, decision rule for lower-tail test.

$H_0: \beta_{0a} = \beta_{0b}$,

$H_A: \beta_{0a} \neq \beta_{0b}$.

If $|t_c| > |t_t| = t_{(\alpha/2, n_a+n_b-4)}$, reject H_0 at α.

For lower-tail test (Figure 2.46),

$H_0: \beta_{0a} \geq \beta_{0b}$,

$H_A: \beta_{0a} < \beta_{0b}$.

If $t_c < t_t = t_{(-\alpha, n_a+n_b-4)}$, reject H_0 at α.

For upper-tail test (Figure 2.47),

$H_0: \beta_{0a} \leq \beta_{0b}$,

$H_A: \beta_{0a} > \beta_{0b}$.

If $t_c > t_t = t_{\alpha, (n_a+n_b-4)}$, reject H_0 at α.

Step 5: Perform statistical evaluation to determine t_c.

Step 6: Draw conclusions based on comparing t_c and t_t.

Let us now work an example where the experimenter wants to compare the initial populations (time $= 0$) for equivalence.

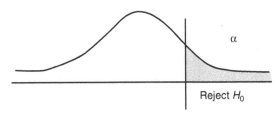

FIGURE 2.47 Step 4, decision rule for upper-tail test.

Step 1: This would again be a two-tail test.

Two Tail:

$H_0: \beta_{0a} = \beta_{0b}$,

$H_A: \beta_{0a} \neq \beta_{0b}$. (The initial populations—y intercepts—are not equivalent.)

Step 2: Let us set α at 0.05, as usual.

Step 3: The test statistic is

$$t_c = \frac{b_{0a} - b_{0b}}{s_{0_{a-b}}}.$$

Step 4: Decision rule (Figure 2.48):

$t_{t(\alpha/2, n_a+n_b-4)} = t_{t(0.05/2, 25+2-4)} \approx 2.021$, from Table B, the Student's t table.

If $|t_c| > |2.021|$, reject H_0.

Step 5: Perform statistical evaluation to derive t_c:

$$t_c = \frac{b_{0a} - b_{0b}}{s_{b_{a-b}}},$$

$b_{0a} = 5.28$,

$b_{0b} = 5.56$,

$$s_{0_{a-b}}^2 = s_{pooled}^2 \left[\frac{1}{n_a} + \frac{1}{n_b} + \frac{\bar{x}_a^2}{(n_a - 1)s_{x_a}^2} + \frac{\bar{x}_b^2}{(n_b - 1)s_{x_b}^2} \right],$$

$$s_x^2 = \frac{\sum_{i=1}^{n} x_i^2 - \frac{\left(\sum_{i=1}^{n} x_i \right)^2}{n}}{n-1} = \frac{33{,}750 - \frac{(750)^2}{25}}{25-1} = 468.75,$$

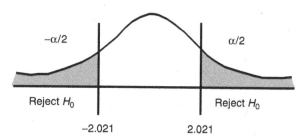

−α/2   α/2

Reject H_0 Reject H_0

−2.021   2.021

FIGURE 2.48 Step 4, decision rule.

$$s^2_{pooled} = \frac{(n_a - 2)MS_{E_a} + (n_b - 2)MS_{E_a}}{n_a + n_b - 4} = \frac{(25 - 2)0.046 + (25 - 2)0.021}{25 + 25 - 4},$$

$$s^2_{pooled} = 0.0335,$$

$$\text{so, } s_{0a-b} = 0.0335 \left[\frac{1}{25} + \frac{1}{25} + \frac{30^2}{24(468.75)} + \frac{30^2}{24(468.75)}\right] = 0.0080,$$

$$s_{0_{a-b}} = 0.090,$$

$$t_c = \frac{5.28 - 5.56}{0.090} = -3.11.$$

Step 6: Because $|t_c| = |3.11| > t_t = |2.021|$, one can reject H_0 at $\alpha = 0.05$. The baseline values are not equivalent.

MULTIPLE REGRESSION

Multiple regression procedures are very easily accomplished using software packages such as MiniTab. However, in much of applied research, they can become less useful for several reasons: more difficult to understand, cost–benefit ratio is often low, and often underlie a poorly thought-out experiment.

MORE DIFFICULT TO UNDERSTAND

As the variable numbers increase, so does the complexity of the statistical model and its comprehension. If comprehension becomes more difficult, interpretation becomes nebulous. For example, if researchers have a four- or five-variable model, visualizing what a fourth or fifth dimension represents is impossible. If the researchers work in industry, no doubt their job will soon be in jeopardy for nonproductivity. The question is not whether the models fit the data better by an r^2 or F test fit, but rather, can the investigators truly comprehend the model's meaning and explain that to others in unequivocal terms? In this author's view, it is far better to use a weaker model (lower r^2 or F value) and understand the relationship between fewer variables than to hide behind a complex model that is applicable only to a specific data set and is not robust enough to hold up to other data collected under similar circumstances.

COST–BENEFIT RATIO LOW

Generally, the more the variables, the greater the experimental costs and the relative value of the extra variables often diminishes. The developed model simply cannot produce valuable and tangible results in developing new drugs, new methods, or new processes with any degree of repeatability. Generally, this is due to lack of robustness. A complex model will tend to not hold true if even minute changes occur in variables.

It is far better to control variables—temperature, weight, mixing, flow, drying, and so on—than to produce a model in an attempt to account for them. In practice, no quality control or assurance group is prepared to track a four-dimensional control chart, and government regulatory agencies would not support them anyway.

POORLY THOUGHT-OUT STUDY

Most multiple regression models applied in research are the result of a poorly controlled experiment or process. When this author first began his industrial career in 1981, he headed a solid dosage validation group. His group's goal was to predict the quality of a drug batch before it was made, by measuring mixing times, drying times, hardness, temperatures, tableting press variability, friability, dissolution rates, compaction, and hardness of similar lots, as well as other variables. Computationally, it was not difficult; time series and regression model development were not difficult either. The final tablet prediction confidence interval was useless. A 500 mg tablet ± 50 mg became 500 ± 800 mg at a 95% confidence interval. Remember then, the more the variables the more the error.

CONCLUSION

Now, the researcher has a general overview of simple linear regression, a very useful tool. However, not all applied problems can be described with simple linear regression. The rest of this book describes more complex regression models.

3 Special Problems in Simple Linear Regression: Serial Correlation and Curve Fitting

AUTOCORRELATION OR SERIAL CORRELATION

Whenever there is a time element in the regression analysis, there is a real danger of the dependent variable correlating with itself. In the literature of statistics, this phenomenon is termed autocorrelation or serial correlation; in this text, we use the latter as descriptive of a situation in which the value, y_i, is dependent on y_{i-1}, which, in turn, is dependent on y_{i-2}. From a statistical perspective, this is problematic because the error term, e_i, is not independent—a requirement of the linear regression model. This interferes with least-squares calculation.

The regression coefficients, b_0 and b_1, although still unbiased, no longer have the minimum variance properties of the least-squares method for determining b_0 and b_1. Hence, the mean square error term MS_E may be underestimated as well as both the standard error of b_0, s_{b_0} and the standard error of b_1, s_{b_1}. The confidence intervals discussed previously (Chapter 2), as well as the tests using the t and F distribution, may no longer be appropriate.

Each $e_i = y_i - \hat{y}_i$ error term is a random variable that is assumed independent of all the other e_i values. However, when the error terms are self- or autocorrelated, the error term is not e_i but $e_{i-1} + d_i$. That is, e_i (error of the ith value) is composed of the previous error term e_{i-1} and a new value called a disturbance, d_i. The d_i value is the independent error term with a mean of 0 and a variance of 1.

When positive serial correlation is present ($r > 0$), the e_i value will be small in pairwise size and positive errors will tend to remain positive and negative errors will tend to be negative, slowly oscillating between positive and negative values (Figure 3.1). The regression parameters, b_0 and b_1, can be thrown off and the error term estimated incorrectly.

Negative serial correlation (Figure 3.1b) tends to display abrupt changes between e_i and e_{i-1}, generally "bouncing" from positive to negative values.

Therefore, any time the y values are collected sequentially over time (x), the researcher must be on guard for serial correlation. The most common

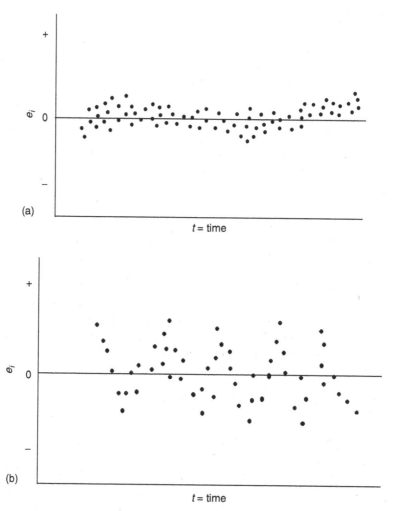

FIGURE 3.1 (a) Positive serial correlation of residuals. (The residuals change sign in gradual oscillation.) (b) Negative serial correlation of residuals. (The residuals bounce between positive and negative, but not randomly.)

serial correlation situation is pairwise correlation detected between residuals e_i vs. e_{i-1}. This is a 1 lag or 1 step apart correlation. However, serial correlation can occur in other lags, such as 2, 3, and so on.

DURBIN–WATSON TEST FOR SERIAL CORRELATION

Whenever researchers perform a regression analysis using data collected over time, they should conduct the Durbin–Watson Test. Most statistical software packages have it as a standard subroutine and it can be chosen for inclusion in the analyses.

More often than not, serial correlation will involve positive correlation, where each e_i value is directly correlated to the e_{i-1} value. In this case, the Durbin–Watson test is a one-sided test, and the population serial correlation component—under the alternative hypothesis—is $P > 0$. The Durbin–Watson formula for 1 lag is

$$D_W = \frac{\sum_{i=2}^{n} (e_i - e_{i-1})^2}{\sum_{i=1}^{n} e_i^2}.$$

For other lags, the change in the formula is straightforward. For example, a 3 lag Durbin–Watson calculation is

$$D_W = \frac{\sum_{i=4}^{n} (e_i - e_{i-3})^2}{\sum_{i=1}^{n} e_i^2}.$$

If $P > 0$, then $e_i = e_{i-1} + d_i$. The Durbin–Watson test can be evaluated using the six-step procedure:

Step 1: Specify the test hypothesis (generally upper-tail or positive correlation).

$H_0: P \leq 0$ (P is the population correlation coefficient),
$H_A: P > 0$; serial correlation is positive.

Step 2: Set n and α.
Often, n is predetermined. The Durbin–Watson table is found in Table E, with three different α levels: $\alpha = 0.05$, $\alpha = 0.025$, and $\alpha = 0.01$; n is the number of values, and k is the number of x predictor variables, taking a value other than 1 only in multiple regression.

Step 3: Write out the Durbin–Watson test statistic for 1 lag

$$D_W = \frac{\sum_{i=2}^{n}(e_i - e_{i-1})^2}{\sum_{i=1}^{n} e_i^2}. \tag{3.1}$$

The e_i values are determined from the regression analysis as $e_i = y_i - \hat{y}_i$. To compute the Durbin–Watson value using 1 lag, see Table 3.1 ($n = 5$). The e_i column is the original column of e_i, derived from $y_i - \hat{y}_i$ and the e_{i-1} column is the same column but "dropped down one value," the position for a lag of 1.

Step 4: Determine the acceptance or rejection of the tabled value.

Using Table E, find the α value, the value of n and k, where, in this case, $k = 1$, because there is only one x predictor variable. Two tabled D_W values are given: d_L and d_U, or d lower and d upper. This is because the actual tabled D_W value is a range, not an exact value.

Because this is an upper-tail test, the decision rule is

If D_W calculated $> d_U$ tabled, reject H_A.
If D_W calculated $< d_L$ tabled, accept H_A.

If D_W calculated is between d_U and d_L ($d_L \leq D_W \leq d_U$), the test is inconclusive and the sample size should be increased.

Note that small values of D_W support H_A because e_i and e_{i-1} are about the same value when serially correlated. Therefore, when e_i and e_{i-1} are correlated, their difference will be small and $P > 0$. Some authors maintain that an n of at least 40 is necessary to use the Durbin–Watson test (e.g., Kutner et al., 2005). It would be great if one could do this, but, in many tests, even 15 measurements are a luxury.

TABLE 3.1
Example of Calculations for Durbin–Watson Test

n	e_i	e_{i-1}	$e_i - e_{i-1}$	e_i^2	$(e_i - e_{i-1})^2$
1	1.2	—	—	1.44	—
2	−1.3	1.2	−2.5	1.69	6.25
3	−1.1	−1.3	0.2	1.21	0.04
4	0.9	−1.1	2.0	0.81	4.00
5	1.0	0.9	0.1	1.00	0.01
				$\Sigma e_i^2 = 6.15$	$\Sigma(e_i - e_{i-1})^2 = 10.30$

Step 5: Perform the D_W calculation.

The computation for D_W is straightforward. Using Table 3.1,

$$D_W = \frac{\sum_{i=2}^{n}(e_i - e_{i-1})^2}{\sum_{i=1}^{n} e_i^2} = \frac{10.30}{6.15} = 1.67.$$

Step 6: Determine the test significance.

Let us do an actual problem, Example 3.1, the data for which are from an actual D value computation for steam sterilization. Biological indicators (strips of paper containing approximately 1×10^6 bacterial spores per strip) were affixed to stainless steel hip joints. In order to calculate a D value, or the time required to reduce the initial population by 1 $\log_{10}$, the adequacy of the regression model must be evaluated. Because b_0 and b_1 are unbiased estimators, even when serial correlation is present, the model $\hat{y} = b_0 + b_1 x + e_i$ may still be useful. However, recall that e_i is now composed of $e_{i-1} + d_i$, where the d_is are $N(0, 1)$.

Given that the error term is composed of $e_{i-1} + d_i$, the MS_E calculation may not be appropriate. Only three hip joints were available and were reused, over time, for the testing. At time 0, spore strips (without hip joints) were heat shocked (spores stimulated to grow by exposure to 150°C water) and the average value recovered was found to be 1.0×10^6. Then, spore strips attached to the hip joints underwent $1, 2, 3, 4$, and 5 min exposures to steam heat in a BIER vessel. Table 3.2 provides the spore populations recovered following three replications at each time of exposure.

A scatterplot of the bacterial populations recovered, which is presented in Figure 3.2, appears to be linear. A linear regression analysis resulted in an R^2 value of 96.1%, which looks good (Table 3.3). Because the data were collected over time, the next step is to graph the e_is to the x_is (Figure 3.3).

Note that the residuals plotted over the time exposures do not appear to be randomly centered around 0, which suggests that the linear model may be inadequate and that positive serial correlation may be present. Table 3.4 provides the actual x_i:y_i data values, the predicted values $\hat{y}_i$ and the residuals e_i.

Although the pattern displayed by the residuals may be due to lack of linear fit (as described in Chapter 2), before any linearizing transformation, the researcher should perform the Durbin–Watson test. Let us do that, using the six-step procedure.

Step 1: Determine the hypothesis.

H_0: $P \leq 0$.
H_A: $P > 0$, where P is the population correlation coefficient.

TABLE 3.2
D-Value Study Results, Example 3.1

n	Exposure Time in Minutes	Log_{10} Microbial Population
1	0	5.7
2	0	5.3
3	0	5.5
4	1	4.2
5	1	4.0
6	1	3.9
7	2	3.5
8	2	3.1
9	2	3.3
10	3	2.4
11	3	2.2
12	3	2.0
13	4	1.9
14	4	1.2
15	4	1.4
16	5	1.0
17	5	0.8
18	5	1.2

Step 2: The sample size is 18 and we set $\alpha = 0.05$.

Step 3: We apply the Durbin–Watson test at 1 lag.

$$D_\text{W} = \frac{\sum\limits_{i=2}^{n} (e_i - e_{i-1})^2}{\sum\limits_{i=1}^{n} e_i^2}.$$

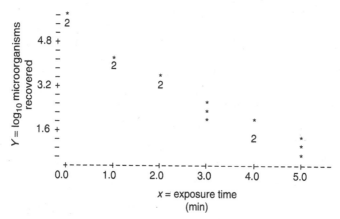

FIGURE 3.2 Regression scatterplot of bacterial populations recovered, Example 3.1.

TABLE 3.3
***D*-Value Regression Analysis, Example 3.1**

Predictor	Coef	St. Dev	*t*-Ratio	*P*
b_0	5.1508	0.1359	37.90	0.000
b_1	−0.89143	0.04488	−19.86	0.000
$s = 0.3252$		R-sq $= 96.1\%$		R-sq(adj) $= 95.9\%$

Analysis of Variance

Source	DF	SS	MS	F	p
Regression	1	41.719	41.719	394.45	0.000
Error	16	1.692	0.106		
Total	17	43.411			

The regression equation is $\hat{y} = 5.15 - 0.891x$.

Step 4: Decision rule:
Using Table E, the Durbin–Watson Table, $n = 18$, $\alpha = 0.05$, $k = 1$, $d_L = 1.16$, and $d_U = 1.39$.
Therefore,

If the computed $D_W > 1.39$, conclude H_0.
If the computed $D_W < 1.16$, accept H_A.
If $1.16 \leq D_W \leq 1.39$, the test is inconclusive and we need more samples.

Step 5: Compute the D_W value.
There are two ways to compute D_W using a computer. One can use a software package, such as MiniTab and attach it to a regression analysis. Table 3.5 shows this.

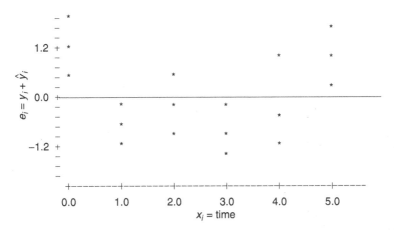

FIGURE 3.3 Plot of e_i residuals over x_i time graph, Example 3.1.

TABLE 3.4
Residuals vs. Predicted Values, Example 3.1

n	x_i (Time)	y_i ($\log_{10}$ Values)	$\hat{y}_i$ (Predicted)	e_i (Residuals)
1	0	5.7	5.15079	0.549206
2	0	5.3	5.15079	0.149206
3	0	5.5	5.15079	0.349206
4	1	4.2	4.25937	−0.059365
5	1	4.0	4.25937	−0.259365
6	1	3.9	4.25937	−0.359365
7	2	3.5	3.36794	0.132063
8	2	3.1	3.36794	0.267937
9	2	3.3	3.36794	−0.067937
10	3	2.4	2.47651	−0.076508
11	3	2.2	2.47651	−0.276508
12	3	2.0	2.47651	−0.476508
13	4	1.9	1.58508	0.314921
14	4	1.2	1.58508	−0.385079
15	4	1.4	1.58508	−0.185079
16	5	1.0	0.69365	0.306349
17	5	0.8	0.69365	0.106349
18	5	1.2	0.69365	0.506349

TABLE 3.5
Regression Analysis with the Durbin–Watson Test,
Example 3.1

Predictor	Coef	St. Dev	t-Ratio	p
b_0	5.1508	0.1359	37.90	0.000
b_1	−0.89143	0.04488	−19.86	0.000

$s = 0.3252$ R-sq $= 96.1\%$ R-sq(adj) $= 95.9\%$

Analysis of Variance

Source	DF	SS	MS	F	p
Regression	1	41.719	41.719	394.45	0.000
Error	16	1.692	0.106		
Total	17	43.411			

Lack-of-fit test $= F = 5.10$, $p = 0.0123$, df $= 12$.
Durbin–Watson statistic $= 1.49881$.
The Durbin–Watson computation is ~1.50.
The regression equation is $\hat{y} = 5.15 - 0.891x$.

If a software package does not have this option, individual columns can be manipulated to derive the test results. Table 3.6 provides an example of this approach.

$$D_W = \sum_{i=2}^{n} \frac{(e_i - e_{i-1})^2}{\sum_{i=1}^{n} e_i^2} = \frac{2.53637}{1.69225} = 1.4988 \approx 1.50.$$

Step 6: Draw the conclusion

Because $D_W = 1.50 > 1.39$, conclude H_0. Serial correlation is not a distinct problem with this D value study at $\alpha = 0.05$.

However, let us revisit the plot of e_i vs. x_i (Figure 3.3). There is reason to suspect that the linear regression model $\hat{y} = b_0 + b_1 x_1$ is not exact. Recall from Chapter 2 that we discussed both pure error and lack of fit in regression. Most statistical software programs have routines to compute these, or the computations can be done easily with the aid of a hand-held calculator.

TABLE 3.6
Durbin–Watson Test Performed Manually, with Computer Manipulation, Example 3.1

n	x_i	y_i	$\hat{y}_i$	e_i	e_{i-1}	$e_i - e_{i-1}$	$(e_i - e_{i-1})^2$	e_i^2
1	0	5.7	5.15079	0.549206	*	*	*	0.301628
2	0	5.3	5.15079	0.149206	0.549206	−0.400000	0.160000	0.022263
3	0	5.5	5.15079	0.349206	0.149206	0.200000	0.040000	0.121945
4	1	4.2	4.25937	−0.059365	0.349206	−0.408571	0.166931	0.003524
5	1	4.0	4.25937	−0.259365	−0.059365	−0.200000	0.040000	0.067270
6	1	3.9	4.25937	−0.359365	−0.259365	−0.100000	0.010000	0.129143
7	2	3.5	3.36794	0.132063	−0.359365	0.419429	0.241502	0.017441
8	2	3.1	3.36794	0.267937	0.132063	−0.400000	0.160000	0.071790
9	2	3.3	3.36794	−0.067937	0.267937	0.200000	0.040000	0.004615
10	3	2.4	2.47651	−0.076508	−0.067937	−0.008571	0.000073	0.005853
11	3	2.2	2.47651	−0.276508	−0.076508	−0.200000	0.040000	0.076457
12	3	2.0	2.47651	−0.476508	−0.276508	−0.200000	0.040000	0.227060
13	4	1.9	1.58508	0.314921	−0.476508	0.791429	0.626359	0.099175
14	4	1.2	1.58508	−0.385079	0.314921	−0.700000	0.490000	0.148286
15	4	1.4	1.58508	−0.185079	−0.385079	0.200000	0.040000	0.034254
16	5	1.0	0.69365	0.306349	−0.185079	0.491429	0.241502	0.093850
17	5	0.8	0.69365	0.106349	0.306349	−0.200000	0.040000	0.011310
18	5	1.2	0.69365	0.506349	0.106349	0.400000	0.160000	0.256390

$$\sum_{i=1}^{18} (e_i - e_{i-1})^2 = 2.53637 \qquad \sum_{i=1}^{18} e_i^2 = 1.69225$$

Recall that the sum of squares term (SS_E) consists of two components if the test is significant: (1) sum of squares pure error (SS_{PE}) and (2) sum of squares lack of fit (SS_{LF}).

$$SS_E = SS_{PE} + SS_{LF},$$

$$y_{ij} - \hat{y}_{ij} = \overbrace{y_{ij} - \bar{y}_j} + \overbrace{\bar{y}_j - \hat{y}_{ij}}.$$

SS_{PE} is attributed to random variability or pure error, and SS_{LF} is attributed to significant failure of the model to fit the data.

In Table 3.5, the lack of fit was calculated as $F_c = 5.10$, which was significant at $\alpha = 0.05$. The test statistic is $F_{\text{lack-of-fit}} = F_{LF} = \frac{MS_{LF}}{MS_{PE}} = 5.10$. If the process must be computed by hand, see Chapter 2 for procedures.

So what is one to do? The solution usually lies in field knowledge, in this case, microbiology. In microbiology, often there is an initial growth spike depicted by the data at $x = 0$ because populations resulting from the heat-shocked spores at $x = 0$, and the sterilized spore samples at $x = $ exposure times 1 min through 5 min do not "line up" straight. In addition, there tends to be a tailing effect, a reduction in the rate of kill as spore populations decline, due to spores that are highly resistant to steam heat. Figure 3.4 shows this. At time 0, the residuals are highly positive ($y - \hat{y} > 0$), so the regression underestimates the actual spore counts at $x = 0$. The same phenomena occur at $x = 5$, probably as a result of a decrease in the spore inactivation rate (Figure 3.4).

The easiest way to correct this is to remove the data where $x = 0$ and $x = 5$. We kept them in this model to evaluate serial correlation because if we

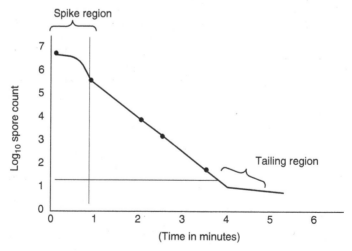

FIGURE 3.4 Graphic display of the spike and tailing.

TABLE 3.7
New Data and Regression Analysis with $x = 0$ and $x = 5$ Omitted,
Example 3.1

n	x_i	y_i	e_i	$\hat{y}_i$
1	1	4.2	0.136667	4.06333
2	1	4.0	−0.063333	4.06333
3	1	3.9	−0.163333	4.06333
4	2	3.5	0.306667	3.19333
5	2	3.1	−0.093333	3.19333
6	2	3.3	0.106667	3.19333
7	3	2.4	0.076667	2.32333
8	3	2.2	−0.123333	2.32333
9	3	2.0	−0.323333	2.32333
10	4	1.9	0.446667	1.45333
11	4	1.2	−0.253333	1.45333
12	4	1.4	−0.053333	1.45333

had removed them before conducting the Durbin–Watson test, then we would have had too small a sample size to use the test. Let us see if eliminating the population counts at $x=0$ and $x=5$ provides an improved fit. Table 3.7 shows these data and Table 3.8 provides the regression analysis.

TABLE 3.8
Modified Regression Analysis, Example 3.1

Predictor	Coef	St. Dev	t-Ratio	p
b_0	4.9333	0.1667	29.60	0.000
b_1	−0.87000	0.06086	−14.29	0.000
$s = 0.2357$		R-sq $= 95.3\%$		R-sq(adj) $= 94.9\%$

Analysis of Variance

Source	DF	SS	MS	F	p
Regression	1	11.353	11.353	204.32	0.000
Error	10	0.556	0.056		
Total	11	11.909			

Unusual Observations

Observation	x	y	$\hat{y}$ fit	St. dev. fit	e_i residual	St. residual
10	4	1.9000	1.4533	0.1139	0.4467	2.16R

Lack-of-fit test $= F = 0.76$, $P = 0.4975$, df (pure error) $= 8$.
R denotes an observation with a large standardized residual.
The regression equation is $\hat{y} = 4.93 - 0.870x$.

Because we removed the three values where $x=0$ and three values where $x=5$, we have only 12 observations now. Although the lack-of-fit problem has vanished, observation 10 ($x=4$, $y=1.9$) has been flagged as suspicious. We leave it as is, however, because a review of records shows that this was an actual value. The new plot of e_i vs. x_i (Figure 3.5) is much better than the data spread portrayed in Figure 3.3, even with only 12 time points, and it is adequate for the research and development study.

Notes:

1. The Durbin–Watson test is very popular, so when discussing time series correlation, most researchers who employ statistics are likely to know it. It is also the most common one found in statistical software.
2. The type of serial correlation most often encountered is positive correlation where e_i and e_{i+1} are fairly close in value (Figure 3.1a). When negative correlation is observed, a large positive value of e_i will be followed by a large negative e_{i+1} value.
3. Negative serial correlation can also be easily evaluated using the six-step procedure:

Step 1: State the hypothesis.

$H_0: P \geq 0$.
$H_A: P < 0$, where P is the population correlation coefficient.

Step 2: Set α and n, as always.

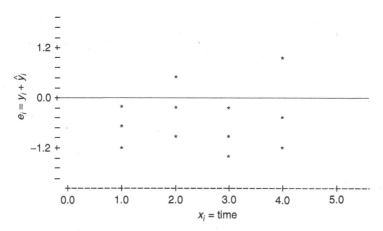

FIGURE 3.5 New e_i vs. x_i graph, not including $x = 0$ and $x = 5$, Example 3.1.

Step 3: The Durbin–Watson value, D_W, is calculated exactly as before. For a lag of 1:

$$D_W = \frac{\sum\limits_{i=2}^{n}(e_i - e_{i-1})^2}{\sum\limits_{i=1}^{n} e_i^2}.$$

Nevertheless, one additional step must be included to determine the final Durbin–Watson test value D'_W. D'_W is computed as $D'_W = 4 - D_W$.

Step 4: Decision rule:

Reject H_0 if $D'_W < d_L$.
Accept H_0 if $D'_W > d_U$.

If $d_L \leq D'_W \leq d_U$, the test is inconclusive, as earlier. Steps 5 and 6 are the same, as for the earlier example. A two-tail test can also be conducted.

Two-Tail Durbin–Watson Test Procedure

Step 1: State the hypothesis.

H_0: $P = 0$.
H_A: $P \neq 0$, or the serial correlation is negative or positive.

Step 2: Set α and n.
The sample size selection does not change, however, because the Durbin–Watson tables (Table E) are one-sided; the actual α level is 2α. That is, if one is using the 0.01 table, it must be reported as $\alpha = 2(0.01)$ or 0.02.

Step 3: Test statistic:
The two-tail test requires performing both an upper- and lower-tail test, that is, calculating both D_W and D'_W.

Step 4: Decision rule:
If either $D_W < d_L$ or $D'_W < d_L$, reject H_0 at 2α. If D_W or D'_W falls between d_U and d_L, the test is inconclusive; so, more samples are needed. If $4 - D_W$ or $D'_W > d_U$, no serial correlation can be detected at 2α.

Step 5: If one computes $d_L < D_W < d_U$, it is still prudent to suspect possible serial correlation, particularly when $n < 40$. So, in drawing statistical conclusions, this should be kept in mind.

Simplified Durbin–Watson Test

Draper and Smith (1998) suggest that, in many practical situations, one can work as if D_L does not exist and, therefore, consider only the D_U value. This is attractive in practice, for example, because it side steps an inadequate sample size problem. Exactly the same computation procedures are used as previously. The test modification is simply as follows:

For positive correlation, H_0: $P > 0$.
The decision to reject H_0 at α occurs if $D_W < d_U$.
For negative correlation, H_A: $P < 0$.
The decision to reject H_0 at α occurs if $4 - D_W < d_U$.
For a two-tail test, H_A: $P \neq 0$.
The decision to reject H_0 occurs if $D_W < d_U$ or if $4 - D_W < d_U$ at 2α.

There is no easy answer as to how reliable the simplified test is, but the author of this chapter finds that the Draper and Smith simplified test works well. However, generally, the researcher is urged to check out the model in depth to be sure a process problem is not occurring or some extra unaccountable variable has been included.

ALTERNATE RUNS TEST IN TIME SERIES

An alternative test that can be used for detecting serial correlation is observing the "+" "−" value runs on the e_i vs. x_i plot. It is particularly useful when one is initially reviewing an e_i vs. x_i plot. As we saw in the data we collected in Example 3.1, there appeared to be a nonrandom pattern of "+" and "−" (Figure 3.3). In a random pattern of e_i values plotted against x_i values in large samples, there will be about $x_n/2$ values, both negative and positive. They will not have an alternating $+ - + - + -$ pattern or a $+ + + - - - -$ run pattern, but vary in $+/-$ sequencing. When one sees $+ - + - + -$ sequences, there is probably a negative correlation and with $+ + + - - - -$ patterns, one will suspect positive correlation. Tables I and J can be used to detect serial correlation. Use the lower-tail (Table I) for positive correlation (too few runs or changes in $+ - -$) and Table J for negative correlation (too many runs or excessive $+ -$ changes).

For example, suppose that 15 data points are available, and the $+/-$ value of each of the e_is was $+ + + + - - - - + + + + + + - -$. We let $n_1 = +$ and $n_2 = -$. There are

$(+ + + +)$	$(- - -)$	$(+ + + + + +)$	$(- -)$
1	2	3	4

four runs of $+/-$ data, with $n_1 = 10$ and $n_2 = 5$. Recall that on an e_i vs. x_i plot, the center point is 0. Those values where $y > \hat{y}$ (positive) will be above the 0 point and those values where $y < \hat{y}$ (negative) will be below it.

Looking at Table I (lower-tail and positive correlation), find n_1, the number of positive e_is and n_2, the number of negative e_is. Using a lower-tail test (i.e., positive correlation, because there are few runs), $n_1 = 10$ and $n_2 = 5$. However, looking at Table I, we see that n_1 must be less than n_2, so we simply exchange them: $n_1 = 5$ and $n_2 = 10$. There are four runs, or $r = 4$. The probability of this pattern being random is ≤ 0.029. There is a good indication of positive correlation.

When n_1 and $n_2 \geq 10$

When larger sample sizes are used, n_1 and $n_2 > 10$, a normal approximation can be made:

$$\bar{x} = \frac{2n_1 n_2}{n_1 + n_2} + 1, \tag{3.2}$$

$$s^2 = \frac{2n_1 n_2 (2n_1 n_2 - n_1 - n_2)}{(n_1 + n_2)^2 (n_1 + n_2 - 1)}. \tag{3.3}$$

A lower-tail test approximation (positive correlation) can be completed using the normal Z tables (Table A), where

$$z_c = \frac{\dot{n} - \bar{x} + \frac{1}{2}}{s} \tag{3.4}$$

and z_c is the calculated z value to find in the tabled normal distribution, for the stated significance level (Table A). $\dot{n}$ is the number of runs, $\bar{x}$ is Equation 3.2, s is the square root of Equation 3.3, and $\frac{1}{2}$ is the correction factor.

If too many runs are present (negative correlation), the same formula is used, but $-\frac{1}{2}$ is used to compensate for an upper-tail test

$$z_c = \frac{\dot{n} - \bar{x} - \frac{1}{2}}{s}. \tag{3.5}$$

Example 3.1 (continued). Let us perform the runs test with the collected D value data.

Step 1: Formulate the hypothesis.
To do so, first determine $\dot{n}$ and then $\bar{x}$.
General rule:

If $\dot{n} < \bar{x}$, use the lower-tail test.
If $\dot{n} > \bar{x}$, use the upper-tail test.

Table 3.9 contains the residual values from Table 3.6.

TABLE 3.9
Residual Values Table with Runs,
Example 3.1

n	e_i (Residuals)	Run Number
1	0.549206	
2	0.149206	1
3	0.349206	
4	−0.059365	
5	−0.259365	2
6	−0.359365	
7	0.132063	3
8	−0.267937	
9	−0.067937	
10	−0.076508	4
11	−0.276508	
12	−0.476508	
13	0.314921	5
14	−0.385079	6
15	−0.185079	
16	0.306349	
17	0.106349	7
18	0.506349	

Let n_1, the number of "+" residuals $= 8$,
n_2, the number of "−" residuals $= 10$,
and $\dot{n} = 7$,

$$\bar{x} = \frac{2n_1 n_2}{n_1 + n_2} + 1 = \frac{2(8)(10)}{8 + 10} + 1 = 9.89.$$

Because $\dot{n} < \bar{x}$, use lower-tail test.

So, H_0: $P \leq 0$.
    H_A: $P > 0$ or positive serial correlation.*

Note: For serial correlation, when $P > 0$, this is a lower-tail test.

Step 2: Determine sample size and α.
    $n = 18$, and we will set $\alpha = 0.05$.

Step 3: Specify the test equation.
Because this is a lower-tail test, we use Equation 3.4.

$$z_c = \frac{\dot{n} - \bar{x} + \frac{1}{2}}{s}.$$

Step 4: State the decision rule.
If $z_c \leq 0.05$, reject H_0.

Step 5: Compute the statistic.
$\bar{x} = 9.89$ (previously computed),

$$s^2 = \frac{2n_1 n_2 (2n_1 n_2 - n_1 - n_2)}{(n_1 + n_2)^2 (n_1 + n_2 - 1)} = \frac{2(8)(10)[2(8)(10) - 8 - 10]}{(8 + 10)^2 (8 + 10 - 1)} = 4.12,$$

$$z_c = \frac{\dot{n} - \bar{x} + \frac{1}{2}}{s} = \frac{7 - 9.89 + \frac{1}{2}}{\sqrt{4.12}} = -1.18.$$

From Table A, where $z_c = 1.18$, the area under the normal curve is $+0.3810$.

Because the Z table includes the value of Z from the mean (center) outward, we must accommodate the negative sign of z_c, -1.18, by subtracting the $+0.3810$ value from 0.5, that is, $0.5 - 0.3810 = 0.1190$. We see that $0.1190 \not< 0.05$ (our value of α). Hence, we cannot reject H_0 at $\alpha = 0.05$.

Technically, the runs test is valid only when the runs are independent. However, in most time series studies, this is violated. A y_i reading will always be after y_{i-1}. For example, in clinical trials of human subjects, blood taken 4 h after ingesting a drug will always occur before an 8 h reading. In practical research and development situations, the runs test works fine, even with clearly time-related correlation studies.

MEASURES TO REMEDY SERIAL CORRELATION PROBLEMS

As previously stated, most serial correlation problems point to the need for another, or several values for the x_i variable. For instance, in Example 3.1, the sterilization hip joint study, looking at the data, the researcher noted that the temperature fluctuation in the steam vessel was $\pm 2.0°C$. In this type of study, a range of $4.0°C$ can be very influential. For example, as x_{i_1}, x_{i_2}, and x_{i_3} are measured, the bier vessel cycles throughout the $\pm 2.0°C$ range. The serial correlation would tend to appear positive due to the very closely related temperature fluctuations. A way to correct this situation partially would be to add another regression variable, x_2, representing temperature. The model would then be

$$\hat{y} = \beta_0 + \beta_1 x_1 + \beta_2 x_2, \tag{3.6}$$

where $\beta_0 = y$ intercept, $\beta_1 =$ slope of thermodeath rate of bacterial spores, $\beta_2 =$ slope of Bier sterilizer temperature.

Alternatively, one can transform regression variables to better randomize the patterns in the residual e_i data. However, generally, it is better to begin the statistical correction process by assigning x_i predictors to variables for which one has already accounted. Often, however, one has already collected the data and has no way of going back to reassign other variables post hoc. In this case, the only option left to the experimenter is a transformation procedure. This, in itself, argues for performing a pilot study before a larger one. If additional variables would be useful, the researcher can repeat the pilot study. Yet, sometimes, one knows an additional variable exists, but that it is measured with so much random error, or noise, that it does not contribute significantly to the SS_R. For example, if, as in Example 3.1, the temperature fluctuates $\pm 4°C$, but the precision of the Bier Vessel is $\pm 2°C$, there may not be enough accurate data collected to warrant it as a separate variable. Again, a transformation may be the solution.

Note that efforts described above would not take care of the major problem, that is x_i, to some degree, is determined by x_{i-1}, which is somewhat determined by x_{i-2}, and so on. Forecasting methods, such as moving averages, are better in these situations.

TRANSFORMATION PROCEDURE (WHEN ADDING MORE PREDICTOR x_i VALUES IS NOT AN OPTION)

When deciding to measure correlated error (e_i) values (lag 1), remember that the y_i values are the cause of this. Hence, any transformation must go to the root problem, the y_is. In the following, we also focus on lag 1 correlation. Other lags can be easily modeled from a 1 lag equation. Equation 3.7 presents the decomposition of y_i, the dependent y_i variable, influenced by y_{i-1}

$$y_i' = y_i - Py_{i-1}, \tag{3.7}$$

where y_i' is the transformed value of y measured at i, y_i is the value of y measured at i, y_{i-1} is the correlated contribution to y_i at $i - 1$ (1 lag) for a dependent variable and P is the population serial correlation coefficient.

Expanding Equation 3.7, in terms of the standard regression model, we have

$$y_i' = (\beta_0 + \beta_1 x_i + e_i) - P(\beta_0 + \beta_1 x_{i-1} + e_{i-1}).$$

and reducing the term algebraically,

$$y_i' = \beta_0(1 - P) + \beta_1(x_i - Px_{i-1}) + (e_i - Pe_{i-1}).$$

If we let $d_i = e_i - Pe_{i-1}$, then

$$y_i' = \beta_0(1-p) + \beta_1(x_i - Px_{i-1}) + d_i,$$

where d_i is the random error component, $N(0, \sigma^2)$.
The final transformation equation for the population is

$$Y_i' = \beta_0' + \beta_1' X_i' + D_i, \tag{3.8}$$

where

$$Y_i' = Y_i - PY_{i-1}, \tag{3.9}$$

$$X_i' = X_i - PX_{i-1}, \tag{3.10}$$

$$\beta_0' = \beta_0(1-P), \tag{3.11}$$

$$\beta_1' = \beta_1. \tag{3.12}$$

With this transformation, the linear regression model, using the ordinary least-squares method of determination, is valid. However, to employ it, we need to know the population serial correlation coefficient, P. We estimate it by r. The population Equation 3.9 through Equation 3.11 will be changed to population estimates:

$$y_i' = y_i - ry_{i-1}, \tag{3.13}$$

$$x_i' = x_i - rx_{i-1}, \tag{3.14}$$

$$b_0' = b_0(1-r). \tag{3.15}$$

The regression model becomes

$$\hat{y}' = b_0' + b_1' x'.$$

Given that the serial correlation is eliminated, the model can be retransformed to the original scale:

$$\hat{y} = b_0 + b_1 x_1.$$

However,

$$b_0 = \frac{b_0'}{1-r} \tag{3.16}$$

and $b_1' = b_1$ or the original slope.

The regression parameters and standard deviations for b_0' and b_1' are

$$s_{b_0} = \frac{s_{b_0}'}{1 - r},$$ (3.17)

$$s_{b_1} = s_{b_1}'.$$ (3.18)

The only problem is "what is r?" There are several ways to determine this.

COCHRANE–ORCUTT PROCEDURE

This very popular method uses a three-step procedure.

Step 1: Estimate the population serial correlation coefficient, P, with the sample correlation coefficient, r. It requires a regression through the origin or the $(0, 0)$ points, using the residuals, instead of y and x, to find the slope. The equation has the form

$$\varepsilon_i = P\varepsilon_{i-1} + D_i,$$ (3.19)

where ε_i is the response variable as in y_i, ε_{i-1} is the predictor variable as in x_i, D_i is the error term, and P is the slope of the regression line through the origin.

The parameter estimators used are e_i, e_{i-1}, d_i, and r. The slope is actually computed as

$$r = \text{slope} = \frac{\sum\limits_{i=2}^{n} e_{i-1}e_i}{\sum\limits_{i=2}^{n} e_{i-1}^2}.$$ (3.20)

Note that $\Sigma e_{i-1}\, e_i$ is not the same numerator term used in the Durbin–Watson test. Here, the e_{i-1}s and e_is are multiplied but, in the Durbin–Watson test, they are subtracted and squared.

Step 2: The second step is to incorporate r into Equation 3.8, the transformed regression equation $Y_i' = \beta_0' + \beta_1' X_1' + D_i$.

For samples, the estimate equation is

$$y_i' = b_0' + b_1' x_1' + d_i,$$

where

$$y_i' = y_i - ry_{i-1},$$ (3.21)

$$x_i' = x_i - rx_{i-1},$$ (3.22)

d_i = error term.

The y_i' and x_i' transformed sample set data are then used to compute a least-squares regression function:

$$\hat{y}' = b_0' + b_1' x'.$$

Step 3: Evaluate the transformed regression equation by using the Durbin–Watson test to determine if it is still significantly serially correlated. If the test shows no serial correlation, the procedure stops. If not, the residuals from the fitted equation are used to repeat the entire process again, and the new regression that results is tested using the Durbin–Watson test, and so on.

Let us now look at a new example (Example 3.2) of data that do have significant serial correlation (Table 3.10).

We perform a standard linear regression and find very high correlation (Table 3.11).

Testing for serial correlation using the Durbin–Watson test, we find, in Table E, that for $n = 18$, $k = 1$, $\alpha = 0.05$, and $d_L = 1.16$.

H_A: $P > 0$, if $D_{W_c} < 1.16$ at $\alpha = 0.05$.

TABLE 3.10
Significant Serial Correlation, Example 3.2

n	x_i	y_i
1	0	6.3
2	0	6.2
3	0	6.4
4	1	5.3
5	1	5.4
6	1	5.5
7	2	4.5
8	2	4.4
9	2	4.4
10	3	3.4
11	3	3.5
12	3	3.6
13	4	2.6
14	4	2.5
15	4	2.4
16	5	1.3
17	5	1.4
18	5	1.5

x_i is the exposure time in minutes; and y_i is the $\log_{10}$ microbial populations.

TABLE 3.11
Regression Analysis, Example 3.2

Predictor	Coef	St. Dev	t-Ratio	p
b_0	6.36032	0.04164	152.73	0.000
b_1	−0.97524	0.01375	−70.90	0.000
$s = 0.09966$		R-sq $= 99.7\%$		R-sq(adj) $= 99.7\%$

Analysis of Variance

Source	DF	SS	MS	F	p
Regression	1	49.932	49.932	5027.13	0.000
Error	16	0.159	0.010		
Total	17	50.091			

Durbin–Watson statistic $= 1.09$.
The regression equation is $\hat{y} = 6.36 - 0.975x$.

Because $D_{W_C} = 1.09 < D_{W_T} = 1.16$, there is significant serial correlation at $\alpha = 0.05$. Instead of adding another x variable, the researcher decides to transform the data using the Cochrane–Orcutt method.

Step 1: Estimate P by the slope r:

$$r = \text{slope} = \frac{\sum_{i=2}^{n} e_{i-1} e_i}{\sum_{i=2}^{n} e_{i-1}^2}. \tag{3.23}$$

To do this, we use MiniTab interactive (Table 3.12)

$$r = \frac{\sum e_{i-1} e_i}{\sum e_{i-1}^2} = \frac{0.0704903}{0.158669} = 0.4443.$$

Step 2: We next fit the transformed data to a new regression form. To do this, we compute (from Table 3.13):

$$y_i' = y_i - r y_{i-1} = y_i - 0.4443 y_{i-1},$$

$$x_i' = x_i - r x_{i-1} = x_i - 0.4443 x_{i-1}.$$

The new x' and y' values are used to perform a least-squares regression analysis.

Step 2 (continued): Regression on y' and x'.

TABLE 3.12
MiniTab Data Display Printout, Example 3.2

n	x_i	y_i	e_i	$\hat{y}_i$	e_{i-1}	$e_i\,e_{i-1}$	e_{i-1}^2
1	0	6.3	−0.060317	6.36032	—	—	—
2	0	6.2	−0.160317	6.36032	−0.060317	0.0096699	0.0036382
3	0	6.4	0.039683	6.36032	−0.160317	−0.0063618	0.0257017
4	1	5.3	−0.085079	5.38508	0.039683	−0.0033762	0.0015747
5	1	5.4	0.014921	5.38508	−0.085079	−0.0012694	0.0072385
6	1	5.5	0.114921	5.38508	0.014921	0.0017147	0.0002226
7	2	4.5	0.090159	4.40984	0.114921	0.0103611	0.0132068
8	2	4.4	−0.009841	4.40984	0.090159	−0.0008873	0.0081286
9	2	4.4	−0.009841	4.40984	−0.009841	0.0000969	0.0000969
10	3	3.4	−0.034603	3.43460	−0.009841	0.0003405	0.0000969
11	3	3.5	0.065397	3.43460	−0.034603	−0.0022629	0.0011974
12	3	3.6	0.165397	3.43460	0.065397	0.0108164	0.0042767
13	4	2.6	0.140635	2.45937	0.165397	0.0232606	0.0273561
14	4	2.5	0.040635	2.45937	0.140635	0.0057147	0.0197782
15	4	2.4	−0.059365	2.45937	0.040635	−0.0024123	0.0016512
16	5	1.3	−0.184127	1.48413	−0.059365	0.0109307	0.0035242
17	5	1.4	−0.084127	1.48413	−0.184127	0.0154900	0.0339027
18	5	1.5	0.015873	1.48413	−0.084127	−0.0013353	0.0070773
					$\Sigma e_i\,e_{i-1} = 0.0704903$		$\Sigma e_{i-1}^2 = 0.158669$

Step 3: We again test for serial correlation using the Durbin–Watson test procedure. Because this is the second computation of the regression equation, we lost one value to the lag adjustment, so $n = 17$. For every iteration, the lag adjustment reduces n by 1.

H_A: $P > 0$, if $D_{W_C} < 1.13$; $d_L = 1.13$, $n = 17$, $\alpha = 0.05$ (Table E).

If $1.13 \leq D_{W_C} \leq 1.39$, undeterminable.
If $D_{W_C} > 1.39$, accept H_0. $d_U = 1.39$, $n = 17$, and $\alpha = 0.05$ (Table E).
$D_{W_C} = 1.64$ (Table 3.14).
Because $D_{W_C} = 1.64$, reject H_A at $\alpha = 0.05$. No significant serial correlation is present. If serial correlation had been present, one would substitute x' and y' for x_i and y_i, recompute r, and perform steps 2 and 3.

Because this iteration removed the serial correlation, we transform the data back to their original scale. This does not need to be done if one wants to use the transformed $x'y'$ values, but this is awkward and difficult for many to understand. The transformation back to y and x is more easily accomplished using Equation series 3.16 and Table 3.14.

TABLE 3.13
Regression Analysis, Example 3.2

n	x_i	y_i	y_{i-1}	$y_i' = y_i - ry_{i-1}$	x_{i-1}	$x_i' = x_i - rx_{i-1}$
1	0	6.3	—	—	—	—
2	0	6.2	6.3	3.40091	0	0.00000
3	0	6.4	6.2	3.64534	0	0.00000
4	1	5.3	6.4	2.45648	0	1.00000
5	1	5.4	5.3	3.04521	1	0.5557
6	1	5.5	5.4	3.10078	1	0.5557
7	2	4.5	5.5	2.05635	1	1.5557
8	2	4.4	4.5	2.40065	2	1.1114
9	2	4.4	4.4	2.44508	2	1.1114
10	3	3.4	4.4	1.44508	2	2.1114
11	3	3.5	3.4	1.98938	3	1.6671
12	3	3.6	3.5	2.04495	3	1.6671
13	4	2.6	3.6	1.00052	3	2.6671
14	4	2.5	2.6	1.34482	4	2.2228
15	4	2.4	2.5	1.28925	4	2.2228
16	5	1.3	2.4	0.23368	4	3.2228
17	5	1.4	1.3	0.82241	5	2.7785
18	5	1.5	1.4	0.87798	5	2.7785

$$b_0 = \frac{b_0'}{1-r} = \frac{3.56202}{1-0.4443} = 6.410,$$

$$b_1 = b_1' = -0.98999.$$

TABLE 3.14
Regression Analysis on Transformed Data, Example 3.2

Predictor	Coef	SE Coef	T	p
b_0	3.56202	0.04218	84.46	0.000
b_1	−0.98999	0.02257	−43.86	0.000
$s = 0.0895447$		R-sq $= 99.2\%$		R-sq(adj) $= 99.2\%$

Analysis of Variance

Source	DF	SS	MS	F	p
Regression	1	15.423	15.423	1923.52	0.000
Residual error	15	0.120	0.008		
Total	16	15.544			

Durbin–Watson statistic $= 1.64164$.
The regression equation is $\hat{y}' = 3.61 - 0.990x'$.

The new regression equation is

$$y = b_0 + b_1 x_1,$$

$$y = 6.410 - 0.98999x.$$

The results from the new regression equation are presented in Table 3.15. The new $\hat{y}$ vs. x plot is presented in Figure 3.6.

The new residual e_i vs. x_i is plotted in Figure 3.7. As can be seen, this procedure is easy and can be extremely valuable in working with serially correlated data.

Note that $s_{(b_0)} = \dfrac{s'_{(b_0)}}{1 - r}$ and

$$s_{(b_1)} = s'_{(b_1)}. \tag{3.24}$$

TABLE 3.15
New Data, Example 3.2

Row	x_i	y_i	$\hat{y}_i^a$	$\hat{y}$
1	0	6.3	6.41000	−0.11000
2	0	6.2	6.41000	−0.21000
3	0	6.4	6.41000	−0.01000
4	1	5.3	5.42001	−0.12001
5	1	5.4	5.42001	−0.02001
6	1	5.5	5.42001	0.07999
7	2	4.5	4.43002	0.06998
8	2	4.4	4.43002	−0.03002
9	2	4.4	4.43002	−0.03002
10	3	3.4	3.44003	−0.04003
11	3	3.5	3.44003	0.05997
12	3	3.6	3.44003	0.15997
13	4	2.6	2.45004	0.14996
14	4	2.5	2.45004	0.04996
15	4	2.4	2.45004	−0.05004
16	5	1.3	1.46005	−0.16005
17	5	1.4	1.46005	−0.06005
18	5	1.5	1.46005	0.03995

[a] $\hat{y}_i = 6.410 - 0.098999x.$

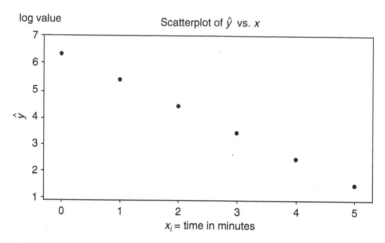

FIGURE 3.6 Scatterplot of $\hat{y}$ vs. x, Example 3.2.

Recall that

$$s_{b_0} = \frac{\sqrt{MS_E\left[\dfrac{1}{n} + \dfrac{\bar{x}^2}{\sum (x_i - \bar{x})^2}\right]}}{1 - r},$$

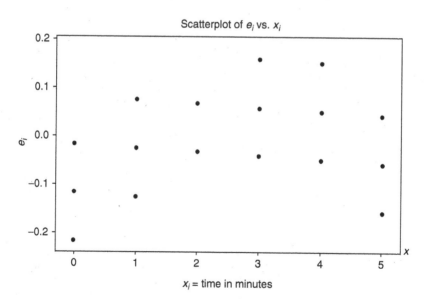

FIGURE 3.7 Scatterplot of e_i vs. x_i, Example 3.2.

$$s_{b_1} = \sqrt{\frac{MS_E}{\sum\limits_{i=1}^{n}(x_i - \bar{x})^2}}.$$

From Table 3.11,

$$s_{b_0} = \frac{0.04164}{1 - 0.4443} = 0.07493,$$

$$s_{b_1} = 0.01375.$$

LAG 1 OR FIRST DIFFERENCE PROCEDURE

Some statisticians prefer an easier method than the Cochrane–Orcutt procedure for removing serial correlation—the first difference procedure. As previously discussed, when serial correlation is present, P, the population correlation coefficient, tends to be large ($P > 0$), so a number of statisticians recommend just setting $P = 1$ and applying the transforming Equation 3.25 (Kutner et al., 2005)

$$Y_i' = \beta_0' + \beta_1 X_i' + D_i, \tag{3.25}$$

where

$$Y' = Y_i - Y_{i-1},$$

$$X' = X_i - X_{i-1},$$

$$D_i = e_i - e_{i-1}.$$

Because $\beta_0 (1 - P) = \beta_0 (1 - 1) = 0$, the regression equation reduces to a regression through the origin:

$$Y_i' = \beta_1 X_i' + D_i \tag{3.26}$$

or, for the sample set

$$\hat{y}_i = b_1 x_i + d_i$$

or, expanded

$$y_i - y_{i-1} = b_1(x_i - x_{i-1}) + (e_i - e_{i-1}). \tag{3.27}$$

The fitted model is

$$\hat{y}_i' = b_1' x', \tag{3.28}$$

which is a regression through the origin, where

$$b_1' = \frac{\sum x_i' y_i'}{\sum x_i'^2}. \tag{3.29}$$

It can easily be transformed back to the original scale, $\hat{y}_i = b_0 + b_1 x$, where

$$b_0 = \bar{y} - b_1' \bar{x} \quad \text{and} \quad b_1 = b_1'.$$

Let us apply this approach to the data from Example 3.2 (Table 3.10). Using MiniTab, we manipulated the x_i and y_i data to provide the necessary transformed data (Table 3.16).

$$x_i' = x_i - x_{i-1} \quad \text{and} \quad y_i' = y_i - y_{i-1}.$$

We can now regress y_i' on x_i', which produces a regression equation nearly through the origin or $b_0 = 0$ (Table 3.17). However, the Durbin–Watson test

TABLE 3.16
MiniTab Transformed Data, Example 3.2

Row	x_i	y_i	x_{i-1}	y_{i-1}	$x_i' = x_i - x_{i-1}$	$y_i' = y_i - y_{i-1}$	$x_i' y_i'$	$x_i'^2$
1	0	6.3	—	—	—	—	—	—
2	0	6.2	0	6.3	0	−0.1	0.0	0
3	0	6.4	0	6.2	0	0.2	0.0	0
4	1	5.3	0	6.4	1	−1.1	−1.1	1
5	1	5.4	1	5.3	0	0.1	0.0	0
6	1	5.5	1	5.4	0	0.1	0.0	0
7	2	4.5	1	5.5	1	−1.0	−1.0	1
8	2	4.4	2	4.5	0	−0.1	0.0	0
9	2	4.4	2	4.4	0	0.0	0.0	0
10	3	3.4	2	4.4	1	−1.0	−1.0	1
11	3	3.5	3	3.4	0	0.1	0.0	0
12	3	3.6	3	3.5	0	0.1	0.0	0
13	4	2.6	3	3.6	1	−1.0	−1.0	1
14	4	2.5	4	2.6	0	−0.1	0.0	0
15	4	2.4	4	2.5	0	−0.1	0.0	0
16	5	1.3	4	2.4	1	−1.1	−1.1	1
17	5	1.4	5	1.3	0	0.1	0.0	0
18	5	1.5	5	1.4	0	0.1	0.0	0
							$\sum x_i' y_i' = -5.2$	$\sum x_i'^2 = 5$

TABLE 3.17
MiniTab Regression Using Transformed Data, Example 3.2

Predictor	Coef	St. Dev	t-Ratio	p
b_0'	0.03333	0.02776	1.20	0.248
b_1'	−1.07333	0.05118	−20.97	0.000
$s = 0.09615$		R-sq = 96.7%		R-sq(adj) = 96.5%

Analysis of Variance

Source	DF	SS	MS	F	P
Regression	1	4.0660	4.0660	439.84	0.000
Error	15	0.1387	0.0092		
Total	16	4.2047			

Durbin–Watson statistic = 1.84936.
The regression equation is $\hat{y}_i' = 0.0333 - 1.07x_i'$.

---

cannot be completed on data when $b_0 = 0$, so we accept the 0.03333 value from Table 3.17 and test the D_W statistic.

Note that the Durbin–Watson test was significant at $D_W = 1.09$ before the first difference transformation was carried out (Table 3.11). Now, the value for D_W is 1.85 (Table 3.17), which is not significant at $\alpha = 0.05$, $n = 17$ (Table E), $d_L = 1.13$, and $d_U = 1.38$, because $D_W = 1.85 > d_U = 1.38$. Hence, the first difference procedure was adequate to correct for the serial correlation.

We can convert $y_i' = b'x_i'$ to the original scale.

$$\hat{y}_i = b_0 + b_1 x_1,$$

where

$$b_0 = \bar{y} - b_1'\bar{x},$$

$$b_1 = b_1' = \frac{\sum x_i' y_i'}{\sum x_i'^2},$$

$$\sum x_i'^2 = 5.0 \text{ (Table 3.16)},$$

$$\sum x_i' y_i' = -5.2 \text{ (Table 3.15)},$$

$$b_1' = \frac{-5.2}{5.0} = -1.04.$$

The transformed equation is used to predict new $\hat{y}_i$ values (Table 3.18). Note that $s_{b_1'} = $ St. dev $= s_{b_1}$ and $s_{b_1} = 0.05118$ (Table 3.17).

TABLE 3.18
Transformed Data Table, Example 3.2

Row	x_i	y_i	$\hat{y}_i$	e_i
1	0	6.3	6.59722	−0.29722
2	0	6.2	6.59722	−0.39722
3	0	6.4	6.59722	−0.19722
4	1	5.3	5.52722	−0.22722
5	1	5.4	5.52722	−0.12722
6	1	5.5	5.52722	−0.02722
7	2	4.5	4.45722	0.04278
8	2	4.4	4.45722	−0.05722
9	2	4.4	4.45722	−0.05722
10	3	3.4	3.38722	0.01278
11	3	3.5	3.38722	0.11278
12	3	3.6	3.38722	0.21278
13	4	2.6	2.31722	0.28278
14	4	2.5	2.31722	0.18278
15	4	2.4	2.31722	0.08278
16	5	1.3	1.24722	0.05278
17	5	1.4	1.24722	0.15278
18	5	1.5	1.24722	0.25278

CURVE FITTING WITH SERIAL CORRELATION

In many practical applications using regression analysis, the data collected are not linear. In these cases, the experimenter must linearize the data by means of a transformation to apply simple linear regression methods. In approaching all regression problems, it is important to plot the y_i, x_i values to see their shape. If the shape of the data is linear, the regression can be performed. It is usually wise, however, to perform a lack-of-fit test after the regression has been conducted and plot the residuals against the x_i values, to see if these appear patternless.

If the y_i, x_i values are definitely nonlinear, a transformation must be performed. Let us see how this is performed in Example 3.3. In a drug-dosing pilot study, the blood levels of an antidepressant drug, R-0515-6, showed the drug elimination profile for five human subjects, presented in Table 3.19.

x represents the hourly blood draw after ingesting R-0515-6. Blood levels were ≈ 30 μg until 4 h, when the elimination phase of the study began and continued for 24 h postdrug dosing. Figure 3.8 provides a diagram of the study results.

Clearly, the rate of eliminating the drug from the blood is not linear, as it begins declining at an increasing rate 6 h after dosing. The regression analysis for the nontransformed data is presented in Table 3.20.

TABLE 3.19
Blood Elimination Profile for R-0515-6, Example 3.3

n	x (hour of sample)	y (µg/mL)
1	4	30.5
2	4	29.8
3	4	30.8
4	4	30.2
5	4	29.9
6	6	20.7
7	6	21.0
8	6	20.3
9	6	20.8
10	6	20.5
11	10	12.5
12	10	12.7
13	10	12.4
14	10	12.7
15	10	12.6
16	15	8.5
17	15	8.6
18	15	8.4
19	15	8.2
20	15	8.5
21	24	2.8
22	24	3.1
23	24	2.7
24	24	2.9
25	24	3.1

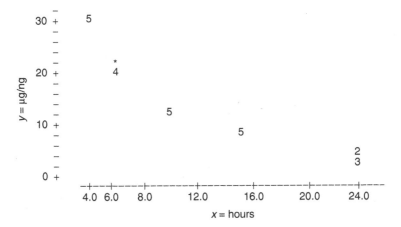

FIGURE 3.8 Drug elimination profile.

TABLE 3.20
Regression Analysis for Nontransformed Data

Predictor	Coef	St. Dev	t-Ratio	p
b_0	29.475	1.516	19.44	0.000
b_1	−1.2294	0.1098	−11.20	0.000
s = 3.935		R-sq = 84.5%		R-sq(adj) = 83.8%

Analysis of Variance

Source	DF	SS	MS	F	p
Regression	1	1940.7	1940.7	125.35	0.000
Error	23	356.1	15.5		
Total	24	2296.8			

The regression equation is $\hat{y} = 29.5 - 1.23x$.

Recall from Chapter 2 the discussion on how to linearize curved data that exhibit patterns as seen in Figure 3.9. Data producing such a pattern are linearized by lowering the power scale of the x and/or y data. We lower the y data and retain the x values in their original form.

Recall

Power	Regression Transformation	None
1	y	Raw
1/2	$\sqrt{y}$	Square root
0	$\log_{10} y$	Logarithm
−1/2	$\sqrt[-1]{y}$	Reciprocal root (minus sign preserves order)

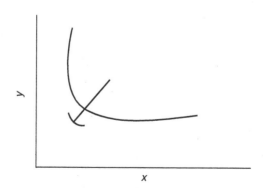

FIGURE 3.9 Curved data patterns.

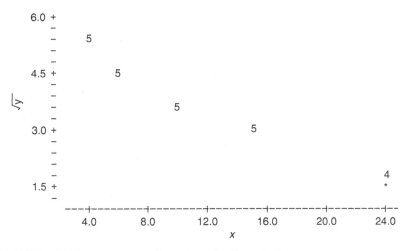

FIGURE 3.10 Square root transformation of y, Example 3.3.

We begin with the square-root transformation (Figure 3.10). Table 3.21 provides the regression analysis on the square-root transformation.

The data, although more linear, still show a definite curve. We, therefore, proceed down in the power scale to a $\log_{10} y$ transformation (Figure 3.11). The regression analysis is presented in Table 3.22. The $\log_{10}$ transformation has nearly linearized the data. The MS_E value is 0.0013, very low, and $R^2 = 99.1\%$. We plot the e_i vs. x values now, because we are very close to finishing. Figure 3.12 shows the residual vs. time plot. Although they are not perfect, this distribution will do for this phase of the analysis.

Figure 3.13 provides the plot of a $-1/\sqrt{y}$ transformation. The $-1/\sqrt{y}$ transformation slightly overcorrects the data and is slightly less precise in fitting the data (Table 3.23). Hence, we go with the $\log_{10}$ transformation.

TABLE 3.21
Square Root of y Regression Analysis, Example 3.3

Predictor	Coef	St. Dev	t-Ratio	p	
b_0	5.7317	0.1268	45.20	0.000	
b_1	−0.177192	0.009184	−19.29	0.000	
$s = 0.3291$		R-sq $= 94.2\%$		R-sq(adj) $= 93.9\%$	

Analysis of Variance

Source	DF	SS	MS	F	p
Regression	1	40.314	40.314	372.23	0.000
Error	23	2.491	0.108		
Total	24	42.805			

The regression equation is $\hat{y} = 5.73 - 0.177x$.

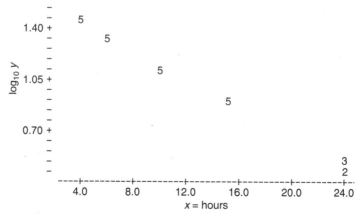

FIGURE 3.11 Log_{10} transformation of y.

Table 3.24 presents the $\log_{10} y$ transformation data. Because these data were collected over time, there is a real danger of serial correlation. Now that we have the appropriate transformation, we conduct a Durbin–Watson positive serial correlation test.

Let us compute the Durbin–Watson test for a lag of 1, using the six-step procedure.

Step 1: State the hypothesis.

$H_0: P \leq 0,$
$H_A: P > 0$ (serial correlation is significant and positive over time).

TABLE 3.22
Log_{10} of y Regression Analysis, Example 3.3

Predictor	Coef	St. Dev	t-Ratio	p
b_0	1.63263	0.01374	118.83	0.000
b_1	−0.0487595	0.0009952	−49.00	0.000
$s = 0.03566$		R-sq $= 99.1\%$		R-sq(adj) $= 99.0\%$

Analysis of Variance

Source	DF	SS	MS	F	p
Regression	1	3.0527	3.0527	2400.59	0.000
Error	23	0.0292	0.0013		
Total	24	3.0819			

Durbin–Watson statistic $= 0.696504$.
The regression equation is $\hat{y} = 1.63 − 0.0488x$.

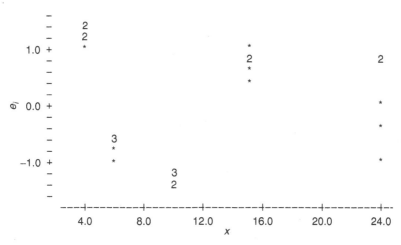

FIGURE 3.12 Residual vs. time $\log_{10} y$ transformation, Example 3.3.

Step 2: Set α and n.

$\alpha = 0.05$,

n already equals 24.

Step 3: The test we use for serial correlation is the Durbin–Watson, where

$$D_W = \frac{\sum\limits_{i=2}^{n} (e_i - e_{i-1})^2}{\sum\limits_{i=1}^{n} e_i^2}.$$

Because some practitioners may not have this test generated automatically via their statistical software, we do it interactively. Table 3.25 provides the necessary data.

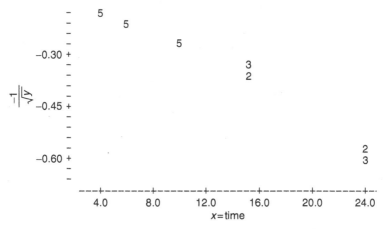

FIGURE 3.13 $-1/\sqrt{y}$ transformation of y, Example 3.3.

TABLE 3.23
Regression Analysis of $-1/\sqrt{y}$ Transformation, Example 3.3

Predictor	Coef	St. Dev	t-Ratio	P
b_0	−0.090875	0.009574	−9.49	0.000
b_1	−0.0196537	0.0009635	−28.34	0.000
$s = 0.02485$		R-sq = 97.2%		R-sq(adj) = 97.1%

Analysis of Variance

Source	DF	SS	MS	F	P
Regression	1	0.49597	0.49597	803.26	0.000
Error	23	0.01420	0.00062		
Total	24	0.51017			

The regression equation is $\hat{y} = -0.0909 - 0.0197x$.

TABLE 3.24
Log_{10} Transformation of y, Example 3.3

Row	x_i	y_i	$\log y_i$	e_i	$\log \hat{y}$
1	4	30.5	1.48430	0.0467101	1.43759
2	4	29.8	1.47422	0.0366266	1.43759
3	4	30.8	1.48855	0.0509610	1.43759
4	4	30.2	1.48001	0.0424172	1.43759
5	4	29.9	1.47567	0.0380815	1.43759
6	6	20.7	1.31597	−0.0241003	1.34007
7	6	21.0	1.32222	−0.0178513	1.34007
8	6	20.3	1.30750	−0.0325746	1.34007
9	6	20.8	1.31806	−0.0220073	1.34007
10	6	20.5	1.31175	−0.0283167	1.34007
11	10	12.5	1.09691	−0.0481224	1.14503
12	10	12.7	1.10380	−0.0412287	1.14503
13	10	12.4	1.09342	−0.0516107	1.14503
14	10	12.7	1.10380	−0.0412287	1.14503
15	10	12.6	1.10037	−0.0446619	1.14503
16	15	8.5	0.92942	0.0281843	0.90123
17	15	8.6	0.93450	0.0332638	0.90123
18	15	8.4	0.92428	0.0230446	0.90123
19	15	8.2	0.91381	0.0125792	0.90123
20	15	8.5	0.92942	0.0281843	0.90123
21	24	2.8	0.44716	−0.0152406	0.46240
22	24	3.1	0.49136	0.0289630	0.46240
23	24	2.7	0.43136	−0.0310349	0.46240
24	24	2.9	0.46240	−0.0000007	0.46240
25	24	3.1	0.49136	0.0289630	0.46240

Durbin–Watson statistic $= 0.696504$.

Step 4: Decision Rule

From Table E, $n = 24$, $\alpha = 0.05$, $k = 1$, $d_L = 1.27$, and $d_U = 1.45$.

Therefore, if $D_{W_C} < d_L = 1.27$, serial correlation is significant at $\alpha = 0.05$.

If $d_L \leq D_W \leq d_U$, the test is inconclusive.

If $D_{W_C} > d_U$, reject H_A at $\alpha = 0.05$.

Step 5:

$$D_{W_C} = \frac{\sum (e_i - e_{i-1})^2}{\sum e_i^2}.$$

By computer manipulation, $D_{W_C} = 0.696504$ (Table 3.24).

By computer manipulation, $D_{W_C} = \dfrac{\sum (e_i - e_{i-1})^2}{\sum e_i^2} = \dfrac{0.0203713}{0.0270661} = 0.7526$

(Table 3.25).

TABLE 3.25
Data for Interactive Calculation of D_W, Example 3.3

Row	e_i	e_{i-1}	$e_i - e_{i-1}$	e_i^2	$(e_i - e_{i-1})^2$
1	0.0467101	—	—	—	—
2	0.0366266	0.0467101	−0.0100836	0.0013415	0.0001017
3	0.0509610	0.0366266	0.0143345	0.0025970	0.0002055
4	0.0424172	0.0509610	−0.0085438	0.0017992	0.0000730
5	0.0380815	0.0424172	−0.0043358	0.0014502	0.0000188
6	−0.0241003	0.0380815	−0.0621817	0.0005808	0.0038666
7	−0.0178513	−0.0241003	0.0062489	0.0003187	0.0000390
8	−0.0325746	−0.0178513	−0.0147233	0.0010611	0.0002168
9	−0.0220073	−0.0325746	0.0105673	0.0004843	0.0001117
10	−0.0283167	−0.0220073	−0.0063095	0.0008018	0.0000398
11	−0.0481224	−0.0283167	−0.0198056	0.0023158	0.0003923
12	−0.0412287	−0.0481224	0.0068937	0.0016998	0.0000475
13	−0.0516107	−0.0412287	−0.0103820	0.0026637	0.0001078
14	−0.0412287	−0.0516107	0.0103820	0.0016998	0.0001078
15	−0.0446619	−0.0412287	−0.0034332	0.0019947	0.0000118
16	0.0281843	−0.0446619	0.0728461	0.0007944	0.0053066
17	0.0332638	0.0281843	0.0050795	0.0011065	0.0000258
18	0.0230446	0.0332638	−0.0102192	0.0005311	0.0001044
19	0.0125792	0.0230466	−0.0104654	0.0001582	0.0001095
20	0.0281843	0.0125792	0.0156051	0.0007944	0.0002435
21	−0.0152406	0.0281843	−0.0434249	0.0002323	0.0018857
22	0.0289630	−0.0152406	0.0442037	0.0008389	0.0019540
23	−0.0310349	0.0289630	−0.0599979	0.0009632	0.0035998
24	−0.0000007	−0.0310349	0.0310342	0.0000000	0.0009631
25	0.0289630	−0.0000007	0.0289637	0.0008389	0.0008389

$$\sum e_i^2 = 0.0270661 \quad \sum (e_i - e_{i-1})^2 = 0.0203713$$

Step 6:
Because $D_{W_c} = 0.75 < 1.27$, reject H_0.
Significant serial correlation exists at $\alpha = 0.05$.

REMEDY

We use the Cochrane–Orcutt procedure to remedy the serial correlation.

Step 1: Estimate

$$\varepsilon_i = P\varepsilon_{i-1} + D_i.$$

We estimate P (population correlation) using r (Equation 3.23)

$$r = \text{slope} = \frac{\displaystyle\sum_{i=2}^{n} e_{i-1}e_i}{\displaystyle\sum_{i=2}^{n} e_{i-1}^2}.$$

Step 2: Fit the transformed model.

$$y_i' = y_i - ry_{i-1} \quad (y_i \text{ and } y_{i-1} \text{ are } \log_{10} y \text{ values}),$$

$$x_i' = x_i - rx_{i-1}.$$

Table 3.26A provides the raw data manipulation needed for determining r

$$r = \frac{\sum e_{i-1}e_i}{\sum e_{i-1}^2} = \frac{0.0175519}{0.0284090} = 0.6178.$$

Table 3.26B provides the data manipulation for determining y' and x', which are, in turn, used to perform a regression analysis. Table 3.27 provides the transformed regression analysis. Therefore, the transformation was successful. The new Durbin–Watson value is $2.29 > d_U = 1.45$, which is not significant for serial correlation at $\alpha = 0.05$. We can now transform the data back to the original scale

$$\hat{y} = b_0 + b_1 x,$$

where

$$b_0 = \frac{b_0'}{1 - r} = \frac{0.62089}{1 - 0.6178} = 1.6245, \tag{3.16}$$

TABLE 3.26A
Manipulation of Raw Data from Table 3.25, Example 3.3

Row	x_i	y_i	e_{i-1}	e_i	$e_{i-1}e_i$	e_{i-1}^2
1	4	1.48430	0.0467101	—	—	—
2	4	1.47422	0.0366266	0.0467101	0.0017108	0.0021818
3	4	1.48855	0.0509610	0.0366266	0.0018665	0.0013415
4	4	1.48001	0.0424172	0.0509610	0.0021616	0.0025970
5	4	1.47567	0.0380815	0.0424172	0.0016153	0.0017992
6	6	1.31597	−0.0241003	0.0380815	−0.0009178	0.0014502
7	6	1.32222	−0.0178513	−0.0241003	0.0004302	0.0005808
8	6	1.30750	−0.0325746	−0.0178513	0.0005815	0.0003187
9	6	1.31806	−0.0220073	−0.0325746	0.0007169	0.0010611
10	6	1.31175	−0.0283167	−0.0220073	0.0006232	0.0004843
11	10	1.09691	−0.0481224	−0.0283167	0.0013627	0.0008018
12	10	1.10380	−0.0412287	−0.0481224	0.0019840	0.0023158
13	10	1.09342	−0.0516107	−0.0412287	0.0021278	0.0016998
14	10	1.10380	−0.0412287	−0.0516107	0.0021278	0.0026637
15	10	1.10037	−0.0446619	−0.0412287	0.0018413	0.0016998
16	15	0.92942	0.0281843	−0.0446619	−0.0012588	0.0019947
17	15	0.93450	0.0332638	0.0281843	0.0009375	0.0007944
18	15	0.92428	0.0230446	0.0332638	0.0007666	0.0011065
19	15	0.91381	0.0125792	0.0230446	0.0002899	0.0005311
20	15	0.92942	0.0281843	0.0125792	0.0003545	0.0001582
21	24	0.44716	−0.0152406	0.0281843	−0.0004295	0.0007944
22	24	0.49136	0.0289630	−0.0152406	−0.0004414	0.0002323
23	24	0.43136	−0.0310349	0.0289630	−0.0008989	0.0008389
24	24	0.46240	−0.0000007	−0.0310349	0.0000000	0.0009632
25	24	0.49136	0.0289630	−0.0000007	−0.0000000	0.0000000

$$\sum e_{i-1}\, e_i = 0.0175519 \quad \sum e_{i-1}^2 = 0.0284090$$

$$b_1 = b_1' = -0.048390.$$

Therefore, $\hat{y} = 1.6245 - 0.048390\, x_i$, which uses the original x_i and y_i in $\log_{10}$ scale

$$s_{b_0} = \frac{s_{b_0}'}{1 - r} = \frac{0.01017}{1 - 0.6178} = 0.0266, \tag{3.17}$$

$$s_{b_1} = s_{b_1}' = 0.001657. \tag{3.18}$$

This analysis was quite involved, but well within the capabilities of the applied researcher.

TABLE 3.26B
Data for Determining y' and x', Example 3.3

Row	x_i	y_i	y_{i-1}	y'_{i-1}	x_{i-1}	x'_i	e_{i-1}	$\hat{y}'_{i-1}$
1	4	1.48430	—	—	—	—	—	—
2	4	1.47422	1.48430	0.557216	4	1.5288	0.0103081	0.546908
3	4	1.48855	1.47422	0.577780	4	1.5288	0.0308722	0.546908
4	4	1.48001	1.48855	0.560380	4	1.5288	0.0134726	0.546908
5	4	1.47567	1.48001	0.561323	4	1.5288	0.0144152	0.546908
6	6	1.31597	1.47567	0.404301	4	3.5288	−0.0458273	0.450128
7	6	1.32222	1.31597	0.509213	6	2.2932	−0.0007057	0.509918
8	6	1.30750	1.32222	0.490629	6	2.2932	−0.0192895	0.509918
9	6	1.31806	1.30750	0.510292	6	2.2932	0.0003738	0.509918
10	6	1.31175	1.31806	0.497454	6	2.2932	−0.0124641	0.509918
11	10	1.09691	1.31175	0.286508	6	6.2932	−0.0298506	0.316359
12	10	1.10380	1.09691	0.426133	10	3.8220	−0.0098074	0.435940
13	10	1.09342	1.10380	0.411492	10	3.8220	−0.0244483	0.435940
14	10	1.10380	1.09342	0.428288	10	3.8220	−0.0076523	0.435940
15	10	1.10037	1.10380	0.418441	10	3.8220	−0.0174995	0.435940
16	15	0.92942	1.10037	0.249610	10	8.8220	0.0556192	0.193991
17	15	0.93450	0.92942	0.360303	15	5.7330	0.0168364	0.343467
18	15	0.92428	0.93450	0.346946	15	5.7330	0.0034791	0.343467
19	15	0.91381	0.92428	0.342794	15	5.7330	−0.0006730	0.343467
20	15	0.92942	0.91381	0.364865	15	5.7330	0.0213976	0.343467
21	24	0.44716	0.92942	−0.127037	15	14.7330	−0.0349954	−0.092042
22	24	0.49136	0.44716	0.215107	24	9.1728	0.0380918	0.177016
23	24	0.43136	0.49136	0.127801	24	9.1728	−0.0492152	0.177016
24	24	0.46240	0.43136	0.195901	24	9.1728	0.0188858	0.177016
25	24	0.49136	0.46240	0.205692	24	9.1728	0.0286765	0.177016

TABLE 3.27
Transformed Regression of y' and x', Example 3.3

Predictor	Coef	SE Coef	t-Ratio	p
b_0	0.62089	0.01017	61.07	0.000
b_1	−0.048390	0.001657	−29.21	0.000
$s = 0.0270948$		R-sq $= 97.5\%$		R-sq(adj) $= 97.4\%$

Analysis of Variance

Source	DF	SS	MS	F	p
Regression	1	0.62636	0.62636	853.21	0.000
Error	22	0.01615	0.00073		
Total	23	0.64251			

Durbin–Watson statistic $= 2.29073$.
The regression equation is $\hat{y}' = 0.621 - 0.0484x'$.

RESIDUAL ANALYSIS $y_i - \hat{y}_i = e_i$

Up to this point, we have looked mainly at residual plots, such as e_i vs. x_i, e_i vs. y_i, and e_i vs. $\hat{y}_i$, to help evaluate how well the regression model fits the data. There is much that can be done with this type of "eye-ball" approach. In fact, the present author uses this procedure in at least 90% of the work he does, but there are times when this approach is not adequate and a more quantitative procedure of residual analysis is required.

Recall that the three most important phenomena uncovered from residual analysis are

1. Serial correlation
2. Model adequacy
3. Outliers

We have already discussed serial correlation and the importance of evaluating the pairwise values when data have been collected over a series of sequential time points. Residual analysis is therefore very important in understanding the correlation and determining when it has been corrected by transformation of the regression model.

Model adequacy is an on-going challenge. It would be easy if one could merely curve-fit each new experiment, but, in practice, this is usually not an option. For example, for a drug formulation stability study of product A, suppose a $\log_{10}$ transformation is used to linearize the data. Decision makers like consistency in that the data for stability studies will always be reported in $\log_{10}$ scale. The use of $\log_{10}$ scale for 1 month, a square root the next, and a negative reciprocal of the square root the next month each may provide the best model but will unduly confuse readers. Moreover, from an applied perspective in industry, statistics is a primary mechanism of communication providing clarity to all. The p-values need to be presented as yes or no, feasible or not feasible, or similar terms, and analysis must be conceptually straightforward enough for business, sales, quality assurance, and production to understand what is presented. The frequent inability of statisticians to deal with cross-disciplinary reality has resulted in failures in the acceptance of statistics by the general management community and even scientists.

Chapter 2 presented the basic model requirements for a simple linear regression. The b_1 or slope must be approximately linear over the entire regression data range. The variance and standard deviation of b_1 must be constant (Figure 3.14).

Nonnormal patterns are presented in Figure 3.15. Nonnormal patterns are often very hard to see on a dataplot of y_i vs. x_i, but analysis of residuals is much more sensitive to nonnormal patterns. For example, Figure 3.16

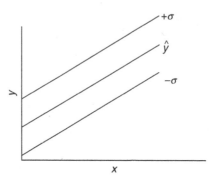

FIGURE 3.14 Variance of the slope is constant.

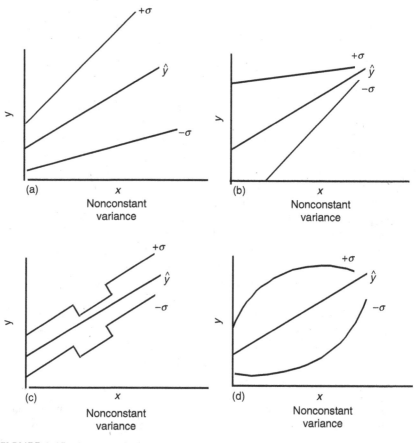

FIGURE 3.15 Nonnormal patterns.

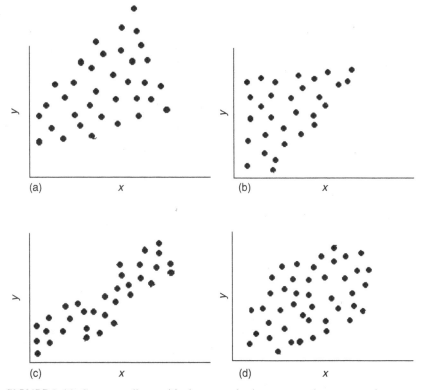

FIGURE 3.16 Corresponding residual patterns in the y_i vs. x_i plots.

illustrates the corresponding residual patterns in the y_i vs. x_i plots presented in Figure 3.15.

We also note that

$$\bar{e} = \frac{\sum\limits_{i=1}^{n} e_i}{n} = 0 \text{ for the } y_i - \hat{y}_i = e_i \text{ data set,} \qquad (3.30)$$

$$s_e^2 = \frac{\sum\limits_{i=1}^{n} e_i^2}{n-2} \text{ for simple linear regressions, } \hat{y} = b_0 + b_1 x_i \qquad (3.31)$$

Note that $\frac{SS_E}{n-2}$ equals s_e^2, if the model $\hat{y} = b_0 + b_1 x_i$ is adequate.

The e_i values are not completely independent variables, for once one has summed $n-1$ of the e_is the next or final e_i value is known because $\Sigma e_i = 0$. However, given $n > k + 1$, the e_is can be treated as independent random variables, where n is the number of e_i values, and k the number of b_is (not including b_0), so $k + 1 = 2$.

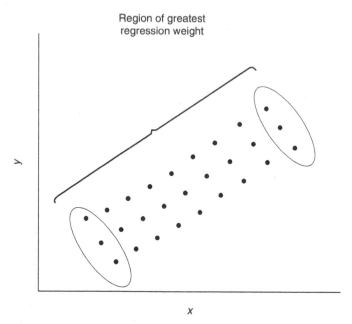

FIGURE 3.17 Region of greatest regression weight.

Outliers present a problem in practice that is often difficult to address. Sometimes, extreme values are removed from the data when they should not be, because they are true values. An outlier is merely an unusually extreme value, large or small, relative to the tendency of the mass of data values. Because outlier values have so much weight, their presence or absence often results in contradictory conclusions. Just as they exert much influence on the mean $\bar{x}$ estimate and the standard deviation, they also may strongly influence the regression parameters, b_0 and b_1. Recall from Chapter 2 that, in regression analysis, the first and last x_i values and their corresponding y_i values have the greatest influence in determining b_1 and b_0 (Figure 3.17).

A better estimate of b_0 and b_1 is usually gained by extending the x_i range. However, what happens when several outliers occur, say, one at the x_1 and another at x_n? Figure 3.18 shows one possibility.

In this case, if the extreme values are left in the regression analysis, the b_0 values will be underestimated because it is on the extreme low end of the x_i values. The x_n extreme value will contribute to overestimating the b_1 value, but what if the outliers, although extreme, are real data? To omit them from an analysis would bias the entire work. What should be done in such a case? This is a real problem.

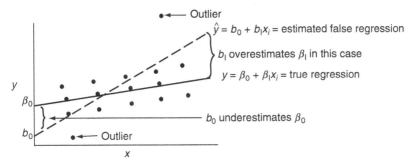

FIGURE 3.18 Estimated regression with outliers.

The applied researcher, then, needs to remove extreme values that are truly nonrepresentational and include extreme values that are representational. The researcher must also discover the phenomena contributing to these values. Rescaling the residuals can be very valuable in helping to identify outliers. Rescaling procedures include standardizing residuals, studentizing residuals, and jackknife residuals.

We consider briefly the process of standardizing residuals, as it applies to linear regression models. Residuals can also be studentized, that is, made to approximate the Student's t distribution, or they can be "jackknifed." The term "jackknife" is one that Tukey (1971) uses for the procedure, in that it is as useful as a "Boy Scout's knife." In general, it is a family of procedures for omitting a group of values, or a single value, from an analysis to examine the effect of the omission on the data body. Studentizing and jackknifing of residuals are procedures applied in multiple regression, often by means of matrix algebra and will be discussed in Chapter 8.

STANDARDIZED RESIDUALS

Sometimes, one can get a clearer picture of the residuals when they are in standardized form. Recall that the standardization used in statistics means the data conform to $\bar{x} = 0$ and $s = 1$. This is because $\Sigma (x - \bar{x}) = 0$ in a sample set, and because 68% of the data are contained within $+$ or $- s$. The standardized residual is

$$z_i = \frac{e_i}{s}, \qquad (3.32)$$

where z_i is the standard normalized residual with a mean of 0, and a variance of 1, $N \approx (0, 1)$, $e_i = y_i - \bar{y}$, $\bar{y}$ is the average rate, and s is the standard deviation of the residuals.

$$s = \sqrt{\frac{\sum (y_i - \hat{y})^2}{n-2}} = \sqrt{\frac{\sum e_i^2}{n-2}} *. \qquad (3.33)$$

Recall that about 68% of the data reside within + or − one standard deviation, 95% within + or − two standard deviations, and 97% within + or − three standard deviations. There should be only a few residuals as extreme as + or − three standard deviations in the residual set.

The method for standardizing the residuals is reasonably straightforward and will not be demonstrated. However, the overall process of residual analysis by studentizing and jackknifing procedures that use hat matrices will be explored in detail in Chapter 8.

---

*The general formula for s when more b_is than b_0 and b_1 are in the model is

$$\sqrt{\frac{\sum_{i=1}^{n}(y_i - \hat{y})^2}{n-p}} = \sqrt{\frac{\sum_{i=1}^{n}e_i^2}{n-p}} = \sqrt{MS_E},$$ where n = sample size; p = number of b_i values estimated, including b_0.

4 Multiple Linear Regression

Multiple linear regression is a direct extension of simple linear regression. In simple linear regression models, only one x predictor variable is present, but in multiple linear regression, there are k predictor values, $x_i, x_2, \ldots, x_k$. For example, a two-variable predictor model is presented in the following equation:

$$Y_i = \beta_0 + \beta_1 x_{i1} + \beta_2 x_{i2} + \varepsilon_i, \tag{4.1}$$

where β_1 is the ith regression slope constant acting on x_{i1}; β_2, the ith regression slope constant acting on x_{i2}; x_{i1}, the ith x value in the first x predictor; x_{i2}, the ith x value in the second x predictor; and ε_i is the ith error term.

A four-variable predictor model is presented in the following equation:

$$Y_i = \beta_0 + \beta_1 x_{i1} + \beta_2 x_{i2} + \beta_3 x_{i3} + \beta_4 x_{i4} + \varepsilon_i. \tag{4.2}$$

We can plot two x_i predictors (a three-dimensional model), but not beyond. A three-dimensional regression function is not a line, but it is a plane (Figure 4.1). All the $E[Y]$ or $\hat{y}$ values fit on that plane. Greater than two x_i predictors move us into four-dimensional space and beyond.

As in Chapter 2, we continue to predict y_i via $\hat{y}_i$, but now, relative to multiple x_i variables. The residual value, e_i, continues to be the difference between y_i and $\hat{y}_i$.

REGRESSION COEFFICIENTS

For the model $\hat{y} = b_0 + b_1 x_1 + b_2 x_2$, the b_0 value continues to be the point on the y axis where x_1 and $x_2 = 0$, but other than that, it has no meaning independent of the b_i values. The slope constant b_1 represents the change in the mean response value $\hat{y}$ when x_2 is held constant. Likewise for b_2, when x_1 is held constant. The b_i coefficients are linear, but the predictor x_i values need not be.

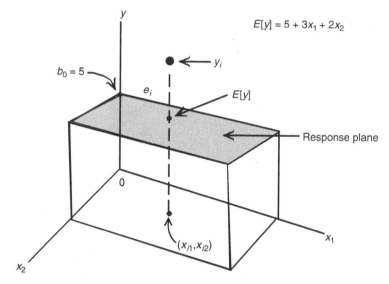

FIGURE 4.1 Regression plane for two-predictor variables.

MULTIPLE REGRESSION ASSUMPTIONS

The multiple linear response variables (y_is) are assumed statistically independent of one another. As in simple linear regression, when data are collected in a series of time intervals, the researcher must be cautious of serial or autocorrelation. The same basic procedures described in Chapter 2 must be followed, as is discussed later.

The variance σ^2 of y is considered constant for any fixed combination of x_i predictor variables. In practice, the assumption is rarely satisfied completely, and small departures usually have no adverse influence on the performance and validity of the regression model.

Additionally, it is assumed that, for any set of predictor values, the corresponding y_is are normally distributed about the regression plane. This is a requirement for general inference making, e.g., confidence intervals, prediction of $\hat{y}$, etc. The predictor variables, x_is, are also considered independent of each other, or additive. Therefore, the value of x_1 does not, in any way, affect or depend on x_2, if they are independent. This is often not the case, so the researcher must check and account for the presence of interaction between the predictor x_i variables.

The general multiple linear regression model for a first-order model, that is, when all the predictor variable x_is are linear, is

$$E[Y] = \beta_0 + \beta_1 x_{i1} + \beta_2 x_{i2} + \cdots + \beta_k x_{ik} + \varepsilon_i,$$

where $E[Y]$ is the expected value of y, k represents the number of predictor variables, $x_1, x_2, \ldots, x_k$, in the model, $\beta_0, \beta_1, \ldots, \beta_k$ are constant regression coefficients, $x_{i_1}, x_{i_2}, \ldots, x_{i_k}$ are fixed independent predictor variables, and ε_i is the error $= y_i - \hat{y}_i$, which are considered independent. They are not completely so, because, if one knows $\sum_{i=1}^{n} y_i$, then y_n is determined, because $\sum_{i=1}^{n} e_i = 0$. The ε_i values are also normally distributed, $N(0, \sigma^2)$.

As additional x_i predictor variables are added to a model, interaction among them is possible. That is, the x_i variables are not independent, so as one builds a regression model, one wants to measure and account for possible interactions.

In this chapter, we focus on x_i variables that are quantitative, but in a later chapter, we add qualitative or dummy variables. These can be very useful in comparing multiple treatments in a single regression model. For example, we may call $x_2 = 0$, if female, and 1, if male, to evaluate drug bioavailability using a single set of data, but two different regressions result.

GENERAL REGRESSION PROCEDURES

Please turn to Appendix II, Matrix Algebra Review, for a brushup on matrix algebra, if required. The multiple regression form is

$$Y = \beta_0 + \beta_1 x_{i1} + \beta_2 x_{i2} + \cdots + \beta_k x_{ik} + \varepsilon_i.$$

We no longer use it exclusively for operational work. Instead, we use the matrix format. Although many statistical software packages offer general routines for the analyses described in this book, some do not. Hence, knowing how to use matrix algebra to perform these tests using interactive statistical software is important. In matrix format,

$$Y = Xb + \varepsilon, \tag{4.3}$$

$$Y = \begin{bmatrix} y_1 \\ y_2 \\ y_3 \\ \vdots \\ y_n \end{bmatrix}, \quad X = \begin{bmatrix} 1 & x_{11} & x_{12} & \cdots & x_{1,k} \\ 1 & x_{21} & x_{22} & \cdots & x_{2,k} \\ 1 & x_{31} & x_{32} & \cdots & x_{3,k} \\ \vdots & \vdots & \vdots & \vdots & \vdots \\ 1 & x_{n1} & x_{n2} & \cdots & x_{n,k} \end{bmatrix}^{*}.$$

Note:

$$b_{k \times 1} = \begin{bmatrix} \beta_0 \\ \beta_1 \\ \beta_2 \\ \vdots \\ \beta_k \end{bmatrix}, \quad \varepsilon_{n \times 1} = \begin{bmatrix} \varepsilon_1 \\ \varepsilon_2 \\ \varepsilon_3 \\ \vdots \\ \varepsilon_n \end{bmatrix},$$

where Y is a vector of the response variable, b is a vector of regression, ε is a vector of error terms, and X is a matrix of the predictor variables.

The least-squares calculation procedure is still performed, but within a matrix algebra format. The general least-squares equation is

$$X'Xb = X'Y. \tag{4.4}$$

Rearranging terms to solve for b, we get

$$b = (X'X)^{-1}X'Y, \tag{4.5}$$

where b is the regression statistical estimate for the β, or population. The fitted or predict values

$$\hat{Y} = Xb \tag{4.6}$$

and the residual values are

$$Y_{n \times 1} - \hat{Y}_{n \times 1} = e_{n \times 1}. \tag{4.7}$$

The variance of b

$$\mathbf{var}\,(b), \text{ or } \sigma^2(b) = \sigma^2[X'X]^{-1}. \tag{4.8}$$

Generally, for σ^2, MS_E is used as its predictor, that is $MS_E = s^2$.

For the matrix, its $MS_E[\underset{p \times p}{X'X}]^{-1}$ diagonals provide the variance of each b_i. This $p \times p$ matrix (read p by p) is called the variance–covariance matrix. The off-diagonal values provide the covariances of each $x_i\, x_j :$ combination.

$$
\begin{bmatrix}
\mathbf{var}\,b_0 & & & & \\
& \mathbf{var}\,b_1 & & & \\
& & \mathbf{var}\,b_2 & & \\
& & & \ddots & \\
& & & & \mathbf{var}\,b_k
\end{bmatrix},
$$

$$\mathbf{var}\,b_i = s^2\{b_i\}.$$

APPLICATION

Let us work an example (Example 4.1). In an antibiotic drug accelerated stability study, 100 mL polypropylene stopper vials were stored at 48°C for 12 weeks. Each week (7 days), three vials were selected at random and evaluated for available mg/mL of the drug, A1-715. The average baseline, or time-zero level was ≈500 mg/mL. The acceptance standard for rate of aging requires that the product be within ±10% of that baseline value at 90 days. The relative humidity was also measured to determine its effect, if any, on the product's integrity.

The chemist is not sure how the data would sort out, so first, y and x_1 are plotted. The researcher knows that time is an important variable but he has no idea if humidity is. The plot of y against x_1 is presented in Figure 4.2.

We know that the product degraded more than 10% (450 mg/mL) over the 12-week period. In addition, in the tenth week of accelerated stability testing, the product degraded at an increasing rate. The chemists want to know the rate of degradation, but this model is not linear. Table 4.2 shows the multiple regression analysis of y on x_1 and x_2 for Example 4.1 (Table 4.1)

Let us discuss Table 4.2. The regression equation in matrix form is $Y = Xb$. Once the values have been determined, the matrix form is simpler to use than is the original linear format, $\hat{y}_i = 506 - 15.2x_i + 33x_2$. $Y = 39 \times 1$ matrix or vector of the mg/mL value, $X = 39 \times 3$ matrix of the x_i response value. There are two x_i response variables, and the first column consisting of 1s corresponds to b_0. $b = 3 \times 1$ matrix (vector) of b_0, b_1, and b_2. Hence, from Table 4.2, the matrix setup is

$$
\begin{array}{ccc}
Y = & X & b \\
\begin{bmatrix} 508 \\ 495 \\ 502 \\ \vdots \\ 288 \end{bmatrix} &
\begin{bmatrix} 1 & 0 & 0.60 \\ 1 & 0 & 0.60 \\ 1 & 0 & 0.60 \\ \vdots & \vdots & \vdots \\ 1 & 12 & 0.76 \end{bmatrix} &
\begin{bmatrix} 506 \\ -15.2 \\ 33 \end{bmatrix}
\end{array},
$$

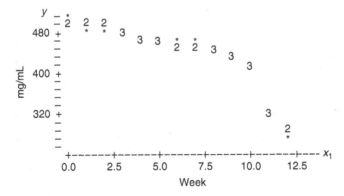

FIGURE 4.2 Potency (y) vs. storage time (x_1).

TABLE 4.1
Data for Example 4.1

n	y	x_1	x_2	
1	508	0	0.60	y = mg/mL A1-715
2	495	0	0.60	x_1 = week of chemical analysis
3	502	0	0.60	x_2 = relative humidity, 1.0 = 100%
4	501	1	0.58	
5	502	1	0.58	
6	483	1	0.58	
7	489	2	0.51	
8	491	2	0.51	
9	487	2	0.51	
10	476	3	0.68	
11	481	3	0.68	
12	472	3	0.68	
13	462	4	0.71	
14	471	4	0.71	
15	463	4	0.71	
16	465	5	0.73	
17	458	5	0.73	
18	462	5	0.73	
19	453	6	0.68	
20	451	6	0.68	
21	460	6	0.68	
22	458	7	0.71	
23	449	7	0.71	
24	451	7	0.71	
25	452	8	0.73	
26	446	8	0.73	
27	442	8	0.73	
28	435	9	0.70	
29	432	9	0.70	
30	437	9	0.70	
31	412	10	0.68	
32	408	10	0.68	
33	409	10	0.68	
34	308	11	0.74	
35	309	11	0.74	
36	305	11	0.74	
37	297	12	0.76	
38	300	12	0.76	
39	288	12	0.76	

TABLE 4.2
Multiple Regression Analysis

Predictor	Coef	St. Dev	t-Ratio	p
b_0	506.34	68.90	7.35	0.000
b_1	−15.236	2.124	−7.17	0.000
b_2	33.3	114.7	0.29	0.773

$s = 32.96$ R-sq $= 75.3\%$ R-sq(adj) $= 73.9\%$

Analysis of Variance

Source	DF	SS	MS	F	p
Regression	2	119,279	59,640	54.91	0.000
Error	36	39,100	1,086		
Total	38	158,380			

Source	DF	SEQ SS
Week	1	119,188
Humid	1	92

Unusual Observations

Obs.	Week	mg/mL	Fit	St dev fit	Residual	St resid
38	12.0	278.00	348.81	9.97	−70.81	−2.25R
39	12.0	285.00	348.81	9.97	−63.81	−2.03R

The regression equation is $\hat{y} = b_0 + b_1x_1 + b_2x_2*$, where x_1 is the analysis week, and x_2 is the relative humidity.

$\hat{y} = 506 - 15.2x_1 + 33x_2$, or mg/mL $= 506 - 15.2$ week $+ 33$ humidity.

where Y is the mg/mL of drug, X (column 2) is the week of analysis, X (column 3) is the relative humidity, and b represents b_0, b_1, and b_2 from the regression equation. The information in the regression analysis is interpreted exactly like that of linear regression, but with added values.

HYPOTHESIS TESTING FOR MULTIPLE REGRESSION

Overall Test

Let us now discuss the analysis of variance (ANOVA) portion of the regression analysis as presented in Table 4.2. The interpretation, again, is like the simple linear model (Table 4.3). Yet, we expand the analysis later to evaluate individual b_is. The matrix computations are

$$SS_R = b'X'Y - \left(\frac{1}{n}\right)Y'JY, \tag{4.9}$$

$J = n \times n \longrightarrow 39 \times 39$ matrix of 1s.

$$SS_E = Y'Y - b'X'Y, \tag{4.10}$$

TABLE 4.3
Structure of the Analysis of Variance

Source	Degrees of Freedom	SS	MS	F
Regression	k	$SS_T - SS_E = SS_R$	$\dfrac{SS_R}{k}$	$F_{c(\alpha;\, k;\, n-k-1)}$
Error	$n - k - 1$	SS_E	$\dfrac{SS_E}{n-k-1}$	
Total	$n - 1$	SS_T		

$$SS_T = Y'Y - \left(\frac{1}{n}\right)Y'JY. \qquad (4.11)$$

The F-test for testing the significance of the full regression is handled the same as for simple linear regression via the six-step procedure.

Step 1: Specify the hypothesis test, which is always a two-tail test.

$H_0: \beta_1 = \beta_2 = 0,$

$H_A:$ At least one β_i is not 0.

(If H_A is accepted, one does not know if all the b_is are significant or only one or two. That requires a partial F-test, which is discussed later.)

Step 2: Specify α and n. (At this point, the sample size and the significance level have been determined by the researcher.) We set $\alpha = 0.05$ and $n = 39$.

Step 3: Write the test statistic to be used.
We simply use $F_c = \frac{MS_R}{MS_E}$, or the basic ANOVA test.

Step 4: Specify the decision rule.
If $F_c > F_T$, reject H_0 at $\alpha = 0.05$. That is, if $F_c > F_T$, at least one b_i is significant at $\alpha = 0.05$

$$F_{T(\alpha;\, k;\, n-k-1)},$$

where n, the sample size is 39; k is the number of predictors (x_is) in the model $= 2$, and $F_{T(0.05;\, 2;\, 39-2-1)}$.
    Using the F table (Table C), $F_{T(0.05;\, 2,\, 36)} = 3.32$.
Decision: If $F_c > 3.32$, reject H_0 at $\alpha = 0.05$. At least one b_i is significant at $\alpha = 0.05$.

Step 5: Compute the F_c value.
From Table 4.2, we see that $F_c = 54.91$.

Step 6: Make the decision.
Because $54.91 > 3.32$, reject H_0 at $\alpha = 0.05$; at least one b_i is significant.

At this point, the researcher could reject the product's stability, for clearly the product does not hold up to the stability requirements. Yet, in the applied sciences, decisions are rarely black and white. Because the product is stable for a number of months, perhaps a better stabilizer could be introduced into the product that reduces the rate at which the active compound degrades. In doing this, the researcher needs a better understanding of the variables of interest. Therefore, the next step is to determine how significant each b_i value is.

Partial *F*-Test

The partial F-test is similar to the F-test, except that individual or subsets of predictor variables are evaluated for their contribution in the model to increase SS_R or, conversely, to decrease SS_E. In the current example, we ask, "what is the contribution of the individual x_1 and x_2 variables?"

To determine this, we can evaluate the model, first with x_1 in the model, then with x_2. We evaluate x_1 in the model, not excluding x_2, but holding it constant, and then we measure it with the sum-of-squares regression (or sum-of-squares error), and vice versa. That is, the sum-of-squares regression is explained by adding x_1 into the model already containing x_2 or $SS_{R(x_1|x_2)}$. The development of this model is straightforward; the $SS_{R(x_k|x_1, x_2, \ldots, x_{k-1})}$ effect of x_k's contribution to the model containing x_{k-1} variables or various other combinations.

For the present two-predictor variable model, let us assume that x_1 is important, and we want to evaluate the contribution of x_2, given x_1 is in the model. The general strategy of partial F-tests is to perform the following:

1. Regression with x_1 only in the model.
2. Regression with x_2 and x_1 in the model.
3. Find the difference between the model containing only x_1 and the model containing x_2, given x_1 is already in the model, $(x_2|x_1)$; this measures the contribution of x_2.
4. A regression model with x_k predictors in the model can be contrasted in a number of ways, e.g., $(x_k|x_{k-1})$ or $(x_k, x_{k-1}, x_{k-2}|x_{k-3}, \ldots)$.
5. The difference between $(x_k|x_1, x_2, x_3, \ldots, x_{k-1})$ and $(x_1, x_2, x_3, \ldots, x_{k-1})$ is the contribution of x_k.

The computational model for the contribution of each extra x_i variable in the model is

Sum-of-squares regression (SS_R) from adding the additional x_i variable = SS_R with the extra x_i variable in the model − SS_R without the extra x_i variable in the model, or
(4.12)

$$SS_{R(x_k|x_1, x_2, ..., x_{k-1})} = SS_{R(x_1, x_2, ..., x_k)} = SS_{R(x_1, x_2, ..., x_{k-1})}.$$
(4.13)

To compute the partial F-test, the following formula is used:

$$F_{c(x_k|x_1, x_2, ..., x_{k-1})} = \frac{\text{Extra sum-of-squares value due to the } x_k\text{s contribution to the model, given } x_1, x_2, ..., x_{k-1} \text{ are in the model}}{\begin{array}{c}\text{Mean square residual for the model} \\ \text{containing all variables } x_1, ..., x_k{}^*\end{array}}$$
(4.14)

$$F_{c(x_k|x_1, x_2, ..., x_{k-1})} = \frac{SS_{R(x_k|x_1, x_2, ..., x_{k-1})}{}^*}{MS_{E(x_1, x_2, ..., x_k)}}.$$
(4.15)

Note: *MS_R is not specified because $MS_R = SS_R$, because of only 1 degree of freedom.

Table 4.4A presents the full regression model; this can be decomposed to Table 4.4B, which presents the partial decomposition of the regression.

Let us perform a partial F-test of the data from Example 4.1.

Step 1: Formulate the test hypothesis.

H_0: x_2 (humidity) does not contribute significantly to the increase of SS_R.
H_A: The above statement is not true.

Step 2: Specify α and n.
Let us set $\alpha = 0.025$, and $n = 39$. Normally, the researcher has a specific reason for the selections, and this needs to be considered.

TABLE 4.4A
Full Model ANOVA

Source	DF	SS
Regression of $x_1, x_2, ..., x_k$	k	$SS_R(x_1, x_2, ..., x_k)$
Residual	$n - k - 1$	$SS_E(x_1, x_2, ..., x_k)$

TABLE 4.4B
A Partial ANOVA

Source	DF	SS	MS_E
x_1	1	$SS_{R(x_1)}$	$SS_{R(x_1)}$
$x_2|x_1$	1	$SS_{R(x_2|x_1)} - SS_{R(x_1)} = SS_{R(x_2|x_1)}$	$SS_{R(x_2|x_1)}$
$x_3|x_1, x_2$	1	$SS_{R(x_1, x_2, x_3)} - SS_{R(x_1, x_2)} =$ $SS_{R(x_3|x_1, x_2)}$	$SS_{R(x_3|x_1, x_2)}$
$\vdots$	$\vdots$	$\vdots$	$\vdots$
$x_k|x_1, x_2, \ldots, x_{k-1}$	1	$SS_{R(x_1, x_2, \ldots, x_k)} - SS_{R(x_1, x_2, \ldots, x_{k-1})} =$ $SS_{R(x_k|x_1, x_2, \ldots, x_{k-1})}$	$SS_{R(x_k|x_1, x_2, \ldots, x_{k-1})}$
Residual	$n-k-1$	$SS_{R(x_1, x_2, \ldots, x_k)}$	$\dfrac{SS_E}{n-k-1}$

Note: k is the number of x predictor variables in the model, excluding b_0 and n is the sample size.

Step 3: Test statistic.
The specific test to evaluate the term of interest is stated here. The F_c in this partial F-test is written as

$$F_c = \frac{SS_{R(x_2|x_1)}}{(MS_{E(x_1x_2)})} = \frac{SS_{R(x_1x_2)} - SS_{R(x_1)}}{(MS_{E(x_1x_2)})}.$$

Step 4: State the decision rule.
This requires the researcher to use the F tables (Table C) with 1 degree of freedom in the numerator and $n - k - 1 = 39 - 2 - 1 = 36$

$$F_T = F_{T(\alpha, 1, n-k-1)} = F_{T(0.025, 1, 36)} = 5.47.$$

So, if $F_c > F_T$ (5.47), reject H_0 at $\alpha = 0.025$.

Step 5: Perform the experiment and collect the results.
We use MiniTab statistical software for our work, but almost any other statistical package does as well.
First, determine the reduced model: $y = b_0 + b_1x_1$, omitting b_2x_2.
Table 4.5 is the ANOVA for the reduced model.

TABLE 4.5
Analysis of Variance Reduced Model, Example 4.1

Source	DF	SS	MS	F	p
Regression	1	119,188	119,188	112.52	0.000
Error	37	39,192	1,059		
Total	38	158,380			

TABLE 4.6
Analysis of Variance Full Model, Example 4.1

Analysis of Variance

Source	DF	SS	MS	F	p
Regression	2	119,279	59,640	54.91	0.000
Error	36	39,100	1,086		
Total	38	158,380			

$$SS_{R(x_1)} = 119,188$$

Second, compute the full model, $y = b_0 + b_1 x_1 + b_2 x_2$; the ANOVA is presented in Table 4.6.

$SS_{R(x_1, x_2)} = 119,279.$

$SS_{R(x_2|x_1)} = SS_{R(x_1, x_2)} - SS_{R(x_1)} = 119,279 - 119,188 = 91.$

$MS_{E(x_1, x_2)} = 1086$ (Table 4.6).

$$F_{c(x_2|x_1)} = \frac{SS_{R(x_2|x_1)}}{MS_{E(x_1|x_2)}} = \frac{91}{1086} = 0.08.$$

Step 6: Decision rule.
Because $F_c = 0.08 < F_T, 5.47$, we cannot reject the H_0 hypothesis at $\alpha = 0.025$. The researcher probably already knew that relative humidity did not influence the stability data substantially, but the calculation was included because it was a variable. The researcher now uses a simple linear regression model.

Note in Table 4.2 that the regression model already had been partitioned by MiniTab. For the convenience of the reader, the pertinent part of Table 4.2 is reproduced later in Table 4.7.

TABLE 4.7
Short Version of Table 4.2

Analysis of Variance

Source	DF	SS	MS	F	p
Regression	2	119,279	59,640	54.91	0.000
Error	36	39,100	1,086		
Total	38	158,380			
Source	DF	SEQ SS			
$SS_{R(x_1)}$week	1	119,188			
$SS_{R(x_2|x_1)}$humid	1	92			

This greatly simplifies the analysis we have just done. In practice, F_c can be taken directly from the table

$$F_c = \frac{SS_{R(x_2|x_1)}}{MS_{E(x_1,x_2)}} = \frac{92}{1086} = 0.0847.$$

Alternative to SS$_R$

The partitioning of SS_R could have been performed in an alternate way: the reduction of SS_E, instead of the increase of SS_R. Both provide the same result, because $SS_{total} = SS_R + SS_E$

$$SS_{E(x_2|x_1)} = SS_{E(x_1)} - SS_{E(x_1,x_2)}.$$

From Table 4.5, we find $SS_{E(x_1)} = 39{,}192$.
From Table 4.6, $SS_{E(x_1,x_2)} = 39{,}100$.
Therefore,

$$SS_{E(x_1)} - SS_{E(x_1,x_2)} = 39{,}192 - 39{,}100 = 92$$
$$SS_{E(x_2|x_1)} = 92.$$

The final model we evaluate is $\hat{y} = b_0 + b_1 x_1$, in which time is the single x_i variable (Table 4.8).

Although we determined that x_2 was not needed, the regression model has other problems. First, the Durbin–Watson statistic $DW_C = 0.24$, $DW_{T(\alpha, k, n)} = DW_{T(\alpha = 0.05, 1, 39)}$, which is ($d_L = 1.43$, and $d_U = 1.54$ in Table E), points to significant serial correlation, a common occurrence in time-series studies (Table 4.8). Second, the data plot y_i vs. x_{1i} is not linear (Figure 4.2). A transformation of the data should be performed. In Chapter 3, we learned how this is completed. First, linearize the data by transformation, and then correct for autocorrelation. However, there may be another problem. The statistical procedure may be straightforward to the researcher, but not to others. If a researcher attempts to transform the data to linearize them, it requires that x_is be raised to the fourth power (x_i^4), and y_is also raised to the fourth power (y_i^4). And even that will not solve our problem, because week 0 and 1 will not transform (Figure 4.3).

Additionally, the values are extremely large and unwieldy. The data should be standardized, via $\frac{x_i - \bar{x}}{s_x}$ and perhaps $\frac{y_i - \bar{y}}{s_y}$, and then linearized. However, such a highly derived process would likely make the data abstract. A preferred way, and a much simpler method, is to perform a piecewise regression, using indicator or dummy variables. We employ that method in a later chapter, where we make separate functions for each linear portion of the data set.

TABLE 4.8
Final Regression Model, Example 4.1

Predictor	Coef	St. Dev	t-Ratio	p
b_0	526.136	9.849	53.42	0.000
b_1	−14.775	1.393	−10.61	0.000
$s = 32.55$		R-sq = 75.3%		R-sq(adj) = 74.6%

Analysis of Variance

Source	DF	SS	MS	F	p
Regression	1	119,188	119,188	112.52	0.000
Error	37	39,192	1,059		
Total	38	158,380			

Unusual Observations

Obs.	Week	mg/mL	Fit	St. Dev fit	Residual	St resid
38	12.0	278.0	348.84	9.85	−70.84	−2.28R
39	12.0	285.00	348.84	9.85	−63.84	−2.06R

The regression equation is mg/mL $= 526 - 14.8$ week; $\hat{y} = b_0 + b_1 x$.
Note: R denotes an observation with a large standardized residual (St resid), Durbin–Watson
statistic $= 0.24$.

The t-Test for the Determination of the β_i Contribution

As an alternative to performing the partial F-test to determine the significance
of the x_i predictors, one can perform t-tests for each β_i, which is automatically
done on the MiniTab regression output (see Table 4.2, t-ratio column). Recall

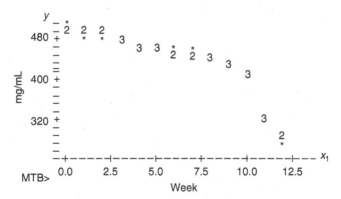

FIGURE 4.3 y^4 and x^4 transformations.

that $Y = \beta_0 + \beta_1 x_1 + \beta_2 x_2 + \cdots + \beta_k x_k$. Each of these β_i values can be evaluated with a t-test.

The test hypothesis can be an upper-, lower-, or two-tail test.

Upper Tail	Lower Tail	Two Tail
H_0: $\beta_i \leq 0$	$\beta_i \geq 0$	$\beta_i = 0$
H_A: $\beta_i > 0$	$\beta_i < 0$	$\beta_i \neq 0$
Reject H_0 if $T_c > T_{t(\alpha;\ n-k-1)}$	$T_c < T_{t(-\alpha;\ n-k-1)}$	$|T_c| > |T_{t(\alpha/2;\ n-k-1)}|$

where k is the present number of x_i predictor variables in the full model (does not include β_0).

$$T_c = \frac{\hat{\beta}_i}{s_{\hat{\beta}_i}}, \text{ or for sample calculations, } t_c = \frac{b_i}{s_{b_i}}, \quad (4.16)$$

where b_i is the regression coefficient for the ith b, and

$$s_{\hat{\beta}_i} = \sqrt{\frac{\text{MS}_E}{\sum (x - \bar{x})^2}}. \quad (4.17)$$

Recall, $\text{MS}_E = \frac{\text{SS}_E}{n-k-1}$ and from Equation 4.10, $\frac{Y'Y - bX'Y}{n-k-1}$.

Fortunately, statistical software programs such as MiniTab already provide these data. Look at Table 4.2; the critical part of that table is presented later in Table 4.9.

Let us perform a two-tail test of β_2 using the data in Example 4.1.

Step 1: First, state the hypothesis.

H_0: $\beta_2 = 0$,
H_A: $\beta_2 \neq 0$.

TABLE 4.9
Short Version of MiniTab Table 4.2

Predictor	Coef	St. Dev	t-Ratio	p
b_0 = Constant	506.34		68.90		7.35	0.000
b_1 = Week	−15.236	$s_{b_i} = $	2.124	$t_c = $	−7.17	0.000
b_2 = Humid	33.3		114.7		0.29	0.773

We are interested in knowing whether β_2 is greater or lesser than 0.

Step 2: Set $\alpha = 0.05$ and $n = 39$.

Step 3: Write the test formula to be used.

$$t_c = \frac{b_2}{s_{b_2}},$$

where

$$s_{b_2} = \sqrt{\frac{MS_E}{\sum (x_2 - \bar{x}_2)^2}}.$$

Step 4: Decision rule (a two-tail test).
  If $|T_c| > |T_{t(\alpha/2; \, n-k-1)}|$, reject H_0 at α.
  $T_t = T_{(0.025; \, 39-2)-1} = T_{(0.025, \, 36)} = 2.042$, from Table B
  If $|T_c| > 2.042$, reject H_0 at $\alpha = 0.05$.

Step 5: Compute the statistic.
  $t_c = \frac{b_2}{s_{b_2}} = \frac{33.3}{114.7} = 0.29$, which is already presented in the t-ratio column
(Table 4.9).

Step 6: Decision rule.
Because $0.29 \not> 2.042$, we cannot reject H_0 at $\alpha = 0.05$. Remove the x_2 values
from the model.
  Let us look at the other b_i values

$b_0: t_c = \frac{b_0}{s_{b_0}} = \frac{506.34}{68.90} = 7.35 > 2.04$, and so, is significant from 0 at $\alpha = 0.05$.

$b_1: t_c = \frac{b_1}{s_{b_1}} = \frac{-15.236}{2.124} = |7.17| > 2.042$, so it, too, is significant at $\alpha = 0.05$.

Multiple Partial F-Tests

At times, a researcher may want to know the relative effects of adding not just
one, but several variables to the model at once. For example, suppose a basic
regression model is $Y = b_0 + b_1 x_1 + b_2 x_2$, and the researcher wants to know
the effects of adding x_3, x_4, and x_5 to the model simultaneously. The procedure
is a direct extension of the partial F-test just examined. It is the sum-
of-squares that results from the addition of x_3, x_4, and x_5 to the model already
containing x_1 and x_2

$$SS_{R(x_3, x_4, x_5 | x_1, x_2)}.$$

To compute $SS_{R(x_3, x_4, x_5 | x_1, x_2)}$, we must subtract the partial model from the full
model.

That is, $SS_{R(x_3,x_4,x_5|x_1,x_2)} = $ full model $-$ partial model

$$SS_{R(x_3,x_4,x_5|x_1,x_2)} = SS_{R(x_1,x_2,x_3,x_4,x_5)} - SS_{R(x_1,x_2)}$$

or equivalently,

$$SS_{E(x_3,x_2,x_4|x_1,x_2)} = SS_{E(x_1,x_2)} - SS_{E(x_1,x_2,x_3,x_4,x_5)}.$$

The general F statistic for this process is

$$F_{c(x_3,x_4,x_5|x_1,x_2)} = \frac{\frac{SS_{R(full)} - SS_{R(partial)}}{k'}}{MS_{E(full)}} \text{ or } \frac{\frac{SS_{E(partial)} - SS_{E(full)}}{k'}}{MS_{E(full)}}. \tag{4.18}$$

The degrees of freedom are k for the numerator, and $n - r - k' - 1$ for the denominator, where k' is the number of x variables added to the model (in this case, x_3, x_4, x_5), or the number of variables in the full model minus the number of variables in the partial model, and r is the number of x variables in the reduced model (x_1, x_2).

Example 4.2. A researcher wishes to predict the quantity of bacterial medium (Tryptic Soy Broth, e.g.) needed to run bioreactors supporting continuous microbial growth over the course of a month. The researcher methodically jots down variable readings that are important in predicting the number of liters of medium that must flow through the system of 10 bioreactors each week—7 days. The researcher had used three predictor x variables in the past: x_1, x_2, and x_3, corresponding to bioreactor temperature °C, $\log_{10}$ microbial population per mm^2 on a test coupon, and the concentration of protein in the medium (1 = standard concentration, 2 = double concentration, etc.). In hopes of becoming more accurate and precise in the predictions, three other variables have been tracked—the calcium/phosphorus (Ca/P) ratio, the nitrogen (N) level, and the heavy metal level. The researcher wants to know whether, on the whole, data on these three additional variables are useful in predicting the amount of media required, when a specific combination of variables is necessary in providing a desired $\log_{10}$ population on coupons. Table 4.10 shows the data.

Step 1: Write out the hypothesis.

H_0: β_4 and β_5 and $\beta_6 = 0$ (i.e., they contribute nothing additive to the model in terms of increasing SS_R or reducing SS_E).

H_A: β_4 and β_5 and $\beta_6 \neq 0$ (their addition contributes to the increase of SS_R and the decrease of SS_E).

Step 2: Set α and n.
Let $\alpha = 0.05$, and $n = 15$ runs.

TABLE 4.10
Data for Example 4.2

Row	Temp °C	$\log_{10}$-count	med-cn	Ca/P	N	Hvy-Mt	L/wk
	x_1	x_2	x_3	x_4	x_5	x_6	Y
1	20	2.1	1.0	1.00	56	4.1	56
2	21	2.0	1.0	0.98	53	4.0	61
3	27	2.4	1.0	1.10	66	4.0	65
4	26	2.0	1.8	1.20	45	5.1	78
5	27	2.1	2.0	1.30	46	5.8	81
6	29	2.8	2.1	1.40	48	5.9	86
7	37	5.1	3.7	1.80	75	3.0	110
8	37	2.0	1.0	0.30	23	5.0	62
9	45	1.0	0.5	0.25	30	5.2	50
10	20	3.7	2.0	2.00	43	1.5	41
11	20	4.1	3.0	3.00	79	0.0	70
12	25	3.0	2.8	1.40	57	3.0	85
13	35	6.3	4.0	3.00	75	0.3	115
14	26	2.1	0.6	1.00	65	0.0	55
15	40	6.0	3.8	2.90	70	0.0	120

Note: Y is the liters of medium used per week, x_1 is the temperature of bioreactor (°C), x_2 is the $\log_{10}$ microbial population per cm^2 of coupon, x_3 is the medium concentration (e.g., $2 = 2x$ standard strength), x_4 is the calcium/phosphorus ratio, x_5 is the nitrogen level, x_6 is the heavy metal concentration ppm (Cd, Cu, Fe).

Step 3: Statistic to use.

$$SS_{R(x_4,x_5,x_6|x_1,x_2,x_3)} = SS_{R(x_1,x_2,x_3,x_4,x_5,x_6)} - SS_{R(x_1,x_2,x_3)}$$

$$F_{c(x_4,x_5,x_6|x_1,x_2,x_3)} = \frac{\frac{SS_{R(full)} - SS_{R(partial)}}{k'}}{MS_{E(full)}} \text{ or } \frac{\frac{SS_{E(partial)} - SS_{E(full)}}{k'}}{MS_{E(full)}}.$$

Step 4: Decision rule.
First, determine $F_{T(\alpha)(k', n-r-k'-1)}$
   $\alpha = 0.05$
   $k' = 3$, for x_4, x_5, and x_6
   $r = 3$, for x_1, x_2, and x_3
   $F_{T (0.05)(3; 15 - 3 - 3 - 1)} = F_{T (0.05, 3, 8)} = 4.07$, from Table C, the F tables
   If $F_c > F_T = 4.07$, reject H_0 at $\alpha = 0.05$. The three variables, x_4, x_5, and x_6
significantly contribute to increasing SS_R and decreasing SS_E.

Step 5: Perform the computation.
As earlier, the full model is first computed (Table 4.11).

TABLE 4.11
Full Model Computation, Example 4.2

Analysis of Variance

Source	DF	SS	MS	F	p
Regression	6	7266.3	1211.1	11.07	0.002
Error	8	875.0	109.4		
Total	14	8141.3			

The regression equation is L/wk $= -23.1 + 0.875$ temp° C $+ 2.56$ $\log_{10}$-ct $+ 14.6$ med-cn $- 5.3$ Ca/P $+ 0.592$ N $+ 3.62$ Hvy-Mt; $R^2 = 89.3\%$.

The reduced model is then computed (Table 4.12)

$$F_{c(x_4, x_5, x_6 | x_1, x_2, x_3)} = \frac{\dfrac{SS_{R(full)} - SS_{R(partial)}}{k'}}{MS_{E(full)}} \text{ or } \frac{\dfrac{SS_{E(partial)} - SS_{E(full)}}{k'}}{MS_{E(full)}},$$

$$F_{c(x_4, x_5, x_6 | x_1, x_2, x_3)} = \frac{\dfrac{7266.3 - 6609.5}{3}}{109.4} \text{ or } \frac{\dfrac{1531.9 - 875.0}{3}}{109.4},$$

$$F_c = 2.00.$$

Step 6: Decision rule.
Because $F_c = 2.00 \not> 4.07$, reject H_A at $\alpha = 0.05$. The addition of the three variables as a whole (x_4, x_5, x_6) does not significantly contribute to increasing SS_R or decreasing SS_E. In addition, note that one need not compute the partial F_c value using both SS_E and SS_R. Use one or the other, as both provide the same result.

Now that we have calculated the partial F test, let us discuss the procedure in greater depth, particularly the decomposition of the sum-of-squares. Recall

TABLE 4.12
Reduced Model Computation, Example 4.2

Analysis of Variance

Source	DF	SS	MS	F	p
Regression	3	6609.5	2203.2	15.82	0.000
Error	11	1531.9	139.3		
Total	14	8141.3			

The regression equation is L/wk $= 19.2 + 0.874$ temp °C $- 2.34$ $\log_{10}$-ct $+ 19.0$ med-cn. $R^2 = 81.2\%$.

that the basic sum-of-squares equation for the regression model is, in terms of ANOVA:

Sum-of-squares total = sum-of-squares due to regression + sum-of-squares due to error, or $SS_T = SS_R + SS_E$

Adding extra predictor x_i variables that increase the SS_R value and decrease SS_E incurs a cost. For each additional predictor x_i variable added, one loses 1 degree of freedom. Given the SS_R value is increased significantly to offset the loss of 1 degree of freedom (or conversely, the SS_E is significantly reduced), as determined by partial F-test, the x_i predictor variable stays in the model. This is the basis of the partial F-test. That is, if $F_c > F_T$, the addition of the extra variable(s) was appropriate.*

Recall that the ANOVA model for a simple linear regression that has only x_1 as a predictor variable is written as $SS_T = SS_{R(x_1)} + SS_{E(x_1)}$. When an additional predictor variable is added to the model, $SS_T = SS_{R(x_1, x_2)} + SS_{E(x_1, x_2)}$, the same interpretation is valid, but with two variables, x_1 and x_2. That is, SS_R is the result of both x_1 and x_2, and likewise for SS_E. As these are derived with both x_1 and x_2 in the model, we have no way of knowing the contribution of either. However, with the partial F-test, we can know this. Now, $SS_T = \underbrace{SS_{R(x_1)} + SS_{R(x_2|x_1)}}_{SS_R} + SS_{E(x_1, x_2)}$, when we decompose SS_R. Now,

we have $SS_{R(x_1)}$ and $SS_{R(x_2)}$, holding x_1 constant. In the case of SS_E, when we decompose it (the alternative method), we account for $SS_{E(x_1)}$ and $SS_{E(x_2|x_1)}$. Instead of increasing the sum-of-squares regression, we now look for a decrease in SS_E.

By decomposing SS_R, we are quickly able to see the contribution of each x_i variable in the model. Suppose that we have the regression $\hat{y} = b_0 + b_1 x_1 + b_2 x_2 + b_3 x_3 + b_4 x_4$, and want to decompose each value to determine its contribution to increasing SS_R. The ANOVA table (Table 4.13) presents the model and annotates the decomposition of SS_R.

Fortunately, statistical software cuts down on the tedious computations. Let us now look at several standard ways to add or subtract x_i predictor variables based on this F-test strategy. Later, we discuss other methods, including those that use R^2. The first method we examine adds to the basic model new x_i predictor variables and tests the contribution of each one. The second method tests the significance of each x_i in the model and then adds

---

*If the F-test is not computed and R^2 is used to judge the significance of adding additional indicator variables, the unwary researcher, seeing R^2 generally increasing with the addition of predictors, may choose an inefficient model. R^2 must be adjusted in multiple regression to

$$R^2_{(adj)} = 1 - \left(\left[\frac{n-1}{n-k-1} \right] \left[\frac{SS_E}{SS_R} \right] \right)$$

where k is the number of predictor x_i variables and n is the sample size.

TABLE 4.13
ANOVA Table of the Decomposition of SS_R

Source (variance)	SS	DF
[a]Regression	$SS_{R(x_1, x_2, x_3, x_4)}$	4
[b]x_1	$SS_{R(x_1)}$	1
$x_2 \| x_1$	$SS_{R(x_2 \| x_1)}$	1
$x_3 \| x_1, x_2$	$SS_{R(x_3, x_1, x_2)}$	1
$x_4 \| x_1, x_2, x_3$	$SS_{R(x_4, x_1, x_2, x_3)}$	1
Error	$SS_{R(x_1, x_2, x_3, x_4)}$	$n - k - 1$
Total	SS_T	$n - 1$

[a]This is the full model where SS_R includes x_1, x_2, x_3, and x_4 and is written as $SS_{R(x_1, x_2, x_3, x_4)}$. It has four degrees of freedom, because there are four predictors in that model.
[b]The decomposition generally begins with x_1, and ends at x_k, as there are k decompositions possible. The sum $\sum_{i=1}^{4} SS_{R(x_i)} = SS_{R(x_1, x_2, x_3, x_4)}$.

new ones using the partial F-test, omitting from the model any x_i that is not significant.

FORWARD SELECTION: PREDICTOR VARIABLES ADDED INTO THE MODEL

In this procedure, x_i predictor variables are added into the model, one at a time. The predictor thought to be most important by the researcher generally is added first, followed by the second, the third, and so on. If the contribution of the predictor value is unknown, one easy way to find out is to run k simple linear regressions, selecting the largest r^2 of the k as x_1, the second largest r^2 as x_2, and so forth.

Let us perform the procedure using the data from Example 4.2 (Table 4.10). This was an evaluation using six x_i variables in predicting the total amount of growth medium for a continuous bioreactor—biofilm—process. The researcher ranked the predictor values in the order of perceived value: x_1, temperature (°C); x_2, $\log_{10}$ microbial count per cm^2 coupon; x_3, medium concentration; x_4, calcium/phosphorous ratio; x_5, nitrogen level, and x_6, heavy metals.

Because x_1 is thought to be the most important predictor x_i value, it is added first. We use the six-step procedure for the model-building process.

Step 1: State the hypothesis.

$H_0: \beta_1 = 0$,
$H_A: \beta_1 \neq 0$ (temperature is a significant predictor of the amount of medium needed).

Step 2: Set α and n.
   $\alpha = 0.05$,
   $n = 15$.

Step 3: Statistic to use.

$$F_c = \frac{MS_{R(x_1)}}{MS_{E(x_1)}}.$$

Step 4: Decision rule.
   If $F_c > F_{T(\alpha;\,1,\,n-2)} = F_{T(0.05;\,1,\,13)} = 4.67$ (from Table C), reject H_0.

Step 5: Perform the ANOVA computation (Table 4.14).

Step 6: Make decision.
Because $F_c = 2.99 \not> F_T = 4.67$, we cannot reject H_0 at $\alpha = 0.05$.

   Despite the surprising result that temperature has little direct effect on the medium requirements, the researcher moves on, using data for x_2 ($\log_{10}$ microbial count) in the model.

Step 1: State the hypothesis.

   $H_0: \beta_2 = 0$,
   $H_A: \beta_2 \neq 0$ ($\log_{10}$ microbial counts on the coupon have a significant effect
      on medium requirements).

Step 2: Set α and n.
   $\alpha = 0.05$,
   $n = 15$.

TABLE 4.14
ANOVA Computation for a Single Predictor Variable, x_1

Predictor	Coef	St. Dev	t-Ratio	p
(Constant) b_0	37.74	22.70	1.66	0.120
(temp °C) b_1	1.3079	0.7564	1.73	0.107
$s = 22.56$		$R\text{-sq} = 18.7\%$		$R\text{-sq(adj)} = 12.4\%$

Analysis of Variance

Source	DF	SS	MS	F	p
Regression $s_{(x1)}$	1	1522.4	1522.4	2.99	0.107
Error	13	6619.0	509.2		
Total	14	8141.3			

The regression equation is L/wk $= 37.7 + 1.31$ temp °C.

Step 3: Statistic to use.

$$F_c = \frac{MS_{R(x_2)}}{MS_{E(x_2)}}.$$

Step 4: Decision rule.
  If $F_c > 4.67$, reject H_0.

Step 5: Perform the computation (Table 4.15).

Step 6: Make decision.
Because $F_c = 19.58 > 4.67$, reject H_0 at $\alpha = 0.05$. The predictor, x_2 ($\log_{10}$ microbial count), is significant in explaining the SS_R and reducing SS_E in the regression equation.

Next, the researcher still suspects that temperature has an effect and does not want to disregard it completely. Hence, $y = b_0 + b_2 x_2 + b_1 x_1$ is the next model to test. (Although, positionally speaking, $b_2 x_2$ is really $b_1 x_1$ now, but to avoid confusion, we keep all variable labels in their original form until we have a final model.)

To do this, we evaluate $SS_{R(x_1|x_2)}$, the sum-of-squares caused by predictor x_1, with x_2 in the model.

Step 1: State the hypothesis.

  H_0: $\beta_1|\beta_2$ in the model $= 0$. (The contribution of x_1, given x_2 in the model, is 0; that is, the slope of b_1 is 0, with b_2 already in the model.)
  H_0: $\beta_1|\beta_2$ in the model $\neq 0$. (The earlier statement is not true.)

TABLE 4.15
ANOVA Computation for a Single Predictor Variable, x_2

Predictor	Coef	St. Dev	t-Ratio	p
(Constant) b_0	39.187	9.199	4.26	0.001
($\log_{10}$-ct) b_2	11.717	2.648	4.42	0.001
$s = 15.81$		R-sq $= 60.1\%$		R-sq(adj) $= 57.0\%$

Analysis of Variance

Source	DF	SS	MS	F	p
Regression x_2	1	4892.7	4892.7	19.58	0.001
Error	13	3248.7	249.9		
Total	14	8141.3			

The regression equation is L/wk $= 39.2 + 11.7 \log_{10}$-ct.

Step 2: Set α and n.
  $\alpha = 0.05$,
  $n = 15$.

Step 3: Statistic to use

$$F_{c(x_1|x_2)} = \frac{SS_{R(x_2, x_1)} - SS_{R(x_2)}}{MS_{E(x_2, x_1)}}.$$

Step 4: Decision rule.
If $F_{T(\alpha; 1, n-p-2)} = F_{T(0.05; 1, 15-1-2)} = F_{T(0.05; 1, 12)}$, where p is the number of x_i variables already in the model (e.g., $x_1|x_2 = p = 1$, $x_1|x_2, x_3 = p = 2$, and $x_1|x_2, x_3, x_4 = p = 3$)
  $F_{T(0.05; 1, 12)} = 4.75$ (Table C).
  If $F_{c(x_1|x_2)} > F_T = 4.75$, reject H_0 at $\alpha = 0.05$.

Step 5: Compute the full model table (Table 4.16).
By Table 4.16, $SS_{R(x_2, x_1)} = 5497.2$ and $MS_{E(x_1, x_2)} = 220.3$.
From the previous table (Table 4.15), $SS_{R(x_2)} = 4892.7$

$$SS_{R(x_1|x_2)} = SS_{R(x_1, x_2)} - SS_{R(x_2)} = 5497.2 - 4892.7 = 604.5.$$
$$F_c = \frac{SS_{R(x_1|x_2)}}{MS_{E(x_1, x_2)}} = \frac{604.5}{220.3} = 2.74.$$

Step 6: Decision rule.
Because $F_c = 2.74 \ngtr 4.75$, we cannot reject H_0 at $\alpha = 0.05$. $x_1 =$ temperature (°C) still does not contribute significantly to the model. Therefore, x_1 is eliminated from the model.
  Next, the researcher likes to evaluate x_3, the media concentration, with x_2 remaining in the model. Using the six-step procedure,

---

TABLE 4.16
Full Model, Predictor Variables x_1 and x_2

Predictor	Coef	St. Dev	t-Ratio	p
Constant	17.53	15.67	1.12	0.285
($\log_{10}$-ct) b_2	10.813	2.546	4.25	0.001
(temp°C) b_1	0.8438	0.5094	1.66	0.124
$s = 14.84$		R-sq = 67.5%		R-sq(adj) = 62.1%

Analysis of Variance

Source	DF	SS	MS	F	p
Regression (x_2, x_1)	2	5497.2	2748.6	12.47	0.001
Error	12	2644.2	220.3		
Total	14	8141.3			

The regression equation is L/wk $= 17.5 + 10.8 \log_{10}$-ct $+ 0.844$ temp °C.

Step 1: State the test hypothesis.

H_0: $\beta_3|\beta_2$ in the model $= 0$. (The addition of x_3 into the model containing x_2 is not useful.)

H_A: $\beta_3|\beta_2$ in the model $\neq 0$.

Step 2: Set α and n.

$\alpha = 0.05$,

$n = 15$.

Step 3: Statistic to use.

$$F_{c(x_3|x_2)} = \frac{SS_{R(x_2, x_3)} - SS_{R(x_2)}}{MS_{E(x_2, x_3)}}.$$

Step 4: Decision rule.

If $F_c > F_{T(\alpha; 1, n-p-2)} = F_{T(0.05; 1, 15-1-2)} = F_{T(0.05; 1, 12)}$, reject H_0.

$F_{T(0.05; 1, 12)} = 4.75$ (Table C).

Step 5: Table 4.17 presents the full model, $\hat{y} = b_0 + b_2 x_2 + b_3 x_3$.

$$SS_{R(x_2, x_3)} = 5961.5, \quad MS_{E(x_2, x_3)} = 181.6,$$
$$SS_{R(x_2)} = 4892.7, \text{ from Table 4.15.}$$
$$SS_{R(x_3|x_2)} = SS_{R(x_2, x_3)} - SS_{R(x_2)}$$
$$= 5961.5 - 4892.7 = 1068.8$$
$$F_{c(x_3|x_2)} = \frac{SS_{R(x_3|x_2)}}{MS_{E(x_2, x_3)}} = \frac{1068.8}{181.6} = 5.886.$$

TABLE 4.17
Full Model, Predictor Variables x_2 and x_3

Predictor	Coef	St. Dev	t-Ratio	p
Constant	41.555	7.904	5.26	0.000
($\log_{10}$-ct) b_2	−1.138	5.760	−0.20	0.847
(med-cn) b_3	18.641	7.685	2.43	0.032
$s = 13.48$		R-sq $= 73.2\%$		R-sq(adj) $= 68.8\%$

Analysis of Variance

Source	DF	SS	MS	F	p
Regression	2	5961.5	2980.8	16.41	0.000
Error	12	2179.8	181.6		
Total	14	8141.3			

The regression equation is L/wk $= 41.6 - 1.14 \log_{10}$-ct $+ 1.86$ med-cn.

Step 6: Decision rule.
Because $F_c = 5.886 > 4.75$, reject H_0 at $\alpha = 0.05$; x_3 contributes significantly to the regression model in which x_2 is present. Therefore, the current model is

$$\hat{y} = b_0 + b_2 x_2 + b_3 x_3.$$

Next, the researcher decides to bring x_4 (calcium/phosphorous ratio) into the model:

$$\hat{y} = b_0 + b_2 x_2 + b_3 x_3 + b_4 x_4.$$

Using the six-step procedure to evaluate x_4,

Step 1: State the hypothesis.

$H_0: \beta_4 | \beta_2, \beta_3 = 0$ (x_4 does not contribute significantly to the model),
$H_A: \beta_4 | \beta_2, \beta_3 \neq 0$.

Step 2: Set α and n.
$\alpha = 0.05$,
$n = 15$.

Step 3: The test statistic.

$$F_{c(x_4 | x_2, x_3)} = \frac{SS_{R(x_2, x_3, x_4)} - SS_{R(x_2, x_3)}}{S_{E(x_2, x_3, x_4)}}.$$

Step 4: Decision rule.
If $F_c > F_{T(\alpha; \, 1, \, n-p-2)} = F_{T(0.05; \, 1, \, 15-2-2)} = F_{T(0.05; \, 1, \, 11)} = 4.84$ (Table C)
If $F_c > 4.84$, reject H_0 at $\alpha = 0.05$.

Step 5: Perform the computation.
Table 4.18 shows the full model, $\hat{y} = b_0 + b_2 x_2 + b_3 x_3 + b_4 x_4$.
From Table 4.18, $SS_{R(x_2, x_1, x_4)} = 6526.3$ and $MS_{E(x_2, x_1, x_4)} = 146.8$.
Table 4.17 gives $SS_{R(x_2, x_3)} = 5961.5$

$$\frac{6526.3 - 5961.5}{146.8} = 3.84.$$

Step 6: Decision rule.
Because $F_c = 3.84 \not> F_T = 4.84$, one cannot reject H_0 at $\alpha = 0.05$. The researcher decides not to include x_4 in the model. Next, the researcher introduces x_5 (nitrogen) into the model:

$$\hat{y} = b_0 + b_2 x_2 + b_3 x_3 + b_5 x_5.$$

TABLE 4.18
Full Model, Predictor Variables x_2, x_3, and x_4

Predictor	Coef	St. Dev	t-Ratio	p
Constant	41.408	7.106	5.83	0.000
($\log_{10}$-ct) b_2	5.039	6.061	0.83	0.423
(med-cn) b_3	21.528	7.064	3.05	0.011
(Ca/P) b_4	−16.515	8.420	−1.96	0.076
$s = 12.12$		R-sq $= 80.2\%$		R-sq(adj) $= 74.8\%$

Analysis of Variance

Source	DF	SS	MS	F	p
Regression	3	6526.3	2175.4	14.82	0.000
Error	11	1615.0	146.8		
Total	14	8141.3			

The regression equation is L/wk $= 41.4 + 5.04 \log_{10}$-ct $+ 21.5$ med-cn $- 16.5$ Ca/P.

Using the six-step procedure for evaluating x_5,

Step 1: State the hypothesis.

$H_0: \beta_5|\beta_2, \beta_3 = 0$. (With x_5, nitrogen, as a predictor, x_5 does not significantly contribute to the model.)
$H_A: \beta_5|\beta_2, \beta_3 \neq 0$.

Step 2: Set α and n.
$\alpha = 0.05$,
$n = 15$.

Step 3: The test statistic.

$$F_{c(x_5|x_2, x_3)} = \frac{SS_{R(x_2, x_3, x_5)} - SS_{R(x_2, x_3)}}{MS_{E(x_2, x_3, x_5)}}.$$

Step 4: Decision rule.
$F_{T(0.05; 1, n-p-1)} = F_{T(0.05; 1, 11)} = 4.84$ (Table C).
If $F_c > 4.84$, reject H_0 at $\alpha = 0.05$.

Step 5: Perform the computation.
Table 4.19 portrays the full model, $\hat{y} = b_0 + b_2 x_2 + b_3 x_3 + b_5 x_5$.
From Table 4.19, $SS_{R(x_2, x_3, x_5)} = 5968.9$, and $SS_{E(x_2, x_3, x_5)} = 197.5$.
Table 4.17 gives $SS_{R(x_2, x_3)} = 5961.5$,

$$SS_{R(x_5|x_2, x_3)} = \frac{5968.9 - 5961.5}{197.5} = 0.04.$$

TABLE 4.19
Full Model, Predictor Variables x_2, x_3, and x_5

Predictor	Coef	St. Dev	t-Ratio	p
Constant	39.57	13.21	3.00	0.012
($\log_{10}$-ct) b_2	−1.633	6.533	−0.25	0.807
(med-cn) b_3	18.723	8.024	2.33	0.040
(N) b_5	0.0607	0.3152	0.19	0.851
$s = 14.05$		R-sq = 73.3%		R-sq(adj) = 66.0%

Analysis of Variance

Source	DF	SS	MS	F	p
Regression	3	5968.9	1989.6	10.07	0.002
Error	11	2172.5	197.5		
Total	14	8141.3			

The regression equation is L/wk $= 39.6 - 1.63 \log_{10}$-ct $+ 18.7$ med-cn $+ 0.061$N.

Step 6: Decision rule.
Because $F_c = 0.04 \not> F_T = 4.84$, one cannot reject H_0 at $\alpha = 0.05$. Therefore, the model continues to be $\hat{y} = b_0 + b_2 x_2 + b_3 x_3$.
Finally, the researcher introduces x_6 (heavy metals) into the model:

$$\hat{y} = b_0 + b_2 x_2 + b_3 x_3 + b_6 x_6.$$

Using the six-step procedure for evaluation x_6,
Step 1: State the test hypothesis.

$H_0: \beta_6 | \beta_2, \beta_3 = 0.$ (x_6 does not contribute significantly to the model.)
$H_A: \beta_6 | \beta_2, \beta_3 \neq 0.$

Step 2: Set α and n.
$\alpha = 0.05,$
$n = 15.$

Step 3: The test statistic.

$$F_{c(x_6|x_2,x_3)} = \frac{SS_{R(x_2,x_3,x_6)} - SS_{R(x_2,x_3)}}{MS_{E(x_2,x_3,x_6)}}.$$

Step 4: Decision rule.
$F_T = 4.84$ (again, from Table C).
If $F_c > 4.84$, reject H_0 at $\alpha = 0.05.$

TABLE 4.20
Full Model, Predictor Variables x_2, x_3, and x_6

Predictor	Coef	St. Dev	t-Ratio	p
Constant b_0	16.26	16.78	0.97	0.353
($\log_{10}$-ct) b_2	7.403	7.398	1.00	0.338
(med-cn) b_3	11.794	8.242	1.43	0.180
(Hvy-Mt) b_6	4.008	2.388	1.68	0.121
$s = 12.56$		R-sq = 78.7%		R-sq(adj) = 72.9%

Analysis of Variance

Source	DF	SS	MS	F	p
Regression	3	6405.8	2135.3	13.53	0.001
Error	11	1735.5	157.8		
Total	14	8141.3			

The regression equation is L/wk = $16.3 + 7.40 \log_{10}$-ct $+ 11.8$ med-cn $+ 4.01$ Hvy-Mt.

Step 5: Perform the statistical computation (Table 4.20).
From Table 4.20, $SS_{R(x_2, x_3, x_6)} = 6405.8$, and $MS_{E(x_2, x_3, x_6)} = 157.8$.
Table 4.17 gives $SS_{R(x_2, x_3)} = 5961.5$,

$$SS_{R(x_6|x_2, x_3)} = \frac{6405.8 - 5961.5}{157.8} = 2.82.$$

Step 6: Decision rule.
Because $F_c = 2.82 \not> F_T = 4.84$, one cannot reject H_0 at $\alpha = 0.05$. Remove x_6 from the model. Hence, the final model is

$$\hat{y} = b_0 + b_2 x_2 + b_3 x_3.$$

The model is now recoded as

$$\hat{y} = b_0 + b_1 x_1 + b_2 x_2,$$

where x_1 is the $\log_{10}$ colony counts and x_2 is medium concentration. The reason for this is that the most important x_i is introduced before those of lesser importance. This method is particularly useful if the researcher has a good idea of the importance or weight of each x_i. Note that, originally, the researcher thought temperature was the most important, but that was not so. Although the researcher collected data for six predictors, only two proved useful. However, the researcher noted in Table 4.17 that the t-ratio or t-value for $\log_{10}$ colony count was no longer significant and was puzzled that the model may be dependent on only the concentration of the medium. The next step is to evaluate $x_1 =$ colony counts with $x_2 =$ media concentration in the model. This step is left to the reader. Many times, when these oddities occur, the researcher must go back to the model and search for other indicator variables perhaps much more important than those included in the model. Additionally, a flag is raised in the researcher's mind by the relatively low value for $r^2_{(adj)}$, 68.8%. Further investigation is needed.

Note that we have not tested the model for fit at this time (linearity of model, serial correlation, etc.), as we combine everything in the model-building chapter.

BACKWARD ELIMINATION: PREDICTORS REMOVED FROM THE MODEL

This method begins with a full set of predictor variables in the model, which, in our case, is six. Each x_i predictor variable in the model is then evaluated as if it were the last one added. Some strategies begin the process at x_k and then x_{k-1}, and so forth. Others begin with x_1 and work toward x_k. This second strategy is the one that we use. We already know that only x_2 and x_3 were accepted in the forward selection method, where we started with one predictor variable and added predictor variables to it. Now we begin with the full model and remove insignificant ones. It continues to be important to value x_1 as the greatest contributor to the model and k as the least. Of course, if one really knew the contribution of each predictor x_i variable, one would not probably do the partial F-test in the first place. One does the best one can with the knowledge available.

Recall that our original model was

$$\hat{y} = b_0 + b_1 x_1 + b_2 x_2 + b_3 x_3 + b_4 x_4 + b_5 x_5 + b_6 x_6,$$

where x_1 is the temperature; x_2, $\log_{10}$ colony count; x_3, medium concentration; x_4, calcium/phosphorus ratio; x_5, nitrogen; and x_6 are the heavy metals.

Let us use the data from Example 4.2 again, and the six-step procedure, to evaluate the variables via the backward elimination procedure, beginning with x_1 and working toward x_k.

Step 1: State the hypothesis.

$H_0: \beta_1|\beta_2, \beta_3, \beta_4, \beta_5, \beta_6 = 0$ (predictor x_1 does not significantly contribute to the regression model, given that $x_2, x_3, x_4, x_5,$ and x_6 are in the model.)

$H_A: \beta_1|\beta_2, \beta_3, \beta_4, \beta_5, \beta_6 \neq 0$.

Step 2: Set α and n.

$\alpha = 0.05$,

$n = 15$.

Step 3: We are evaluating $SS_{R(x_1|x_2,x_3,x_4,x_5,x_6)}$, so

$$SS_{R(x_1|x_2,x_3,x_4,x_5,x_6)} = SS_{R(x_1,x_2,x_3,x_4,x_5,x_6)} - SS_{R(x_2,x_3,x_4,x_5,x_6)}.$$

The tests statistic is $F_{c(x_1|x_2,x_3,x_4,x_5,x_6)} = \dfrac{SS_{R(x_1,x_2,x_3,x_4,x_5,x_6)} - SS_{R(x_2,x_3,x_4,x_5,x_6)}}{MS_{E(x_1,x_2,x_3,x_4,x_5,x_6)}}.$

Step 4: Decision rule.

If $F_c > F_{T(\alpha, 1, n - p - 2)}$,
$p = 5$,
$F_{T(0.05; 1, 15 - 5 - 2)} = F_{T(0.05; 1, 8)} = 5.32$ (Table C),
If $F_c > 5.32$, reject H_0 at $\alpha = 0.05$.

Step 5: Perform the computation (Table 4.21). The full model is presented in Table 4.21, and the reduced in Table 4.22.
From Table 4.21, $SS_{R(x_1, x_2, x_3, x_4, x_5, x_6)} = 7266.3$, and $MS_{E(x_1, x_2, x_3, x_4, x_5, x_6)} = 109.4$
From Table 4.22, $SS_{R(x_1, x_2, x_3, x_4, x_5, x6)} = 6914.3$

$$F_{c(x_1|x_2,x_3,x_4,x_5,x_6)} = \frac{7266.3 - 6914.3}{109.4} = 3.22.$$

Step 6: Decision rule.
Because $F_c = 3.22 \ngtr = 5.32 = F_T$, one cannot reject H_0 at $\alpha = 0.05$. Therefore, drop x_1 from the model, because its contribution to the model is not significant. The new full model is

---

TABLE 4.21
Full Model, Predictor Variables x_1, x_2, x_3, x_4, x_5, and x_6

Predictor	Coef	St. Dev	t-Ratio	p	
Constant b_0	−23.15	26.51	−0.87	0.408	
(temp°C) b_1	0.8749	0.4877	1.79	0.111	
($\log_{10}$-ct) b_2	2.562	6.919	0.37	0.721	
(med-cn) b_3	14.567	7.927	1.84	0.103	
(Ca/P) b_4	−5.35	10.56	−0.51	0.626	
(N) b_5	0.5915	0.2816	2.10	0.069	
(Hvy-Mt) b_6	3.625	2.517	1.44	0.188	
$s = 10.46$		R-sq = 89.3%		R-sq(adj) = 81.2%	

Analysis of Variance

Source	DF	SS	MS	F	p
Regression	6	7266.3	1211.1	11.07	0.002
Error	8	875.0	109.4		
Total	14	8141.3			

The regression equation is L/wk = $-23.1 + 0.875$ temp °C $+ 2.56 \log_{10}$-ct $+ 14.6$ med-cn $- 5.3$ Ca/P $+ 0.592$ N $+ 3.62$ Hvy-Mt.

TABLE 4.22
Reduced Model, Predictor Variables x_2, x_3, x_4, x_5, and x_6

Predictor	Coef	St. Dev	t-Ratio	p
Constant b_0	5.40	23.67	0.23	0.825
($\log_{10}$-ct) b_2	8.163	6.894	1.18	0.267
(med-cn) b_3	16.132	8.797	1.83	0.100
(Ca/P) b_4	−15.30	10.03	−1.53	0.161
(N) b_5	0.4467	0.3011	1.48	0.172
(Hvy-Mt) b_6	3.389	2.806	1.21	0.258
$s = 11.68$		R-sq = 84.9%		R-sq(adj) = 76.6%

Analysis of Variance

Source	DF	SS	MS	F	p
Regression	5	6914.3	1382.9	10.14	0.002
Error	9	1227.0	136.3		
Total	14	8141.3			

The regression equation is L/wk = 5.4 + 8.16 $\log_{10}$-ct + 16.1 med-cn − 15.3Ca/P + 0.447N + 3.39 Hvy-Mt.

$$\hat{y} = b_0 + b_2 x_2 + b_3 x_3 + b_4 x_4 + b_5 x_5 + b_6 x_6.$$

We now test x_2.

Step 1: State the test hypothesis.

$H_0: \beta_1 | \beta_2, \beta_3, \beta_4, \beta_5, \beta_6 = 0,$

$H_A: \beta_1 | \beta_2, \beta_3, \beta_4, \beta_5, \beta_6 \neq 0.$

Step 2: Set α and n.
$\alpha = 0.05,$
$n = 15.$

Step 3: Write the test statistic
The test statistic is $F_{c(x_2 | x_3, x_4, x_5, x_6)} = \dfrac{SS_{R(x_2, x_3, x_4, x_5, x_6)} - SS_{R(x_3, x_4, x_5, x_6)}}{MS_{E(x_2, x_3, x_4, x_5, x_6)}}.$

Step 4: Decision rule.

$F_{T(0.05; n-p-2)} = F_{T(0.05; 1, 15-4-2)} = F_{T(0.05; 1, 9)} = 5.12$ (Table C).
Therefore, if $F_c > 5.12$, reject H_0 at $\alpha = 0.05$.

Step 5: Perform the computation (Table 4.23).
The full model is presented in Table 4.23, and the reduced one in Table 4.24.
From Table 4.23, $SS_{R(x_2, x_3, x_4, x_5, x_6)} = 6914.3$, and $MS_{E(x_2, x_3, x_4, x_5, x_6)} = 136.3$.
From Table 4.24, $SS_{R(x_3, x_4, x_5, x_6)} = 6723.2$

TABLE 4.23
Full Model, Predictor Variables x_2, x_3, x_4, x_5, and x_6

Predictor	Coef	St. Dev	t-Ratio	p
Constant b_0	5.40	23.67	0.23	0.825
($\log_{10}$-ct) b_2	8.163	6.894	1.18	0.267
(med-cn) b_3	16.132	8.797	1.83	0.100
(Ca/P) b_4	−15.30	10.03	−1.53	0.161
(N) b_5	0.4467	0.3011	1.48	0.172
(Hvy-Mt) b_6	3.389	2.806	1.21	0.258
$s = 11.68$		R-sq = 84.9%		R-sq(adj) = 76.6%

Analysis of Variance

Source	DF	SS	MS	F	p
Regression	5	6914.3	1382.9	10.14	0.002
Error	9	1227.0	136.3		
Total	14	8141.3			

The regression equation is L/wk = 5.4 + 8.16 $\log_{10}$-ct + 16.1 med-cn − 15.3 Ca/P + 0.447 N + 3.39 Hvy-Mt.

$$F_{c(x_1 | x_3, x_4, x_5, x_6)} = \frac{6914.3 - 6723.2}{136.3} = 1.40.$$

Step 6: Decision rule.
Because $F_c = 1.40 \not> F_T = 5.12$, one cannot reject H_0 at $\alpha = 0.05$. Thus, omit x_2 ($\log_{10}$ colony counts) from the model. Now observe what has happened.

TABLE 4.24
Reduced Model, Predictor Variables x_3, x_4, x_5, and x_6

Predictor	Coef	St. Dev	t-Ratio	p
Constant b_0	19.07	21.08	0.90	0.387
(med-cn) b_3	24.136	5.742	4.20	0.002
(Ca/P) b_4	−14.47	10.20	−1.42	0.186
(N) b_5	0.4403	0.3071	1.43	0.182
(Hvy-Mt) b_6	1.687	2.458	0.69	0.508
$s = 11.91$		R-sq = 82.6%		R-sq(adj) = 75.6%

Analysis of Variance

Source	DF	SS	MS	F	p
Regression	4	6723.2	1680.8	11.85	0.001
Error	10	1418.2	141.8		
Total	14	8141.3			

The regression equation is L/wk = 19.1 + 24.1 med-cn − 14.5 Ca/P + 0.440 N + 1.69 Hvy-Mt.

In the forward selection method, x_2 was significant. Now, its contribution is diluted by the x_4, x_5, and x_6 variables, with a very different regression equation, and having lost 3 degrees of freedom. Obviously, the two methods may not produce equivalent results. This is often due to model inadequacies, such as x_is, themselves that are correlated, a problem we address in later chapters. The new full model is

$$\hat{y} = b_0 + b_3 x_3 + b_4 x_4 + b_5 x_5 + b_6 x_6.$$

Let us evaluate the effect of x_3 (medium concentration).

Step 1: State the test hypothesis.

$H_0: \beta_3 | \beta_4, \beta_5, \beta_6 = 0,$

$H_A: \beta_3 | \beta_4, \beta_5, \beta_6 \neq 0.$

Step 2: Set α and n.
$\alpha = 0.05,$
$n = 15.$

Step 3: The test statistic is

$$F_{c(x_3 | x_4, x_5, x_6)} = \frac{SS_{R(x_3, x_4, x_5, x_6)} - SS_{R(x_4, x_5, x_6)}}{MS_{E(x_3, x_4, x_5, x_6)}}.$$

Step 4: Decision rule.
$F_{T(\alpha; n-p-2)} = T_{T(0.05; 1, 15-3-2)} = F_{T(0.05, 1, 10)} = 4.96.$
If $F_c > 4.96$, reject H_0 at $\alpha = 0.05$.

Step 5: Perform the computation (Table 4.25).
The full model is presented in Table 4.25, and the reduced model in Table 4.26. From Table 4.25,

$$SS_{R(x_3, x_4, x_5, x_6)} = 6723.2 \quad \text{and} \quad MS_{E(x_3, x_4, x_5, x_6)} = 141.8.$$

From Table 4.26, $SS_{R(x_4, x_5, x_6)} = 4217.3$

$$F_{c(x_3 | x_4, x_5, x_6)} = \frac{6723.2 - 4217.3}{141.8} = 17.67.$$

Step 6: Decision rule.
Because $F_c = 17.67 > F_T = 4.96$, reject H_0 at $\alpha = 0.05$, and retain x_3 in the model.
The new full model is

$$\hat{y} = b_0 + b_3 x_3 + b_4 x_4 + b_5 x_5 + b_6 x_6.$$

TABLE 4.25
Full Model, Predictor Variables x_3, x_4, x_5, and x_6

Predictor	Coef	St. Dev	t-Ratio	p
Constant b_0	19.07	21.08	0.90	0.387
(med-cn) b_3	24.136	5.742	4.20	0.002
(Ca/P) b_4	−14.47	10.20	−1.42	0.186
(N) b_5	0.4403	0.3071	1.43	0.182
(Hvy-Mt) b_6	1.687	2.458	0.69	0.508
$s = 11.91$		R-sq $= 82.6\%$		R-sq(adj) $= 75.6\%$

Analysis of Variance

Source	DF	SS	MS	F	p
Regression	4	6723.2	1680.8	11.85	0.001
Error	10	1418.2	141.8		
Total	14	8141.3			

The regression equation is L/wk $= 19.1 + 241$ med-cn $- 14.5$ Ca/P $+ 0.440$ N $+ 1.69$ Hvy-Mt.

The next iteration is with x_4.

Step 1: State the test hypothesis.

$$H_0: \beta_4 | \beta_3, \beta_5, \beta_6 = 0,$$
$$H_A: \beta_4 | \beta_3, \beta_5, \beta_6 \neq 0.$$

TABLE 4.26
Reduced Model, Predictor Variables x_4, x_5, and x_6

Predictor	Coef	St. Dev	t-Ratio	p
Constant b_0	−4.15	32.26	−0.13	0.900
(Ca/P) b_4	19.963	9.640	2.07	0.063
(N) b_5	0.5591	0.4850	1.15	0.273
(Hvy-Mt) b_6	5.988	3.544	1.69	0.119
$s = 18.89$		R-sq $= 51.8\%$		R-sq(adj) $= 38.7\%$

Analysis of Variance

Source	DF	SS	MS	F	p
Regression	3	4217.3	1405.8	3.94	0.039
Error	11	3924.1	356.7		
Total	14	8141.3			

The regression equation is L/wk $= -4.2 + 20.0$ Ca/P $+ 0.559$ N $+ 5.99$ Hvy-Mt.

Step 2: Set α and n.
  $\alpha = 0.05$,
  $n = 15$.

Step 3: The test statistic is

$$F_{c(x_4|x_3, x_5, x_6)} = \frac{SS_{R(x_3, x_4, x_5, x_6)} - SS_{R(x_3, x_5, x_6)}}{MS_{E(x_3, x_4, x_5, x_6)}}.$$

Step 4: Decision rule.
  $F_T = 4.96$, as before.
  If $F_c > 4.96$, reject H_0 at $\alpha = 0.05$.

Step 5: Perform the computation.
Table 4.25 contains the full model, and Table 4.27 contains the reduced model.
  From Table 4.25, $SS_{R(x_3, x_4, x_5, x_6)} = 6723.2$, and $MS_{E(x_3, x_4, x_5, x_6)} = 141.8$.
  From Table 4.27, $SS_{R(x_3, x_5, x_6)} = 6437.8$

$$F_{c(x_4|x_3, x_5, x_6)} = \frac{6723.2 - 6437.8}{141.8} = 2.01.$$

Step 6: Decision rule.
Because $F_c = 2.01 \not> F_T = 4.96$, one cannot reject H_0 at $\alpha = 0.05$. Hence, x_4 is dropped out of the model. The new full model is

$$\hat{y} = b_0 + b_3 x_3 + b_5 x_5 + b_6 x_6.$$

TABLE 4.27
Reduced Model, Predictor Variables x_3, x_5, and x_6

Predictor	Coef	St. Dev	t-Ratio	p
Constant b_0	9.33	20.82	0.45	0.663
(med-cn) b_3	17.595	3.575	4.92	0.000
(N) b_5	0.3472	0.3135	1.11	0.292
(Hvy-Mt) b_6	3.698	2.098	1.76	0.106
$s = 12.44$		R-sq = 79.1%		R-sq(adj) = 73.4%

Analysis of Variance

Source	DF	SS	MS	F	p
Regression	3	6437.8	2145.9	13.86	0.000
Error	11	1703.6	154.9		
Total	14	8141.3			

The regression equation is L/wk $= 9.3 + 17.6$ med-cn $+ 0.347$ N $+ 3.70$ Hvy-Mt.

Next, x_5 is evaluated.

Step 1: State the hypothesis.

$$H_0: \beta_5 | \beta_3, \beta_6 = 0,$$

$$H_A: \beta_5 | \beta_3, \beta_6 \neq 0.$$

Step 2: Set α and n.
$\alpha = 0.05,$
$n = 15.$

Step 3: The test statistic is

$$F_{c(x_5 | x_3, x_6)} = \frac{SS_{R(x_3, x_5, x_6)} - SS_{R(x_3, x_6)}}{MS_{E(x_3, x_5, x_6)}}.$$

Step 4: Decision rule.

$$F_T = F_{T(\alpha, 1, n-p-2)} = F_{T(0.05, 1, 15-2-2)} = F_{T(0.05, 1, 11)} = 4.84.$$

If $F_c > 4.84$, reject H_0 at $\alpha = 0.05$.

Step 5: Perform the computation.
Table 4.28 is the full model, and Table 4.29 is the reduced model.
From Table 4.28, $SS_{R(x_3, x_5, x_6)} = 6437.8$ and $MS_{E(x_3, x_5, x_6)} = 154.9$.
From Table 4.29, $SS_{R(x_3, x_6)} = 6247.8$

TABLE 4.28
Full Model, Predictor Variables x_3, x_5, and x_6

Predictor	Coef	St. Dev	t-Ratio	p
Constant b_0	9.33	20.82	0.45	0.663
(med-cn) b_3	17.595	3.575	4.92	0.000
(N) b_5	0.3472	0.3135	1.11	0.292
(Hvy-Mt) b_6	3.698	2.098	1.76	0.106
$s = 12.44$		R-sq = 79.1%		R-sq(adj) = 73.4%

Analysis of Variance

Source	DF	SS	MS	F	p
Regression	3	6437.8	2145.9	13.86	0.000
Error	11	1703.6	154.9		
Total	14	8141.3			

The regression equation is L/wk = 9.3 + 17.6 med-cn + 0.347 N + 3.70 Hvy-Mt.

TABLE 4.29
Reduced Model, Predictor Variables x_3 and x_6

Predictor	Coef	St. Dev	t-Ratio	p
Constant b_0	29.11	10.80	2.70	0.019
(med-cn) b_3	19.388	3.218	6.03	0.000
(Hvy-Mt) b_6	2.363	1.733	1.36	0.198
$s = 12.56$		R-sq $= 76.7\%$		R-sq(adj) $= 72.9\%$

Analysis of Variance

Source	DF	SS	MS	F	p
Regression	2	6247.8	3123.9	19.80	0.000
Error	12	1893.5	157.8		

The regression equation is L/wk $= 29.1 + 19.4$ med-cn $+ 2.36$ Hvy-Mt.

$$F_{c(x_5|x_3, x_6)} = \frac{6437.8 - 6247.8}{154.9} = 1.23.$$

Step 6: Decision rule.
Because $F_c = 1.23 \not> F_T = 4.84$, one cannot reject H_0 at $\alpha = 0.05$. Therefore, drop x_5 from the model. The new full model is

$$\hat{y} = b_0 + b_3 x_3 + b_6 x_6.$$

Now we test x_6.
Step 1: State the test hypothesis.

$$H_0: \beta_6 | \beta_3 = 0,$$

$$H_A: \beta_6 | \beta_3 \neq 0.$$

Step 2: Set α and n.
$\alpha = 0.05$,
$n = 15$.

Step 3: The test statistic is

$$F_{c(x_6|x_3)} = \frac{SS_{R(x_3, x_6)} - SS_{R(x_3)}}{MS_{E(x_3, x_6)}}.$$

Step 4: Decision rule.
$F_T = F_{T(\alpha, 1, n-p-2)} = F_{T(0.05, 1, 15-1-2)} = F_{T(0.05, 1, 12)} = 4.75.$
If $F_c > 4.75$, reject H_0 at $\alpha = 0.05$.

TABLE 4.30
Full Model, Predictor Variables x_3 and x_6

Predictor	Coef	St. Dev	t-Ratio	p
Constant b_0	29.11	10.80	2.70	0.019
(med-cn) b_3	19.388	3.218	6.03	0.000
(Hvy-Mt) b_6	2.363	1.733	1.36	0.198
$s = 12.56$		R-sq $= 76.7\%$		R-sq(adj) $= 72.9\%$

Analysis of Variance

Source	DF	SS	MS	F	p
Regression	2	6247.8	3123.9	19.80	0.000
Error	12	1893.5	157.8		
Total	14	8141.3			

The regression equation is L/wk $= 29.1 + 19.4$ med-cn $+ 2.36$ Hvy-Mt.

Step 5: Perform the computation.
Table 4.30 is the full model, and Table 4.31 is the reduced model.
From Table 4.30, $SS_{R(x_3, x_6)} = 6247.8$, and $MS_{E(x_3, x_6)} = 157.8$.
From Table 4.31, $SS_{R(x_3)} = 5954.5$

$$F_{c(x_6|x_3)} = \frac{6247.8 - 5954.5}{157.8} = 1.86.$$

Step 6: Decision rule.
Because $F_c = 1.86 \not> F_T = 4.75$, one cannot reject H_0 at $\alpha = 0.05$. The appropriate model is

$$\hat{y} = b_0 + b_3 x_3.$$

TABLE 4.31
Reduced Model, Predictor Variable x_3

Predictor	Coef	St. Dev	t-Ratio	p
Constant b_0	40.833	6.745	6.05	0.000
(med-cn) b_3	17.244	2.898	5.95	0.000
$s = 12.97$		R-sq $= 73.1\%$		R-sq(adj) $= 71.1\%$

Analysis of Variance

Source	DF	SS	MS	F	p
Regression	1	5954.5	5954.5	35.40	0.000
Error	13	2186.9	168.2		
Total	14	8141.3			

The regression equation is L/wk $= 40.8 + 17.2$ med-cn.

DISCUSSION

Note that, with Method 1, forward selection, we have the model (Table 4.17):

$$\hat{y} = b_0 + b_2x_2 + b_3x_3,$$
$$\hat{y} = 41.56 - 1.138x_2 + 18.641x_3,$$
$$R^2 = 73.2.$$

For Method 2, Backward Elimination, we have, from Table 4.31

$$\hat{y} = b_0 + b_3x_3,$$
$$\hat{y} = 4.833x_2 + 17.244x_3,$$
$$R^2 = 73.1.$$

Which one is true? Both are true, but partially. Note that the difference between these models is the $\log_{10}$ population variable, x_2. One model has it, the other does not. Most microbiologists would feel the need for x_2 in the model, because they are familiar with the parameter. Given that everything in future studies is conducted in the same way, either model would work. However, there is probably an inadequacy in the data. In order to evaluate x_i predictor variables adequately, there should be a wide range of values in each x_i. Arguably, in this example, no x_i predictor had a wide range of data collected. Hence, measuring the true contribution of each x_i variable was not possible. However, obtaining the necessary data is usually very expensive, in practice. Therefore, to use this model is probably okay, given that the x_i variables in the models remain within the range of measurements of the current study to be valid. That is, there should be no extrapolation outside the ranges.

There is, more than likely, a bigger problem—a correlation between x_i variables, which is a common occurrence in experimental procedures. Recall that we set up the bioreactor experiment to predict the amount of medium used, given a known $\log_{10}$ colony count and medium concentration. Because there is a relationship between all or some of the independent prediction variables, x_i, they influence one another to varying degrees, making their placement in the model configuration important. The preferred way of recognizing codependence of the variables is by having interaction terms in the model, a topic to be discussed in a later chapter.

Y ESTIMATE POINT AND INTERVAL: MEAN

At times, the researcher wants to predict y_i, based on specific x_i values. In estimating a mean response for Y, one needs to specify a vector of x_i values within the range in which the $\hat{y}$ model was constructed. For example, in Example 4.2, looking at the regression equation that resulted when the x_i were added to the model (forward selection), we finished with

$$\hat{y} = b_0 + b_2 x_2 + b_3 x_3.$$

Now, let us call $x_2 = x_1$ and $x_3 = x_2$.
The new model is

$$\hat{y} = b_0 + b_1 x_1 + b_2 x_2 = 41.56 - 1.138 x_1 + 18.641 x_2,$$

where x_1 is the $\log_{10}$ colony count, x_2 is the medium concentration, and y is the liters of media.

We use matrix algebra to perform this example, so the reader will have experience in its utilization, a requirement of some statistical software packages. If a review of matrix algebra is needed, please refer to Appendix II.

To predict the $\hat{y}$ value, set the x_i values at, say, $x_1 = 3.7$ $\log_{10} x_2 = 1.8$ concentration in column vector form. The calculation is

$$\boldsymbol{x}_p = \boldsymbol{x} \text{ predicted} = \begin{bmatrix} x_0 \\ x_1 \\ x_2 \end{bmatrix} = \begin{bmatrix} 1 \\ 3.7 \\ 1.8 \end{bmatrix}.$$

$$\scriptstyle 3 \times 1$$

The matrix equation is $E[\hat{Y}] = \boldsymbol{x}_p' \boldsymbol{\beta}$, estimated by $\hat{Y} = \boldsymbol{x}_p' \boldsymbol{\beta}$,   (4.19)
where the subscript p denotes prediction.

$$\hat{Y} = \boldsymbol{x}_p' \boldsymbol{b} = \begin{bmatrix} 1 & 3.7 & 1.8 \end{bmatrix} \underset{1 \times 3}{\begin{bmatrix} 41.55 \\ -1.138 \\ 18.641 \end{bmatrix}}$$

$$\scriptstyle 1 \times 3$$

$$= 1(41.55) + 3.7(-1.138) + 1.8(18.641) = 70.89.$$

Therefore, 70.89 L of medium is needed. The variance of this estimate is

$$\sigma^2[\hat{Y}_p] = \boldsymbol{x}_p' \sigma^2[\boldsymbol{b}] \boldsymbol{x}_p,$$ (4.20)

which is estimated by

$$s_{\hat{y}}^2 = \text{MSE}\left(\boldsymbol{x}_p' (\boldsymbol{X}'\boldsymbol{X})^{-1} \boldsymbol{x}_p\right).$$ (4.21)

The $1 - \alpha$ confidence interval is

$$\hat{Y}_p \pm t_{(\alpha/2; n-k-1)} s_{\hat{y}},$$ (4.22)

where k is the number of x_i predictors in the model, excluding b_0.

Let us work an example (Example 4.3). In evaluating the effectiveness of a new oral antimicrobial drug, the amount of drug available at the target site, the human bladder, in $\mu g/mL = y$ of blood serum. The drug uptake is dependent on the number of attachment polymers, x_1. The uptake of the drug in the bladder is thought to be mediated by the amount of $\alpha - 1, 3$ promixin available in the blood stream, $x_2 = \mu g/mL$.

In an animal study, 25 replicates were conducted to generate data for x_1 and x_2. The investigator wants to determine the regression equation and confidence intervals for a specific x_1, x_2 configuration. To calculate the slopes for x_1 and x_2, we use the formula

$$b = (X'X)^{-1}X'Y. \tag{4.23}$$

We perform this entire analysis using matrix manipulation (Table 4.32 and Table 4.33). Table 4.35 lists the b_i coefficients.

TABLE 4.32
X Matrix Table, Example 4.3

$$X_{25\times3} = \begin{bmatrix} x_0 & x_1 & x_2 \\ 1.0 & 70.3 & 214.0 \\ 1.0 & 60.0 & 92.0 \\ 1.0 & 57.0 & 454.0 \\ 1.0 & 52.0 & 455.0 \\ 1.0 & 50.0 & 413.0 \\ 1.0 & 55.0 & 81.0 \\ 1.0 & 58.0 & 435.0 \\ 1.0 & 69.0 & 136.0 \\ 1.0 & 76.0 & 208.0 \\ 1.0 & 62.0 & 369.0 \\ 1.0 & 51.0 & 3345.0 \\ 1.0 & 53.0 & 362.0 \\ 1.0 & 51.0 & 105.0 \\ 1.0 & 56.0 & 126.0 \\ 1.0 & 56.0 & 291.0 \\ 1.0 & 69.0 & 204.0 \\ 1.0 & 56.0 & 626.0 \\ 1.0 & 50.0 & 1064.0 \\ 1.0 & 44.0 & 700.0 \\ 1.0 & 55.0 & 382.0 \\ 1.0 & 56.0 & 776.0 \\ 1.0 & 51.0 & 182.0 \\ 1.0 & 56.0 & 47.0 \\ 1.0 & 48.0 & 45.0 \\ 1.0 & 48.0 & 391.0 \end{bmatrix}$$

TABLE 4.33
Y Matrix Table, Example 4.3

$$Y_{25 \times 1} = \begin{bmatrix} 11 \\ 13 \\ 12 \\ 17 \\ 57 \\ 37 \\ 30 \\ 15 \\ 11 \\ 25 \\ 111 \\ 29 \\ 18 \\ 9 \\ 31 \\ 10 \\ 48 \\ 36 \\ 30 \\ 15 \\ 57 \\ 15 \\ 12 \\ 27 \\ 12 \end{bmatrix}$$

Let us predict $\hat{Y}$ if $x_1 = 61$ and $x_2 = 113$.

$$x_p = \begin{bmatrix} 1 \\ 61 \\ 113 \end{bmatrix},$$

$$\hat{Y} = x'_p b = \begin{bmatrix} 16 & 11 & 13 \end{bmatrix} \begin{bmatrix} 36.6985 \\ -0.3921 \\ 0.0281 \end{bmatrix}$$

$$= 1(36.6985) + 61(-0.3921) + 113(0.0281) = 15.96.$$

One does not necessarily need matrix algebra for this. The computation can also be carried out as

$$\hat{y} = b_0 + b_1 x_1 + b_2 x_2 = 36.6985(x_0) - 0.3921(x_1) + 0.0281(x_2).$$

TABLE 4.34
Inverse Values, $(X'X)^{-1}$

$$(X'X)^{-1}_{3 \times 3} = \begin{bmatrix} 2.53821 & -0.04288 & -0.00018 \\ -0.04288 & 0.00074 & 0.00000 \\ -0.00018 & 0.00000 & 0.00000 \end{bmatrix}$$

To calculate, $s^2 = \text{MS}_E = \dfrac{Y'Y - b'X'Y}{n - k - 1} = \dfrac{\text{SS}_E}{n - k - 1}$,   (4.24)

$Y'Y = 31,056$ and $b'X'Y = 27,860.4$,

$\text{SS}_E = Y'Y - b'X'Y = 31,056 - 27,860.4 = 3,195.6$,

$\text{MS}_E = \dfrac{\text{SS}_E}{n - k - 1} = \dfrac{3195.6}{25 - 2 - 1} = 145.2545$,

$s_{\hat{y}}^2 = \text{MS}_E \left(x_p'(X'X)^{-1} x_p \right)$.

$$x_p'(X'X)^{-1} x_p = \begin{bmatrix} 1 & 61 & 113 \end{bmatrix} \begin{bmatrix} 2.53821 & -0.04288 & -0.00018 \\ -0.04288 & 0.00074 & 0.00000 \\ -0.00018 & 0.00000 & 0.00000 \end{bmatrix} \begin{bmatrix} 1 \\ 61 \\ 113 \end{bmatrix}$$

$= 0.0613$

$s_{\hat{y}}^2 = 145.2545(0.0613)$,

$s_{\hat{y}}^2 = 8.9052$,

$s_{\hat{y}} = 2.9842$.

The $1 - \alpha$ confidence interval for $\hat{Y}$ is

$$\hat{Y} \pm t_{(\alpha/2,\, n-k-1)} s_{\hat{y}}.$$

Let us use $\alpha = 0.05$.

$n - k - 1 = 25 - 2 - 1 = 22$.

TABLE 4.35
Coefficients for the Slopes, Example 4.3

$$b = (X'X)^{-1} X'Y = \begin{bmatrix} 36.6985 \\ -0.3921 \\ 0.0281 \end{bmatrix} \begin{matrix} = b_0 \\ = b_1 \\ = b_2 \end{matrix}$$

TABLE 4.36
$(X'X)^{-1}$, Example 4.3

$$(X'X)^{-1} = \begin{bmatrix} 2.53821 & -0.04288 & -0.00018 \\ -0.04288 & 0.00074 & 0.00000 \\ -0.00018 & 0.00000 & 0.00000 \end{bmatrix}$$

From Table B (Student's t Table), $t_T = (df = 22, \alpha/2 = 0.025) = 2.074$
   $15.95 \pm 2.074(2.9842)$
   15.95 ± 6.1891
   $9.76 \le \mu \le 22.14$ is the 95% mean confidence interval of $\hat{y}$ when $x_1 = 61$, $x_2 = 113$.

CONFIDENCE INTERVAL ESTIMATION OF THE β_iS

The confidence interval for a β_i value at $1 - \alpha$ confidence is

$$\beta_i = b_i \pm t_{(\alpha/2,\, n-k-1)} s_{b_i}, \tag{4.25}$$

where

$$s_{b_i}^2 = MS_E (X'X)^{-1} \tag{4.26}$$

Using the data in Example 4.3,
   $MS_E = 145.2545$, and Table 4.36 presents the $(X'X)^{-1}$ matrix:
   Table 4.37 is $MS_E (X'X)^{-1}$
   where the diagonals are $s_{b_0}^2$, $s_{b_1}^2$, and $s_{b_2}^2$.
So,

$$s_{b_0}^2 = 368.686 \rightarrow s_{b_0} = 19.20$$
$$s_{b_1}^2 = 0.108 \rightarrow s_{b_1} = 0.3286$$
$$s_{b_2}^2 = 0.0 \rightarrow s_{b_2} = 0.003911$$

Because there is no variability in b_2, we should be concerned. Looking at Table 4.38, we see that the slope of b_2 is very small (0.0281), and the

TABLE 4.37
Variance, Example 4.3

$$s_{b_i}^2 = MS_E(X'X)^{-1} = \begin{bmatrix} 368.686 & -6.228 & -0.026 \\ -6.228 & 0.108 & 0.000 \\ -0.026 & 0.000 & 0.000 \end{bmatrix}$$

TABLE 4.38
Slope Values, b_i, Example 4.3

$$b = \begin{bmatrix} 36.6985 \\ -0.3921 \\ 0.0281 \end{bmatrix} \begin{matrix} = b_0 \\ = b_1 \\ = b_2 \end{matrix}$$

variability is too small for the program to pick up. However, is this the only problem, or even the real problem? Other effects may be present, such as the x_i predictor variable correlated with other x_i predictor variables, a topic to be discussed later in this book.

Sometimes, it is easier not to perform the computation via matrix manipulation, because there is a significant round-off error. Performing the same calculations using the standard regression model, Table 4.39 provides the results.

Note, from Table 4.39, s_{b_i} are again in the "St dev" column and b_i in the "Coef" column.

Therefore,

$$\beta_0 = b_0 \pm t_{(\alpha/2, n-k-1)}s_{b_0}, \text{ where } t_{(0.025, 25-2-1)} = 2.074 \text{ (Table B)}$$
$$= 36.70 \pm 2.074(19.20)$$
$$= 36.70 \pm 39.82$$
$$-3.12 \le \beta_0 \le 76.52 \text{ at } \alpha = 0.05.$$

TABLE 4.39
Standard Regression Model, Example 4.3

Predictor	Coef	St. Dev	t-Ratio	p
Constant b_0	36.70	19.20	1.91	0.069
b_1	−0.3921	0.3283	−1.19	0.245
b_2	0.028092	0.003911	7.18	0.000
s = 12.05		R-sq = 73.6%	R-sq(adj) = 71.2%	

Analysis of Variance

Source	DF	SS	MS	F	p
Regression	2	8926.5	4463.3	30.73	0.000
Error	22	3195.7	145.3		
Total	24	12122.2			

The regression equation is $\hat{y} = 36.7 - 0.392x_1 + 0.0281x_2$.

We can conclude that β_0 is 0 via a 95% confidence interval (interval contains zero).

$$\beta_1 = b_1 \pm t_{(\alpha/2,\, n-k-1)} s_{b_1}$$
$$= -0.3921 \pm 2.074(0.3283)$$
$$-1.0730 \le \beta_1 \le 0.2888.$$

We can also conclude that β_1 is zero, via a 95% confidence interval.

$$\beta_2 = b_2 \pm t_{(\alpha/2,\, n-k-1)} s_{b_2}$$
$$= 0.028092 \pm 2.074(0.003911)$$
$$= 0.02092 \pm 0.0081$$
$$0.0128 \le \beta_2 \le 0.0290 \text{ at } \alpha = 0.05.$$

We can conclude, because this 95% confidence interval does not contain 0, that β_2 is statistically significant, but with a slope so slight that it has no practical significance. We return to this problem in Chapter 10, which deals with model-building techniques.

There is a knotty issue in multiple regression with using the Student's t-test for >1 independent predictors. That is, because more than one test was conducted, for example, $0.95^3 = 0.857$ confidence. To adjust for this, the user can undertake a correction process, such as the Bonferroni joint confidence procedure. In our example, there are b_{k+1} parameters, if one includes b_0. Not all of them need to be tested, but whatever that test number is, we call it as g, where $g \le k + 1$. The Bonferroni method is $\beta_1 = b_i \pm t_{(\alpha/2g;\, n-k-1)} s_{b_i}$. This is the same formula as the previous one, using the t-table, except that α is divided by $2g$, where g is the number of contrasts.

In addition, note that ANOVA can be used to evaluate specific regression parameter components. For example, to evaluate b_1 by itself, we want to test x_1 by itself. If it is significant, we test $x_2|x_1$, otherwise x_2 alone. Table 4.40 gives a sequential SS_R of each variable.

TABLE 4.40
Sequential Component Analysis of Variance from Table 4.39

Source	DF	SEQ SS
x_1	1	1431.3
x_2	1	7495.3
where		
x_1 SEQ SS $= SS_{R(x_1)}$		
x_2 SEQ SS $= SS_{R(x_2|x_1)}$		

To test $F_{c(x_1)}$, we need to add $SS_{R(x_2|x_1)}$ into $SS_{E(x_1, x_2)}$ to provide $SS_{E(x_1)}$.

$$SS_{R(x_2|x_1)} = 7495.3 \text{ (from Table 4.40)}$$
$$+ SS_{R(x_1, x_2)} = 3195.7 \text{ (from Table 4.39)}$$
$$= SS_{E(x_1)} = 10691.0 \text{ and}$$
$$MS_{E(x_1)} = \frac{10691.0}{25 - 1 - 1} = 464.83$$
$$F_{c(x_1)} = \frac{SS_{R(x_1)}}{MS_{E(x_1)}} = \frac{1431.3}{464.83} = 3.08$$
$$F_{T(0.05, 1, 23)} = 4.28$$

Because $F_c = 3.08 \not> F_T = 4.28$, x_1 is not significant in the model at $\alpha = 0.5$. Hence, we do not need β_1 in the model and can merely compute the data with x_2 in the model (Table 4.41).

PREDICTING ONE OR SEVERAL NEW OBSERVATIONS

To predict a new observation, or observations, the procedure is an extension of simple linear regression. For any

$$\hat{Y}_p = b_0 + b_1 x_1 + \cdots + b_k x_k.$$

The $1 - \alpha$ confidence interval of $\hat{Y}$ is predicted as

$$\hat{Y}_p \pm t_{(\alpha/2, n-k-1)} s_p, \tag{4.27}$$

TABLE 4.41
Reduced Regression Model, Example 4.3

Predictor	Coef	St. Dev	t-Ratio	p
Constant b_0	14.044	3.000	4.68	0.000
b_2	0.029289	0.003815	7.68	0.000
$s = 12.16$		R-sq = 71.9%		R-sq(adj) = 70.7%

Analysis of Variance

Source	DF	SS	MS	F	p
Regression	1	8719.4	8719.4	58.93	0.000
Error	23	3402.9	148.0		
Total	24	12122.2			

The regression equation is $\hat{y} = 14.0 + 0.0293 x_2$.

$$s_p^2 = MS_E + s_{\hat{y}}^2 = MS_E\left(1 + x_p'(X'X)^{-1}x_p\right).\qquad(4.28)$$

For example, using the data in Table 4.39, suppose $x_1 = 57$ and $x_2 = 103$. Then, $x_p' = [1\ 57\ 103]$ and $MS_E = 145.3$. First, $(X_p'(X'X)^{-1}X_p)$ is computed using the inverse values for $(X'X)^{-1}$ in Table 4.34 (Table 4.42). Then, 1 is added to the result, and then multiplied times MS_E.

$$1 + x_p'(X'X)^{-1}x_p = 1 + 0.0527 = 1.0577.$$

Next, multiply 1.0577 by $MS_E = 145.2545 = 146.312$,

$$s_p^2 = 146.312 \text{ and } \sqrt{146.312} = s_p = 12.096,$$
$$\hat{Y}_p = x_p'b,$$

$$x_p' = [1 \quad 57 \quad 103] \times b = \begin{bmatrix} 36.70 \\ -0.3921 \\ 0.028092 \end{bmatrix} = 17.24,$$

$$\hat{Y}_p = 17.24.$$

For $\alpha = 0.05$, $n = 25$, $k = 2$, and $df = n - k - 1 = 25 - 2 - 1 = 22$.

$$t_{(0.025,\ 22)} = 2.074, \text{ from Table B.}$$
$$17.24 \pm 2.074(s_p)$$
$$17.24 \pm 2.074(12.096)$$
$$17.24 \pm 25.09$$
$$-7.85 \le \hat{Y}_p \le 42.33$$

The prediction of a new value with a 95% CI is too wide to be useful in this case. If the researcher fails to do some of the routine diagnostics and gets zero included in the interval, the researcher needs to go back and check the adequacy of the model. We do that in later chapters.

TABLE 4.42
Computation for $(x_p'\ (X'X)^{-1}\ x_p)$, Using the Inverse Values for $(X'X)^{-1}$

$$x_p'(X'X)x_p = [1\quad 57\quad 103] \times \begin{bmatrix} 2.53821 & -0.04288 & -0.00018 \\ -0.04288 & 0.00074 & 0.00000 \\ -0.00018 & 0.00000 & 0.00000 \end{bmatrix} \times \begin{bmatrix} 1 \\ 57 \\ 103 \end{bmatrix} = 0.0527$$

NEW MEAN VECTOR PREDICTION

The same basic procedure used to predict a new observation is used to predict the average expected y value, given the x_i values remain the same. Essentially, this is to predict the mean $1 - \alpha$ confidence interval in an experiment.

The formula is

$$\hat{Y}_{\bar{p}} \pm t_{(\alpha/2,\, n-k-1)} s_{\bar{p}},$$

where

$$s_{\bar{p}}^2 = \frac{MS_E}{q} + s^2 = MS_E \left(\frac{1}{q} + x_p'(X'X)^{-1} x_p \right),$$

and q is the number of repeat prediction observations at a specific x_i vector. For example, using the Example 4.3 data and letting $q = 2$, or two predictions of y, we want to determine the $1 - \alpha$ confidence interval for $\hat{Y}$ in terms of the average value of the two predictors.

$\alpha = 0.05$ and $MS_E = 145.2545$

s^2 was computed from Table 4.42 and is $0.0527 = x_p'\, (X'X)^{-1} x_p$.

$$s_{\bar{p}}^2 = MS_E \left(\frac{1}{q} + x_p'(X'X)^{-1} x_p \right) = 145.2545 \left(\frac{0.0527}{2} \right)$$

$$s_{\bar{p}}^2 = 145.2545(0.0264) = 3.84 \text{ and } s_{\bar{p}} = 1.96.$$

Therefore,

$$\hat{Y}_p \pm t_{(0.025,\, 22)} s_{\bar{p}} = 17.24 \pm (2.074)1.96 = 17.24 \pm 4.06$$
$$13.18 \leq \hat{\bar{y}}_{\bar{p}} \leq 21.30.$$

PREDICTING ℓ NEW OBSERVATIONS

From Chapter 2 (linear regression), we used the Scheffe and Bonferroni simultaneous methods. The Scheffe method, for a $1 - \alpha$ simultaneous CI is

$$\hat{Y}_p \pm s' s_p,$$

where

$$s' = \ell F_{t(\alpha;\, \ell,\, n-k-1)},$$

in which ℓ is the number of x_p predictions made and k is the number of b_is in the model, excluding b_0.

$$s_p^2 = \mathrm{MS_E}\left(1 + x_p'(X'X)^{-1}x_p\right) \tag{4.29}$$

The Bonferroni method for $1 - \alpha$ simultaneous CIs is

$$\hat{Y}_p \pm B's_p,$$

where

$$B' = t_{(\alpha/2;\, 2\ell,\, n-k-1)},$$

$$s_p^2 = \mathrm{MS_E}\left(x_p'(X'X)^{-1}x_p\right).$$

ENTIRE REGRESSION SURFACE CONFIDENCE REGION

The $1 - \alpha$ entire confidence region can be computed using the Working–Hotelling confidence band procedure with x_p

$$\hat{Y}_p \pm Ws_p,$$

where

$$s_p = \mathrm{MS_E}\left(x_p'(X'X)^{-1}x_p\right) \text{ and}$$

$$W^2 = (k+1)F_{T(\alpha,\, k+1,\, n-k-1)}.$$

In Chapter 10, we review our investigations of variables in multiple regression models, using computerization software to perform all the procedures we have just learned, and more.

5 Correlation Analysis in Multiple Regression

Correlation models differ from regression models in that each variable (y_is and x_is) plays a symmetrical role, with neither variable designated as a response or predictor variable. They are viewed as relational, instead of predictive in this process. Correlation models can be very useful for making inferences about any one variable relative to another, or to a group of variables. We use the correlation models in terms of y and single or multiple x_is.

Multiple regression's use of the correlation coefficient, r, and the coefficient of determination r^2 are direct extensions of simple linear regression correlation models already discussed. The difference is, in multiple regression, that multiple x_i predictor variables, as a group, are correlated with the response variable, y. Recall that the correlation coefficient, r, by itself, has no exact interpretation, except that the closer the value of r is to 0, weaker the linear relationship between y and x_is, whereas the closer to 1, stronger the linear relationship. On the other hand, r^2 can be interpreted more directly. The coefficient of determination, say $r^2 = 0.80$, means the multiple x_i predictor variables in the model explain 80% of the y term's variability. As given in Equation 5.1, r and r^2 are very much related to the sum of squares in the analysis of variance (ANOVA) models that were used to evaluate the relationship of SS_R to SS_E in Chapter 4:

$$r^2 = \frac{SS_T - SS_E}{SS_T} = \frac{SS_R}{SS_T}. \tag{5.1}$$

For example, let
$SS_R = 5000,$
$SS_E = 200,$
$SS_T = 5200.$

Then

$$r^2 = \frac{5200 - 200}{5200} = 0.96$$

Like the F_c value, r^2 increases as predictor variables, x_is, are introduced into the regression model, regardless of the actual contribution of the added x_is. Note, however, unlike F_c, that r^2 increases toward the value of 1, which is its size limit. Hence, as briefly discussed in Chapter 4, many statisticians recommend using the adjusted R^2, or $R^2_{(adj)}$, instead of R^2. For samples, we use the lower-case term $r^2_{(adj)}$

$$r^2_{(adj)} = 1 - \frac{\frac{(SS_T - SS_R)}{(n - k - 1)}}{\frac{SS_T}{(n - 1)}} = 1 - \frac{\frac{(SS_E)}{(n - k - 1)}}{\frac{SS_T}{(n - 1)}} = 1 - \frac{MS_E}{MS_T}, \quad (5.2)$$

where k is the number of b_is, excluding b_0. $\frac{SS_T}{(n-1)}$ or MS_T is a constant, no matter how many predictor x_i variables are in the model, so the model is penalized by a lowering of the $r^2_{(adj)}$ value when adding x_i predictors that are not significantly contributing to lowering the SS_E value or, conversely, increasing SS_R. Normally, MS_T is not computed, but it is easier to write when compared with $\frac{SS_T}{n-1}$.

In Example 4.1 of the previous chapter, we looked at the data recovered from a stability study in which the mg/mL of a drug product was predicted over time based on two x_i predictor variables, x_1, the week and x_2, the humidity. Table 4.2 provided the basic regression analysis data, including R^2 and $R^2_{(adj)}$, via MiniTab

$$R^2_{(y, x_1, x_2)} = \frac{SS_T - SS_E}{SS_T} = \frac{158,380 - 39,100}{158,380} = 0.753$$

or (75.3%) and

$$R^2_{(y, x_1, x_2)(adj)} = 1 - \frac{MS_E}{MS_T} = 1 - \frac{1086}{4168} = 0.739 \text{ or } (73.9\%).$$

Hence, R^2 in the multiple linear regression model that predicts y from two independent predictor variables, x_1 and x_2, explains 75.3% or when adjusted, 73.9% of the variability in the model. The other $1 - 0.753 = 0.247$ is unexplained error. In addition, note that a fit of $r^2 = 50\%$ would infer that the prediction of y based on x and x_2 is no better than $\bar{y}$.

Multiple Correlation Coefficient
It is often less ambiguous to denote the multiple correlation coefficient, as per Kleinbaum et al. (1998), as simply the square root of the multiple coefficient of determination,

$$r^2_{(y|x_1, x_2, ..., x_k)}. \quad (5.3)$$

The nonmatrix calculation formula is

$$r_{(y|x_1, x_2, ..., x_k)} = \frac{\sum_{i=1}^{n}(y_i - \bar{y})^2 - \sum(y_i - \hat{y}_i)^2}{\sum_{i=1}^{n}(y_i - \bar{y})^2} = \frac{SS_T - SS_E}{SS_T}. \quad (5.4)$$

However, it is far easier to use the sum-of-squares equation (Equation 5.1). Also, $\sqrt{r^2}$ is always positive, $0 \leq r \leq 1$. As in Chapter 4, with the ANOVA table for $SS_{R(x_1, x_2, \ldots, x_k)}$, the sum of squares caused by the regression included all the x_i values in the model. Therefore, $r_{(y|x_1, x_2, \ldots, x_k)}$ indicates the correlation of y relative to $x_1, x_2, \ldots, x_k$, present in the model. Usually in multiple regression analysis, a correlation matrix is provided in the computer printout of basic statistics. The correlation matrix is symmetrical with the diagonals of 1, so many computer programs provide only half of the complex matrix, due to that symmetry,

$$
\begin{array}{cccc}
y & x_1 & x_2 & y_k \\
\end{array}
$$
$$
\begin{bmatrix}
1 & r_{y,1} & r_{y,2} & \cdots & r_{y,k} \\
 & 1 & r_{1,2} & \cdots & r_{1,k} \\
 & & & \vdots & \vdots & \vdots \\
 & & & & 1
\end{bmatrix}.
$$

$$
r_{k \times k} =
\begin{array}{c}
y \\
x_1 \\
\\
x_k
\end{array}
\begin{array}{cccccc}
y & x_1 & x_2 & & x_k \\
\end{array}
\begin{bmatrix}
1 & r_{y,1} & r_{y,2} & \cdots & r_{y,k} \\
r_{y1} & 1 & r_{1,2} & \cdots & r_{1,k} \\
\vdots & \vdots & \vdots & \vdots & \vdots \\
r_{y,k} & r_{1,k} & r_{2,k} & \cdots & 1
\end{bmatrix}.
$$

One can also employ partial correlation coefficient values to determine the contribution to increased r or r^2 values. This is analogous to partial F-tests in the ANOVA table evaluation in Chapter 4. The multiple r and r^2 values are also related to the sum of squares encountered in Chapter 4, in that, as r or r^2 increases, so does SS_R, and SS_E decreases.

Partial Correlation Coefficients

A partial multiple correlation coefficient measures the linear relationship between the response variable, y, and one x_i predictor variable or several x_i predictor variables, while controlling the effects of the other x_i predictor variables in the model. Take, for example, the model:

$$
Y = \beta_0 + \beta_1 x_1 + \beta_2 x_2 + \beta_3 x_3 + \beta_4 x_4.
$$

Suppose that the researcher wants to measure the correlation between y and x_2 with the other x_i variables held constant. The partial correlation coefficient would be written as

$$
r_{(y, x_2 | x_1, x_3, x_4)}. \tag{5.5}
$$

Let us continue to use the data evaluated in Chapter 4, because the correlation and F-tests are related. Many computer software packages provide output data for the partial F-tests, as well as partial correlation data when using regression models. However, if they do not, the calculations can still be made. We do not present the ANOVA tables from Chapter 4, but present the data required to construct partial correlation coefficients. We quickly see that the testing for partial regression significance conducted on the ANOVA tables in Chapter 4 provided data exactly equivalent to those from using correlation coefficients.

Several general formulas are used to determine the partial coefficients, and they are direct extensions of the F_c partial sum-of-squares computations. The population partial coefficient of determination equation for y on x_2 with x_1, x_3, x_4 in the model is

$$R^2_{(y,x_2|x_1,x_3,x_4)} = \frac{\sigma^2_{(y|x_1,x_3,x_4)} - \sigma^2_{(y|x_1,x_2,x_3,x_4)}}{\sigma^2_{(y|x_1,x_3,x_4)}}. \tag{5.6}$$

The sample formula for the partial coefficient of determination is

$$r^2_{(y,x_2|x_1,x_3,x_4)} = \frac{SS_{E(partial)} - SS_{E(full)}}{SS_{E(partial)}} = \frac{SS_{E(x_1,x_3,x_4)} - SS_{E(x_1,x_2,x_3,x_4)}}{SS_{E(x_1,x_3,x_4)}}, \tag{5.7}$$

$r^2_{(y,x_2|x_1,x_3,x_4)}$ is interpreted in these examples as the amount of variability explained or accounted for between y and x_2 when $x_1, x_3,$ and x_4 are held constant. Then, as mentioned earlier, the partial correlation coefficient is merely the square root of the partial coefficient of determination:

$$r_{(y,x_2|x_1,x_3,x_4)} = \sqrt{r^2_{(y,x_2|x_1,x_3,x_4)}}.$$

In testing for significance, it is easier to evaluate r than r^2, but for intuitive interpretation, r^2 is directly applicable.

The t test can be used to test the significance of the x_i predictor variable in contributing to r, with the other px_i predictor variables held constant. The test formula is

$$t_c = \frac{r\sqrt{n - p - 1}}{\sqrt{1 - r^2}}, \tag{5.8}$$

where n is the sample size, r is the partial correlation value, r^2 is the partial coefficient of determination, and p is the number of x_i variables held constant (not to be mistaken for its other use as representing all b_is in the model, including b_0):

$$t_T = t_{(\alpha/2;\, n-p-1)}. \tag{5.9}$$

PROCEDURE FOR TESTING PARTIAL CORRELATION COEFFICIENTS

The partial correlation coefficient testing can be accomplished via the standard six-step method. Let us hold x_1 constant and measure the contribution of x_2, the humidity, as presented in Example 4.1 (Table 4.5 and Table 4.6).

Step 1: Write out the hypothesis.
H_0: $P_{(y,x_2|x_1)} = 0$. The correlation of y and x_2 with x_1 in the model, but held constant, is 0.
H_A: $P_{(y,x_2 \mid x_1)} \neq 0$. The above is not true.

Step 2: Set α and n.
n was already set at 39 in Example 4.1, and let us use $\alpha = 0.05$.

Step 3: Write out the r^2 computation and test statistic in the sum-of-squares format. We are evaluating x_2, so the test statistic is

$$r^2_{(y,x_2|x_1)} = \frac{SS_{E(partial)} - SS_{E(full)}}{SS_{E(partial)}} = \frac{SS_{E(x_1)} - SS_{E(x_1,x_2)}}{SS_{E(x_1)}}.$$

Step 4: Decision rule.
In the correlation test, $t_T = t_{(\alpha/2, n-p-1)}$, where p is the number of b_i values held constant in the model: $t_T = t_{(0.05/2; 39-1-1)} = t_{(0.025; 37)} = 2.042$ from the Student's t table (Table B). If $t_T > 2.042$, reject H_0 at $\alpha = 0.05$.

Step 5: Compute.
From Table 4.5, we see the value for $SS_{E(x_1)} = 39{,}192$ and, from Table 4.6, we see that $SS_{E(x_1,x_2)} = 39{,}100$. Using Equation 5.7,

$$r^2_{(y,x_2|x_1)} = \frac{SS_{E(x_1)} - SS_{E(x,x_2)}}{SS_{E(x_1)}} = \frac{39{,}192 - 39{,}100}{39{,}192} = 0.0023,$$

from which it can be interpreted directly that x_2 essentially contributes nothing. The partial correlation coefficient is $r_{(y,x_2|x_1)} = \sqrt{0.0023} = 0.0480$. Using Equation 5.9, the test statistic is

$$t_c = \frac{r\sqrt{n-p-1}}{\sqrt{1-r^2}} = \frac{0.0480(\sqrt{39-2})}{\sqrt{1-0.0023}} = 0.2923.$$

Step 6: Decision.
Because $t_c = 0.2923 \not> t_T = 2.042$, one cannot reject H_0 at $\alpha = 0.05$. The contribution of x_2 to the increased correlation of the model, by its inclusion, is 0.

Multiple Partial Correlation

As noted earlier, the multiple partial coefficient of determination, r^2, usually is more of interest than the multiple partial correlation coefficient, because of its direct applicability. That is, an $r^2 = 0.83$ explains 83% of the variability. An $r = 0.83$ cannot be directly interpreted, except the closer to 0 the value is, the smaller the association; the closer r is to 1, the greater the association. The coefficient of determination computation is straightforward. From the model, $Y = \beta_0 + \beta_1 x_1 + \beta_2 x_2 + \beta_3 x_3 + \beta_4 x_4$, suppose that the researcher wants to compute $r^2_{(y, x_3, x_4 | x_1, x_2)}$, or the joint contribution of x_3 and x_4 to the model with x_1 and x_2 held constant. The form would be

$$r^2_{(y, x_3, x_4 | x_1, x_2)} = \frac{r^2_{(y | x_1, x_2, x_3, x_4)} - r^2_{(y | x_1, x_2)}}{1 - r^2_{(y | x_1, x_2)}}.$$

However, the multiple partial coefficient of determination generally is not as useful as the F-test. If the multiple partial F-test is used to evaluate the multiple contribution of independent predictor values, while holding the others (in this case x_1, x_2) constant, the general formula is

$$F_{c(y, x_i, x_j, \dots | x_a, x_b, \dots)} = \frac{\dfrac{SS_{E(x_a, x_b, \dots)} - SS_{E(x_i, x_j, \dots, x_a, x_b, \dots)}}{k}}{MS_{E(x_i, x_j, \dots, x_a, x_b, \dots)}},$$

where k is the number of x_i independent variables evaluated with y and not held constant. For the discussion given earlier,

$$F_{c(y, x_3, x_4 | x_1, x_2)} = \frac{\dfrac{SS_{E(x_1, x_2)} - SS_{E(x_1, x_2, x_3, x_4)}}{k}}{MS_{E(x_1, x_2, x_3, x_4)}}, \qquad (5.10)$$

where k is the number of independent variables being evaluated with $y = 2$. However, the calculation is not the actual r^2, but the sum of squares are equivalent. Hence, to test r^2, we use F_c.

The test hypothesis is

$H_0: P^2_{(y, x_3, x_4 | x_1, x_2)} = 0$. That is, the correlation between y and x_3, x_4, while x_1, x_2 are held constant, is 0.

$H_1: P^2_{(y, x_3, x_4 | x_1, x_2)} \neq 0$. The above is not true.

$$F_c = \frac{\dfrac{SS_{E(x_3, x_4)} - SS_{E(x_1, x_2, x_3, x_4)}}{2}}{MS_{E(x_1, x_2, x_3, x_4)}},$$

and the F_T tabled value is

$$F_{T(\alpha; k, n-k-p-1)},$$

where k is the number of x_is being correlated with y (not held constant), p is the number of x_is being held constant, and n is the sample size.

R^2 USED TO DETERMINE HOW MANY x_i VARIABLES TO INCLUDE IN THE MODEL

A simple way to help determine how many independent x_i variables to keep in the regression model can be completed with an r^2 analysis. We learn other, more efficient ways later in this book, but this is "quick and dirty." As each x_i predictor variable is added to the model, 1 degree of freedom is lost. The goal, then, is to find the minimum value of MS_E, in spite of the loss of degrees of freedom. To do this, we use the test formula:

$$x = \frac{1 - r^2}{(n - k - 1)^2}, \tag{5.11}$$

where k is the number of b_is, excluding b_0. The model we select is at the point where x is minimal. Suppose we have

$$Y = \beta_0 + \beta_1 x_1 + \beta_2 x_2 + \beta_3 x_3 + \beta_4 x_4 + \beta_5 x_5 + \beta_6 x_6 + \beta_7 x_7 + \beta_8 x_8 + \beta_9 x_9 + \beta_{10} x_{10}.$$

TABLE 5.1
Regression Table, R^2 Prediction of Number of x_i Values

k (number of b_is excluding b_0)	New Independent x_i Variable	r^2	$1 - r^2$	$n - k - 1$ ([a]degrees of freedom)	$x = \dfrac{1 - r^2}{(n - k - 1)^2}$
1	x_1	0.302	0.698	32	0.000682
2	x_2	0.400	0.600	31	0.000624
3	x_3	0.476	0.524	30	0.000582
4	x_4	0.557	0.443	29	0.000527
5	x_5	0.604	0.396	28	0.000505
6	x_6	0.650	0.350	27	0.000480
7	x_7	0.689	0.311	26	0.000460
8	x_8	0.703	0.297	25	0.000475
9	x_9	0.716	0.284	24	0.000493
10	x_{10}	0.724	0.276	23	0.000522

[a]$n = 34.$

In this procedure, we begin with x_i and add x_is through x_{10}. The procedure is straightforward; simply perform a regression on each model:

$$y = b_0 + b_1 x_1 = x_1 \text{ for } x_1,$$
$$y = b_0 + b_1 x_1 + b_2 x_2 = x_2 \text{ for } x_2,$$
$$\vdots$$
$$y = b_0 + b_1 x_1 + b_2 x_2 + \ldots + b_{10} x_{10} \text{ for } x_{10}.$$

and make a regression table (Table 5.1), using, in this case, figurative data.

From this table, we see that the predictor x_i model that includes $x_1, x_2, x_3, x_4, x_5, x_6, x_7$ provides the smallest x value; that is, it is the model where x is minimized. The r^2 and $1 - r^2$ values increase and decrease, respectively, for each additional x_i variable, but beyond seven variables, the increase in r^2 and decrease in $1 - r^2$ are not enough to offset the effects of reducing the degrees of freedom.

6 Some Important Issues in Multiple Linear Regression

COLLINEARITY AND MULTIPLE COLLINEARITY

Collinearity means that some independent predictor variables (x_i) are mutually correlated with each other, resulting in ill-conditioned data. Correlated or ill-conditioned predictor variables usually lead to unreliable b_i regression coefficients. Sometimes, the predictor variables (x_i) are so strongly correlated that a $(X'X)^{-1}$ matrix cannot be computed, because there is no unique solution. If x_i variables are not correlated, their position (first or last) in the regression equation does not matter. However, real world data are usually not perfect and often are correlated to some degree. We have seen that adding or removing x_is can change the entire regression equation, even to the extent that different x_i predictors that are significant in one model are not in another. This is because, when two or more predictors, x_i and x_j, are correlated, the contribution of each will be greater the sooner it goes into the model.

When the independent x_i variables are uncorrelated, their individual contribution to SS_R is additive. Take, for example, the model

$$\hat{y} = b_0 + b_1 x_1 + b_2 x_2. \tag{6.1}$$

Both predictor variables, x_1 and x_2, will contribute the same, that is, have the same SS_R value, if the model is

$$\hat{y} = b_0 + b_1 x_1 \tag{6.2}$$

or

$$\hat{y} = b_0 + b_2 x_2 \tag{6.3}$$

or

$$\hat{y} = b_0 + b_1 x_2 + b_2 x_1 \tag{6.4}$$

as does Equation 6.1.

TABLE 6.1A
Data from Example 4.2, the Bioreactor Experiment

Row	Temp (°C)	log$_{10}$-count	med-cn	Ca/Ph	N	Hvy-Mt	L/wk
	x_1	x_2	x_3	x_4	x_5	x_6	Y
1	20	2.1	1.0	1.00	56	4.1	56
2	21	2.0	1.0	0.98	53	4.0	61
3	27	2.4	1.0	1.10	66	4.0	65
4	26	2.0	1.8	1.20	45	5.1	78
5	27	2.1	2.0	1.30	46	5.8	81
6	29	2.8	2.1	1.40	48	5.9	86
7	37	5.1	3.7	1.80	75	3.0	110
8	37	2.0	1.0	0.30	23	5.0	62
9	45	1.0	0.5	0.25	30	5.2	50
10	20	3.7	2.0	2.00	43	1.5	41
11	20	4.1	3.0	3.00	79	0.0	70
12	25	3.0	2.8	1.40	57	3.0	85
13	35	6.3	4.0	3.00	75	0.3	115
14	26	2.1	0.6	1.00	65	0.0	55
15	40	6.0	3.8	2.90	70	0.0	120

Because the x_i variables—some or all—are correlated, it does not mean the model cannot be used. Yet, a real problem can occur when trying to model a group of data, in that the estimated b_i values can vary widely from one sample set to another, preventing the researcher from presenting one common model. Some of the variables may not even prove to be significant, when the researcher knows that they actually are. This is what happened with the x_2 variable, the $\log_{10}$ colony count, in the bioreactor experiment given in Chapter 4. In addition, the interpretation of the b_i values is no longer completely true because of the correlation between x_i variables.

To illustrate this point, let us use the data from Table 4.10 (Example 4.2, the bioreactor experiment) to regress the $\log_{10}$ colony counts (x_2) on the media concentration (x_3). For convenience, the data from Table 4.2 are presented in Table 6.1A. We let $y = x_2$, so $x_2 = b_0 + b_3 x_3$. Table 6.1B provides the regression analysis.

The coefficient of determination is $r^2 = 84.6\%$ between x_2 and x_1 and the F_c value $= 71.63$, $P < 0.0001$. A plot of the $\log_{10}$ colony counts, x_2, vs. media concentration, x_3, is presented in Figure 6.1. Plainly, the two variables are collinear; the greater the media concentration, the greater the $\log_{10}$ colony counts.

MEASURING MULTIPLE COLLINEARITY

There are several general approaches a researcher can take in measuring and evaluating collinearity between the predictor variables (x_i). First, the researcher

TABLE 6.1B
Regression Analysis of Two Predictor Variables, x_2 and x_3

Predictor	Coef	St. Dev	t-Ratio	P
b_0	0.6341	0.3375	1.88	0.083
b_3	1.2273	0.1450	8.46	0.000
$s = 0.6489$		R-sq $= 84.6\%$		R-sq(adj) $= 83.5\%$

Analysis of Variance

Source	DF	SS	MS	F	P
Regression	1	30.163	30.163	71.63	0.000
Error	13	5.475	0.421		
Total	14	35.637			

The regression equation is $x_2 = 0.634 + 1.23x_3$.

can compute a series of coefficients of determination between the x_i predictors. Given a model, say, $y = b_0 + b_1x_1 + b_2x_2 + b_3x_3 + b_4x_4$, each x_i variable is evaluated with the others, x_1 vs. x_2, x_1 vs. x_3, x_1 vs. x_4, x_2 vs. x_3, x_2 vs. x_4, and x_3 vs. x_4; that is, $r^2_{(x_1, x_2)}$, $r^2_{(x_1, x_3)}$, $r^2_{(x_1, x_4)}$, $r^2_{(x_2, x_3)}$, $r^2_{(x_2, x_4)}$, and $r^2_{(x_3, x_4)}$. The goal is to see if any of the r^2 values are exceptionally high. But, what is exceptionally high correlation? Generally, the answer is an r^2 of 0.90 or greater.

Alternatively, one can perform a series of partial correlations or partial coefficients of determination between an x_i and the other x_i variables that are held constant; that is, $r^2_{(x_1 \mid x_2, x_3, x_4)}$, $r^2_{(x_2 \mid x_1, x_3, x_4)}$, $r^2_{(x_3 \mid x_1, x_2, x_3)}$, and $r^2_{(x_4 \mid x_1, x_2, x_3)}$. Again, we are looking for high correlations.

A more formal and often used approach to measuring correlation between predictor variables is the variance inflation factor (VIF) value. It is computed as

$$\text{VIF}_{ij} = \frac{1}{1 - r^2_{ij}}, \qquad (6.5)$$

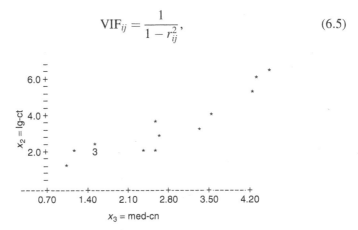

FIGURE 6.1 Plot of $\log_{10}$ colony count vs. media concentration predictor variables x_2 and x_3.

where r_{ij}^2 is the coefficient of determination for any two predictor variables, x_i and x_j, r_{ij}^2 should be 0, if there is no correlation or collinearity between x_i, x_j pairs. Any $VIF_{ij} > 10$ is of concern to the researcher, because it corresponds to a coefficient of determination of $r_{ij}^2 > 0.90$.

If $r^2 = 0.9$, the correlation coefficient is $r_{ij} = 0.95$. One may wonder why one would calculate a VIF if merely looking for an $r^2 \geq 0.90$? That is because many regression software programs automatically compute the VIF and no partial coefficients of determination. Some statisticians prefer, instead, to use the tolerance factor (TF), measuring unaccounted-for variability.

$$TF_{ij} = \frac{1}{VIF_{ij}} = 1 - r_{ij}^2. \tag{6.6}$$

TF measures the other way; that is, when r^2 approaches 1, TF goes to 0. Whether one uses r^2, VIF, or TF, it really does not matter; it is personal preference.

Examining the data given in Table 6.1B, we see $r_{(x_2, x_3)}^2 = 84.6\%$.

$$VIF = \frac{1}{1 - r_{(x_2, x_3)}^2} = \frac{1}{1 - 0.846} = 6.49,$$

which, though relatively high, is not greater than 10. $TF = 1 - r_{(x_2, x_3)}^2 = 1 - 0.846 = 0.154$. The coefficient of determination $(r_{(x_2, x_3)}^2)$ measures the accounted-for variability and $1 - r_{(x_2, x_3)}^2$ the unaccounted-for variability measures.

Other clues for detecting multicollinearity between the predictor variables (x_i) include:

1. Regression b_i coefficients that one senses have the wrong signs, based on one's prior experience.
2. The researcher's perceived importance of the predictor variables (x_i) does not hold, based on partial F tests.
3. When the removal or addition of an x_i variable makes a great change in the fitted model.
4. If high correlation exists among all possible pairs of x_i variables.

Please also note that improper scaling in regression analysis can produce great losses in computational accuracy, even giving a coefficient the wrong sign. For example, using raw microbial data such as colony count ranges of 30–1,537,097 can be very problematic, because there is such an extreme range. When $\log_{10}$ scaling is used, for example, the problem usually disappears. Also, scaling procedures may include normalizing the data with the formula,

$$x' = \frac{x_i - \bar{x}}{s}.$$

TABLE 6.2
Correlation Form Matrix of x Values

		x_1	x_2	x_3	x_4	x_5	x_6
	x_1	1.00183*	0.21487	0.18753	−0.08280	−0.17521	0.07961
	x_2	0.21487	1.00163	0.92117	0.89584	0.69533	−0.68588
$r_{xx} =$	x_3	0.18753	0.92117	1.00095	0.86033	0.62444	−0.48927
	x_4	−0.08280	0.89584	0.86033	0.74784	1.00062	−0.69729
	x_5	−0.17521	0.69533	0.62444	0.74784	1.00062	−0.69729
	x_6	0.07961	−0.68588	−0.48927	−0.73460	−0.69729	1.00121

*Note: The correlations of $x_1, x_1, x_2, x_2, \ldots$ presented in the diagonal $= 1.00$. This is not exact, in this case, because of rounding error. Note also, because the table is symmetrical about that diagonal, only the values above or below the diagonals need be used.

This situation, in Example 4.2, occurs when using multiple x_i variables: x_1 is the temperature of bioreactor (°C); x_2, the $\log_{10}$ microbial population; x_3, the medium concentration; and so forth. The ranges between x_1, x_2, and x_3 are too great.

By creating a correlation matrix of the x_i predictor variables, one can often observe directly if any of the $x_i x_j$ predictor variables are correlated. Values in the correlation matrix of 0.90 and up flag potential correlation problems, but they probably are not severe until $r > 0.95$. If there are only two x_i predictor variables, the correlation matrix is very direct; just read the x_i vs. x_j row column $= r_x x_j$, the correlation between the two $x_i x_j$ variables. When there are more than two x_i variables, then partial correlation analysis is of more use, because the other x_i variables are in the model. Nevertheless, the correlation matrix of the x_i variables is a good place to do a quick number scan, particularly if it is already printed out via the statistical software. For example, using the data from Table 6.1A, given in Example 4.2 (bioreactor problem), Table 6.2 presents the $r_x x_j$ correlation matrix of the x_i variables.

Therefore, several suspects are $r_{x2, x3} = 0.92$ and perhaps $r_{x2, x4} = 0.90$. These are intuitive statements, not requiring anything at the present except a mental note.

EIGEN (λ) ANALYSIS

Another way to evaluate multiple collinearity is by computing the eigen (λ) values of x_i predictor variable correlation matrices. An eigenvalue, λ, is a root value of an $X'X$ matrix. The smaller that value, the greater the correlation between columns of X, or the x_i predictor variables. Eigen (λ) values exist so long as $|A - \lambda I| = 0$. A is a square matrix and I is an identity matrix, and λ is the eigenvalue. For example,

$$A = \begin{bmatrix} 1 & 2 \\ 8 & 1 \end{bmatrix} - \lambda \begin{bmatrix} 1 & 0 \\ 0 & 1 \end{bmatrix} = \begin{bmatrix} 1 & 2 \\ 8 & 1 \end{bmatrix} - \begin{bmatrix} 1-\lambda & 0 \\ 0 & 1-\lambda \end{bmatrix} = \begin{bmatrix} 1-\lambda & 2 \\ 8 & 1-\lambda \end{bmatrix}.$$

The cross product of the matrix is

$$(1-\lambda)^2 - 16 = (1-\lambda^2) - 16 = 0,$$
$$(1-\lambda)(1-\lambda) - 16 = 0,$$
$$1 - \lambda - \lambda + \lambda^2 - 16 = 0,$$
$$\lambda^2 - 2\lambda - 15 = 0.$$

When $\lambda = -3$,

$$1 - 2(-3) + (-3)^2 - 16 = 0,$$
$$(-3)^2 - 2(-3) - 15 = 0,$$

and when $\lambda = 5$,

$$(5)^2 - 2(5) - 15 = 0.$$

Hence, the two eigenvalues are $[-3, 5]$

For more complex matrices, the use of a statistical software program is essential. The sum of the eigen (λ) values always sums to the number of eigenvalues. In the earlier example, there are two eigenvalues, and they sum to $-3 + 5 = 2$.

Eigen (λ) values are connected to principal component analyses (found on most statistical software programs) and are derived from the predictor x_i variables in correlation matrix form. The b_0 parameter is usually ignored, because of centering and scaling the data. For example, the equation $y = b_0 + b_1 x_1 + b_2 x_2 + \cdots + b_k x_k$ is centered via the process of subtracting the mean from the actual values of each predictor variable. $y_i - \bar{y} = b_1(x_{i_1} - \bar{x}_1) + b_2(x_{i_2} - \bar{x}_2) + \cdots + b_k(x_{i_k} - \bar{x}_k)$, where $b_0 = \bar{y}$. The equation is next scaled, or standardized:

$$\frac{y_i - \bar{y}}{s_y} = b_1 \left(\frac{s_1}{s_y}\right) \frac{(x_{i_1} - \bar{x}_1)}{s_1} + b_2 \left(\frac{s_2}{s_y}\right) \frac{(x_{i_2} - \bar{x}_2)}{s_2} + \cdots + b_k \left(\frac{s_k}{s_y}\right) \frac{(x_{i_k} - \bar{x}_k)}{s_k}.$$

The principal components are actually a set of new variables, which are linear combinations of the original x_i predictors. The principal components have two characteristics: (1) they are not correlated with one another and (2) each has a maximum variance, given they are uncorrelated. The eigenvalues are the variances of the principal components. The larger the eigen (λ) value, the more important is the principal component in representing the information in the x_i predictors. When eigen (λ) values approach 0, collinearity is present around the original x_i predictor scale, where 0 represents perfect collinearity.

Eigen (λ) values are important in several methods of evaluating multicollinearity, which we discuss. These include the following:

1. The condition index (CI)
2. The condition number (CN)
3. The variance proportions

CONDITION INDEX

CI can be computed for each eigen (λ) value. First, the eigenvalues are listed from largest to smallest, where $\lambda_1 =$ the largest eigenvalue, and $\lambda_j =$ the smallest. Hence, $\lambda_1 = \lambda_{\max}$. CI is simple; the $\lambda_{\max}$ is divided by each λ_j value. That is, $\text{CI} = \dfrac{\lambda_{\max}}{\lambda_j}$, where $j = 1, 2, \ldots, k$.

Using the MiniTab output for regression of the data from Example 4.2 (Table 6.1A), the bioreactor example, the original full model was

$$\hat{y} = b_0 + b_1 x_1 + b_2 x_2 + b_3 x_3 + b_4 x_4 + b_5 x_5 + b_6 x_6,$$

where y is the liters of media per week; x_1 is the temperature of bioreactor (°C); x_2 the $\log_{10}$ microbial colony counts per cm^2 per coupon; x_3, the media concentration; x_4, the calcium and phosphorous ratio; x_5, the nitrogen level; and x_6 is the heavy metal concentration. The regression analysis is recreated in Table 6.3.

Table 6.4 consists of the computed eigen (λ) values as presented in MiniTab. The condition indices are computed as

$$\text{CI}_j = \frac{\lambda_{\max}}{\lambda_j},$$

where $\lambda_j = 1, 2, \ldots, k$, and $\lambda_1 = \lambda_{\max}$, or the largest eigenvalue, and λ_k is the smallest eigenvalue. Some authors use CI as the square root of

TABLE 6.3
MiniTab Output of Actual Computations, Table 6.1A Data

Predictor	Coef	St. Dev	t-Ratio	P	VIF
b_0	−23.15	26.51	−0.87	0.408	
Temp (°C)	0.8749	0.4877	1.79	0.111	1.9
Lg-ct	2.562	6.919	0.37	0.721	15.6
Med-cn	14.567	7.927	1.84	0.103	11.5
Ca/Ph	−5.35	10.56	−0.51	0.626	11.1
N	0.5915	0.2816	2.10	0.069	2.8
Hvy-Mt	3.625	2.517	1.44	0.188	4.0
s = 10.46		R-sq = 89.3%		R-sq(adj) = 81.2%	

Analysis of Variance

Source	DF	SS	MS	F	P
Regression	6	7266.3	1211.1	11.07	0.002
Error	8	875.0	109.4		
Total	14	8141.3			

Note: The regression equation is L/wk = −23.1 + 0.875 temp °C + 2.56 $\log_{10}$-ct + 14.6 med-cn − 5.3 Ca/Ph + 0.592 N + 3.62 Hvy-Mt.

$$\frac{\lambda_{\max}}{\lambda_j} \quad \text{or} \quad CI_j = \sqrt{\frac{\lambda_{\max}}{\lambda_j}}.$$

It is suggested that those who are unfamiliar compute both, until they find their preference.

TABLE 6.4
Eigen Analysis of the Correlation Matrix

	x_1	x_2	x_3	x_4	x_5	x_6
Eigenvalue (λ_j)	3.9552	1.1782	0.4825	0.2810	0.0612	0.0419
[a]Proportion	0.659	0.196	0.080	0.047	0.010	0.007
[b]Cumulative	0.659	0.856	0.936	0.983	0.993	1.000

Note: $\Sigma \lambda_j = 3.9552 + 1.1782 + \cdots + 0.0419 = 6$, and ranked from left to right, $\lambda_{\max} = 3.9552$ at x_j.
[a]Proportion is ratio of $\dfrac{\lambda_j}{\Sigma \lambda_j} = \dfrac{3.9552}{6.000} = 0.6592$ for x_1.
[b]Cumulative is the sum of proportions. For example, cumulative for x_3 would equal the sum of proportions at x_1, x_2, and x_3, or $0.659 + 0.196 + 0.08 = 0.936$.

CI = Variance Ratio	$\sqrt{CI}$ = Standard Deviation Ratio
$CI_1 = \dfrac{\lambda_{max}}{\lambda_1} = \dfrac{3.9552}{3.9552} = 1$	1
$CI_1 = \dfrac{\lambda_{max}}{\lambda_2} = \dfrac{3.9552}{1.1782} = 3.36$	1.83
$CI_1 = \dfrac{\lambda_{max}}{\lambda_3} = \dfrac{3.9552}{0.4825} = 8.20$	2.86
$CI_1 = \dfrac{\lambda_{max}}{\lambda_4} = \dfrac{3.9552}{0.2810} = 14.08$	3.75
$CI_1 = \dfrac{\lambda_{max}}{\lambda_5} = \dfrac{3.9552}{0.0612} = 64.63$	8.04
$CI_1 = \dfrac{\lambda_{max}}{\lambda_6} = \dfrac{3.9552}{0.0419} = 94.40$	9.72

Eigen (λ) values represent variances; CIs are ratios of the variances, and $\sqrt{CI}$, the standard deviation ratios. The larger the ratio, the greater the problem of multicollinearity, but how large is large? We consider this in a moment.

CONDITION NUMBER

The CN is the largest variance ratio and is calculated by dividing λ_{max} by λ_k, the smallest λ value. For these data,

$$CN = \frac{\lambda_{max}}{\lambda_{min}} = \frac{3.9552}{0.0419} = 94.40$$

for a CN variance ratio, and 9.72 for a $\sqrt{CN}$ standard deviation. Condition numbers less than 100 imply no multiple collinearity; between 100 and 1000, moderate collinearity; and over 1000, severe collinearity. Belsley et al. (1980) recommend that a $\sqrt{CN}$ of >30 be interpreted to mean moderate to severe collinearity is present. The $\sqrt{CN}$ number here is 9.72, so the multiple collinearity between the x_i predictor variables is not excessive.

VARIANCE PROPORTION

Another useful tool is the variance proportion for each x_i, which is the proportion of the total variance of its b_i estimate, for a particular principal component. Note that in Table 6.4, the first column is

	x_1
Eigen (λ) value	3.9552
Proportion	0.659
Cumulative	0.659

The eigen (λ) value is the variance of the principal component. A principal component analysis is simply a new value of the x_i predictors that are linear combinations of the original x_i predictors. Eigenvalues approaching 0 indicate collinearity. As eigenvalues decrease, CIs increase. The variance proportion is the amount of total variability explained by the principal component eigenvalue of the predictor variable, x_1, which is 65.9%, in this case. The cumulative row is the contribution of several or all the eigenvalues to and including a specific x_i predictor. The sum of all the proportions will equal 1. The sum of the eigenvalues equals the number of eigenvalues. Looking at Table 6.4, we note that, while the eigenvalues range from 3.96 to 0.04, they are not out of line. An area of possible interest is x_5 and x_6, because the eigenvalues are about five to seven times smaller than that of x_4. We also note that the contribution to the variability of the model is greatest for x_1 and x_2 and declines considerably through the remaining variables.

STATISTICAL METHODS TO OFFSET SERIOUS COLLINEARITY

When collinearity is severe, regression procedures must be modified. Two ways to do this are (1) rescaling the data (2) using ridge regression.

RESCALING THE DATA FOR REGRESSION

Rescaling of the data should be performed, particularly when some predictor variable values have large ranges, relative to other predictor variables. For example, the model $\hat{y} = b_0 + b_1 x_1 + b_2 x_2 + \cdots + b_k x_k$ rescaled is

$$\frac{y - \bar{y}}{s_y} = b_1' \left(\frac{x_{i_1} - \bar{x}_1}{s_1} \right) + b_2' \left(\frac{x_{i_2} - \bar{x}_2}{s_2} \right) + \cdots + b_k' \left(\frac{x_{i_k} - \bar{x}_k}{s_k} \right),$$

where the computed b_j' values are

$$b_j' = b_j \left(\frac{s_j}{s_y} \right) \quad \text{and} \quad s_j = \sqrt{\frac{\sum (x_{ij} - \bar{x}_j)^2}{n_j - 1}}$$

for each of the j through k predictor variables, and

$$s_y = \sqrt{\frac{\sum (y - \bar{y})^2}{n - 1}}.$$

Once the data have been rescaled, perform the regression analysis and check again for collinearity. If it is present, move to ridge regression.

RIDGE REGRESSION

Ridge regression is also used extensively to remedy multicollinearity between the x_i predictor variables. It does this by modifying the least-squares method of computing the b_i coefficients with the addition of a biasing component.

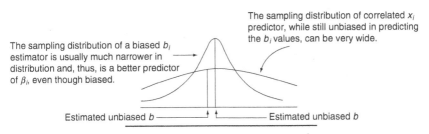

The sampling distribution of correlated x_i predictor, while still unbiased in predicting the b_i values, can be very wide.

The sampling distribution of a biased b_i estimator is usually much narrower in distribution and, thus, is a better predictor of β_i, even though biased.

Estimated unbiased b ———————— Estimated unbiased b

FIGURE 6.2 Biased estimators of b_i in ridge regression.

Serious collinearity often makes the confidence intervals for the b_is too wide to be practical. In ridge regression, the β_i estimates are biased purposely, but even so, will provide a much tighter confidence interval in which the true β_i value resides, though it is biased.

The probability of b_i^b (b_i biased), as it is closer to the actual population β_i parameter than b_i^u (b_i unbiased), is greater using ridge regression, because the confidence interval for the biased estimator is tighter (Figure 6.2). Hence, the rationale of ridge regression is simply that, if a biased estimator can provide a more precise estimate than can an unbiased one, yet still include the true β_i, it should be used. In actual field conditions, multicollinearity problems are common, and although regression models' predicted b_is are valid, the variance of those b_i values may be too high to be useful, when using the least-squares approach to fit the model. Recall the least-squares procedure, which is an unbiased estimate of the population β_i values, is of the form

$$\beta = (X'X)^{-1}X'Y. \tag{6.7}$$

The ridge regression procedure modifies the least-squares regression equation by introducing a constant (c) where $c \geq 0$. Generally, c is $0 \leq c \leq 1$. The population ridge regression equation, then, is in correlation form

$$\widehat{\beta}^r = (X'X + cI)^{-1}X'Y, \tag{6.8}$$

where c is the constant, the ridge estimator, I is the identity matrix in which the diagonal values are 1 and the off-diagonals are 0,

$$I = \begin{bmatrix} 1 & 0 & \cdots & 0 \\ 0 & 1 & \cdots & 0 \\ \vdots & \vdots & \cdots & \vdots \\ 0 & 0 & \cdots & 1 \end{bmatrix}$$

$\widehat{b}_i^r$ are the regression coefficients, linearly transformed by the biasing constant, c. The error term of the population ridge estimator, $\widehat{\beta}^r$ is

Mean square error =	Var($\widehat{\boldsymbol{\beta}}^r$)	+	(bias in $\widehat{\boldsymbol{\beta}}^r$)^2
	↓		↓
	due to variability of the data		due to the biasing effect of the ridge estimator constant

Note that when $c = 0$, the $c\boldsymbol{I}$ matrix drops out of the equation, returning the ridge procedure back to the normal least-squares equation. That is, when $c = 0$, $(\boldsymbol{X'X} + c\boldsymbol{I})^{-1} \boldsymbol{X'Y} = (\boldsymbol{X'X})^{-1} \boldsymbol{X'Y}$.

As c increases in value (moves toward 1.0), the bias of $\boldsymbol{b}^r$ increases, but the variability decreases. The goal is to fit the $\boldsymbol{b}^r$ estimators so that the decrease in variance is not offset by the increase in bias. Although the $\boldsymbol{b}^r$ estimates will not be usually the best or most accurate fit, they will stabilize the $\boldsymbol{b}^r$ parameter estimates.

Setting the c value is a trial-and-error process. Although c is generally a value between 0 and 1, many statisticians urge the researcher to assess 20 to 25 values of c. As c increases from 0 to 1, its effect on the regression parameters can vary dramatically. The selection procedure for a c value requires a ridge trace to find a c value where the b_i^r values are stabilized.

VIF values, previously discussed, are helpful in determining the best c value to use.

RIDGE REGRESSION PROCEDURE

To employ the ridge regression, first (Step 1), the values are transformed to correlation form. Correlation for the y_i value is

$$y_i^* = \frac{1}{\sqrt{n-1}} \left(\frac{y_i - \bar{y}}{s_y} \right), \quad \text{where } s_y = \sqrt{\frac{\sum (y - \bar{y})^2}{n-1}}.$$

The $\boldsymbol{Y}^*$ vector in correlation form is presented in Table 6.5.

The x_i values for each predictor variable are next transformed to correlation form using

$$x_{i_k}^* = \frac{1}{\sqrt{n-1}} \left(\frac{x_{i_k} - \bar{x}_k}{s_{x_k}} \right)$$

For example, referring to data from Table 6.1A, the first x_i in the data for the x_1 variable is

$$x_{11}^* = \frac{1}{\sqrt{15-1}} \left(\frac{20 - 29.00}{7.97} \right) = -0.3018.$$

TABLE 6.5
Y* Vector in Correlation Form

$$
Y^* = \begin{bmatrix}
-0.218075 \\
-0.162642 \\
-0.118295 \\
0.025832 \\
0.059092 \\
0.114525 \\
0.380606 \\
-0.151555 \\
-0.284595 \\
-0.384375 \\
-0.062862 \\
0.103439 \\
0.436039 \\
-0.229162 \\
0.491473
\end{bmatrix}
$$

The entire $15 \times 6X$ matrix is presented in Table 6.6. The transpose of X^* as $X^{*'}$ is presented in Table 6.7, a 6×15 matrix. The actual correlation matrix is presented in Table 6.8.

TABLE 6.6
Entire $15 \times 6X$ Matrix Correlation, Table 6.1A Data

$$
X^*_{15 \times 6} = \begin{bmatrix}
-0.301844 & -0.169765 & -0.227965 & -0.154258 & 0.009667 & 0.117154 \\
-0.268306 & -0.186523 & -0.227965 & -0.160319 & -0.038669 & 0.105114 \\
-0.067077 & -0.119489 & -0.227965 & -0.123952 & 0.170788 & 0.105114 \\
-0.100615 & -0.186523 & -0.049169 & -0.093646 & -0.167566 & 0.237560 \\
-0.067077 & -0.169765 & -0.004470 & -0.063340 & -0.151454 & 0.321844 \\
0.000000 & -0.052454 & 0.017880 & -0.033034 & -0.119230 & 0.333884 \\
0.268306 & 0.332994 & 0.375472 & 0.088191 & 0.315797 & -0.015291 \\
0.268306 & -0.186523 & -0.227965 & -0.366401 & -0.522033 & 0.225519 \\
0.536612 & -0.354110 & -0.339712 & -0.381554 & -0.409248 & 0.249600 \\
-0.301844 & 0.098373 & -0.004470 & 0.148803 & -0.199790 & -0.195900 \\
-0.301844 & 0.165408 & 0.219025 & 0.451864 & 0.380246 & -0.376508 \\
-0.134153 & -0.018937 & 0.174326 & -0.033034 & 0.025779 & -0.015291 \\
0.201230 & 0.534097 & 0.442520 & 0.451864 & 0.315797 & -0.340386 \\
-0.100615 & -0.169765 & -0.317363 & -0.154258 & 0.154676 & -0.376508 \\
0.368921 & 0.483821 & 0.397821 & 0.421558 & 0.235237 & -0.376508
\end{bmatrix}
$$

TABLE 6.7
Transposed $X^{*'}$ Matrix Correlation, Table 6.1A Data

$$X_{6\times15}^{*'} =$$

-0.301844	-0.268306	-0.067077	-0.100615	-0.067077	0.000000	0.268306	0.268306	0.536612	-0.301844	-0.301844	-0.134153	0.201230	-0.100615	0.368921
-0.169765	-0.186523	-0.119489	-0.186523	-0.169765	-0.052454	0.332994	-0.186523	-0.354110	0.098373	0.165408	-0.018937	0.534097	-0.169765	0.483821
-0.227965	-0.227965	-0.227965	-0.049169	-0.004470	0.017880	0.375472	-0.227965	-0.339712	-0.004470	0.219025	0.174326	0.442520	-0.317363	0.397821
-0.154258	-0.160319	-0.123952	-0.093646	-0.063340	-0.033034	0.088191	-0.366401	-0.381554	0.148803	0.451864	-0.033034	0.451864	-0.154258	0.421558
0.009667	-0.038669	0.170788	-0.167566	-0.151454	-0.119230	0.315797	-0.522033	-0.409248	-0.199790	0.380246	0.025779	0.315797	0.154676	0.235237
0.117154	0.105114	0.105114	0.237560	0.321844	0.333884	-0.015291	0.225519	0.249600	-0.195900	-0.376508	-0.015291	-0.340386	-0.376508	-0.376508

TABLE 6.8
$X^{*\prime}X^* = r_{xx}$ **Correlation Matrix,* Table 6.1A Data**

$$X^{*\prime}X^* = r_{xx} = \begin{bmatrix} 1.00109 & 0.21471 & 0.18739 & -0.082736 & -0.175081 & 0.07955 \\ 0.21471 & 1.00088 & 0.92049 & 0.895167 & 0.694807 & -0.68536 \\ 0.18739 & 0.92049 & 1.00020 & 0.859690 & 0.623977 & -0.48890 \\ -0.08274 & 0.89517 & 0.85969 & 0.999449 & 0.747278 & -0.73405 \\ -0.17508 & 0.69481 & 0.62398 & 0.747278 & 0.999876 & -0.69677 \\ 0.07955 & -0.68536 & -0.48890 & -0.734054 & -0.696765 & 1.00046 \end{bmatrix}$$

*Note: This correlation form and the correlation form in Table 6.2 should be identical. They differ here because Table 6.2 was done in an autoselection of MiniTab and Table 6.8 was done via manual matrix manipulation using MiniTab.

The Y^* correlation form matrix must then be correlated with each x_i variable to form an r_{yx} matrix. The easiest way to do this is by computing the matrix, $X^{*\prime}Y^* = r_{yx}$ (Table 6.9). The next step (Step 2) is to generate sets of b^r data for the various c values chosen using the equation, $b^r = (r_{xx} + cI)^{-1} r_{yx}$, where r_{xx} = Table 6.8, which we call M_1 for Matrix 1. It will be used repeatedly with different values of c, as reproduced in Table 6.10.

(y, x_1) = correlation of temp °C and L/wk = 0.432808,
(y, x_2) = correlation of lg-ct and L/wk = 0.775829,
(y, x_3) = correlation of med-cn and L/wk = 0.855591,
(y, x_4) = correlation of Ca/Ph and L/wk = 0.612664,
(y, x_5) = correlation of N and L/wk = 0.546250,
(y, x_6) = correlation of Hvy-Mt and L/wk = −0.252518.
We call this r_{yx} matrix as M_2.

TABLE 6.9
$X^{*\prime}Y^* = r_{yx}$ **Matrix**

$$X^{*\prime}Y^* = r_{yx} = \begin{bmatrix} 0.432808 \\ 0.775829 \\ 0.855591 \\ 0.612664 \\ 0.546250 \\ -0.252518 \end{bmatrix}$$

TABLE 6.10
$r_{xx} = M_1$ **Matrix**

$$
M_1 = \begin{bmatrix}
1.00109 & 0.21471 & 0.18739 & -0.082736 & -0.175081 & 0.07955 \\
0.21471 & 1.00088 & 0.92049 & 0.895167 & 0.694807 & -0.68536 \\
0.18739 & 0.92049 & 1.00020 & 0.859690 & 0.623977 & -0.48890 \\
-0.08274 & 0.89517 & 0.85969 & 0.999449 & 0.747278 & -0.73405 \\
-0.17508 & 0.69481 & 0.62398 & 0.747278 & 0.999876 & -0.69677 \\
0.07955 & -0.68536 & -0.48890 & -0.734054 & -0.696765 & 1.00046
\end{bmatrix}
$$

*Note that the diagonals are not exactly 1.000, due to round off error. Note that in Table 6.9, $X^{*'}Y^* = r_{yx}$, which is in correlation form of $(y, x_1), (y, x_2), \ldots, (y, x_6)$.

$$
r_{yx} = M_2 = \begin{bmatrix}
0.432808 \\
0.775829 \\
0.855591 \\
0.612664 \\
0.546250 \\
-0.252518
\end{bmatrix}.
$$

In Step 3, we construct I matrix with the same dimensions as M_1, which is 6×6. So $I = I_{6 \times 6}$, as the identity matrix.

$$
I = M_3 = \begin{bmatrix}
1 & 0 & 0 & 0 & 0 & 0 \\
0 & 1 & 0 & 0 & 0 & 0 \\
0 & 0 & 1 & 0 & 0 & 0 \\
0 & 0 & 0 & 1 & 0 & 0 \\
0 & 0 & 0 & 0 & 1 & 0 \\
0 & 0 & 0 & 0 & 0 & 1
\end{bmatrix}.
$$

And, finally, the c values are arbitrarily set. We use 15 values.

$$
\begin{aligned}
c_i & \\
c_1 &= 0.002 \\
c_2 &= 0.004 \\
c_3 &= 0.006 \\
c_4 &= 0.008 \\
c_5 &= 0.01 \\
c_6 &= 0.02 \\
c_7 &= 0.03 \\
c_8 &= 0.04 \\
c_9 &= 0.05 \\
c_{10} &= 0.10
\end{aligned}
$$

$$c_{11} = 0.20$$
$$c_{12} = 0.30$$
$$c_{13} = 0.40$$
$$c_{14} = 0.50$$
$$c_{15} = 1.00$$

For actual practice, it is suggested that one assesses more than 15 values of c, between 20 and 25. We perform the calculations manually.

The MiniTab matrix sequence will be

$$b^r = [r_{xx} + cI]^{-1}r_{yx},$$
$$b^r = [M_1 + c_iM_3]^{-1}M_2. \tag{6.9}$$

Let us continue with the bioreactor example, Example 4.2.

When $c_1 = 0.002$, $b^r = \begin{bmatrix} 0.289974 \\ 0.174390 \\ 0.710936 \\ -0.186128 \\ 0.404726 \\ 0.336056 \end{bmatrix} \begin{matrix} = b_1^r \\ = b_2^r \\ = b_3^r \\ = b_4^r \\ = b_5^r \\ = b_6^r \end{matrix}$; when $c_2 = 0.004$, $b^r = \begin{bmatrix} 0.290658 \\ 0.178783 \\ 0.700115 \\ -0.177250 \\ 0.402442 \\ 0.337967 \end{bmatrix}$;

When $c_3 = 0.006$, $b^r = \begin{bmatrix} 0.291280 \\ 0.182719 \\ 0.690048 \\ -0.168892 \\ 0.400170 \\ 0.339559 \end{bmatrix}$; when $c_4 = 0.008$, $b^r = \begin{bmatrix} 0.291845 \\ 0.186262 \\ 0.680652 \\ -0.161008 \\ 0.397910 \\ 0.340871 \end{bmatrix}$;

When $c_5 = 0.01$, $b^r = \begin{bmatrix} 0.292356 \\ 0.189461 \\ 0.671854 \\ -0.153557 \\ 0.395665 \\ 0.341934 \end{bmatrix}$; when $c_6 = 0.02$, $b^r = \begin{bmatrix} 0.294222 \\ 0.201617 \\ 0.634958 \\ -0.121655 \\ 0.384697 \\ 0.344385 \end{bmatrix}$;

When $c_7 = 0.03$, $b^r = \begin{bmatrix} 0.295188 \\ 0.209556 \\ 0.606500 \\ -0.096498 \\ 0.374212 \\ 0.343577 \end{bmatrix}$; when $c_8 = 0.04$, $b^r = \begin{bmatrix} 0.295510 \\ 0.215000 \\ 0.583598 \\ -0.076085 \\ 0.364243 \\ 0.340801 \end{bmatrix}$;

When $c_9 = 0.05, b^r = \begin{bmatrix} 0.295363 \\ 0.218864 \\ 0.564570 \\ -0.059148 \\ 0.354788 \\ 0.336797 \end{bmatrix}$; when $c_{10} = 0.01, b^r = \begin{bmatrix} 0.290869 \\ 0.227214 \\ 0.500677 \\ -0.004375 \\ 0.314521 \\ 0.309674 \end{bmatrix}$;

When $c_{11} = 0.20, b^r = \begin{bmatrix} 0.276211 \\ 0.227515 \\ 0.432292 \\ -0.044859 \\ 0.259265 \\ 0.255204 \end{bmatrix}$; when $c_{12} = 0.30, b^r = \begin{bmatrix} 0.261073 \\ 0.222857 \\ 0.390445 \\ 0.067336 \\ 0.223772 \\ 0.211990 \end{bmatrix}$;

When $c_{13} = 0.40, b^r = \begin{bmatrix} 0.246982 \\ 0.217031 \\ 0.359922 \\ 0.079653 \\ 0.199222 \\ 0.178388 \end{bmatrix}$; when $c_{14} = 0.50, b^r = \begin{bmatrix} 0.234114 \\ 0.210979 \\ 0.335864 \\ 0.086986 \\ 0.181255 \\ 0.151822 \end{bmatrix}$;

When $c_{15} = 1.000, b^r = \begin{bmatrix} 0.184920 \\ 0.183733 \\ 0.260660 \\ 0.097330 \\ 0.134102 \\ 0.075490 \end{bmatrix}$.

Note that each of the c_i values is chosen arbitrarily by the researcher. The next step (Step 4) is to plot the ridge trace data (Table 6.11). The b_i^r values are rounded to three places to the right of the decimal point.

If there are only a few b_i^r variables, they can all be plotted on the same graph. If there are, say, more than four and if they have the same curvature, it is better to plot them individually first, then perform a multiplot of all b_i^r values vs. the c values.

The ridge trace data will first be graphed b_i^i vs. c, then plotted multiply. Figure 6.3 presents b_i^r vs. c. Figure 6.4 presents b_2^r vs. c. Figure 6.5 presents b_3^r vs. c. Figure 6.6 presents b_4^r vs. c. Figure 6.7 presents b_5^r vs. c. Figure 6.8 presents b_6^r vs. c. Putting it all together, we get Figure 6.9, the complete ridge trace plot.

The next step (Step 5), using the complete ridge trace plot, is to pick the smallest value c, in which the betas, b_i^r, are stable—that is, no longer oscillating wildly or with high rates of change. In practice, the job will be

TABLE 6.11
b_r and c Values

c	b_1^r	b_2^r	b_3^r	b_4^r	b_5^r	b_6^r
0.002	0.290	0.174	0.711	−0.186	0.405	0.336
0.004	0.291	0.179	0.700	−0.177	0.402	0.338
0.006	0.291	0.183	0.690	−0.169	0.400	0.310
0.008	0.292	0.186	0.681	−0.161	0.398	0.341
0.010	0.292	0.189	0.672	−0.154	0.396	0.342
0.020	0.294	0.202	0.635	−0.122	0.385	0.344
0.030	0.295	0.210	0.607	−0.096	0.374	0.344
0.040	0.296	0.215	0.584	−0.076	0.364	0.341
0.050	0.295	0.219	0.565	−0.059	0.355	0.337
0.100	0.291	0.227	0.501	−0.004	0.315	0.310
0.200	0.276	0.228	0.432	0.045	0.259	0.255
0.300	0.261	0.223	0.390	0.067	0.224	0.212
0.400	0.247	0.217	0.360	0.080	0.199	0.178
0.500	0.234	0.211	0.336	0.087	0.181	0.152
1.000	0.185	0.184	0.261	0.097	0.134	0.075

much easier if the researcher omits the x_i predictors that, earlier on, were found not to contribute significantly to the regression model, as indicated by increases in SS_R or decreases in SS_E. But for our purposes, we assume all are

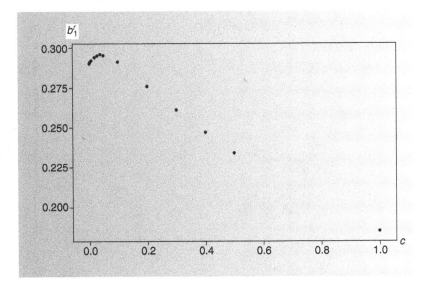

FIGURE 6.3 b_1^r vs. c.

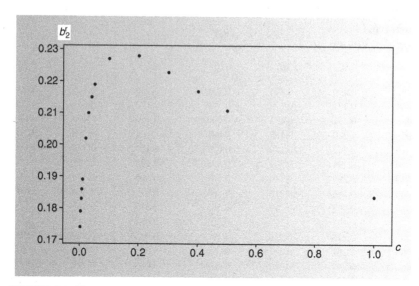

FIGURE 6.4 b_2^r vs. c.

important, and we must select a c value to represent all six b_i^rs. So, where is the ridge trace plot first stable? Choosing too small a c value does not reduce the instability of the model, but selecting too large a c value can add too much bias, limiting the value of the b_i^rs in modeling the experiment. Some

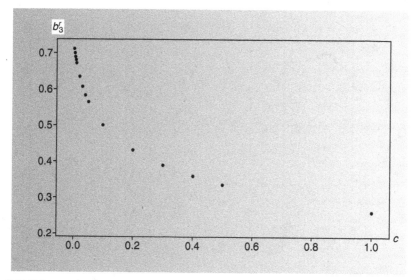

FIGURE 6.5 b_3^r vs. c.

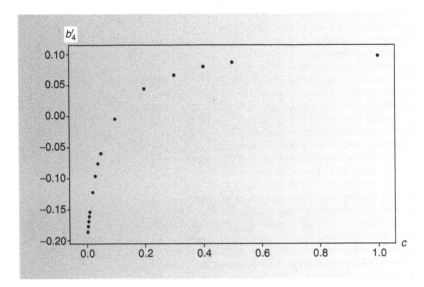

FIGURE 6.6 b_4^r vs. c.

researchers select the c values intuitively; others (Hoerl et al., 1975) suggest a formal procedure.

We employ a formal procedure, computed by iteration, to find the most appropriate value of c to use, and we term that value c'. That is, a series of

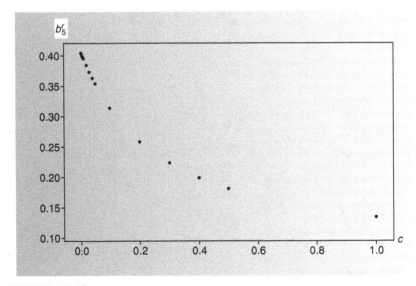

FIGURE 6.7 b_5^r vs. c.

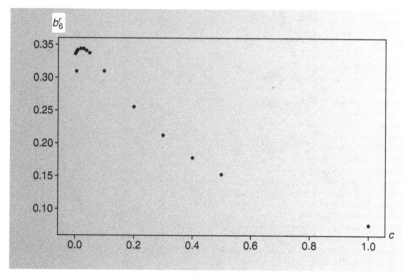

FIGURE 6.8 b_6^r vs. c.

iterations will be performed, until we find the first iterative value of c that satisfies Equation 6.10 (Hoerl and Kennard, 1976):

$$\frac{c_i - c_{i-1}}{c_{i-1}} \leq 20T^{-1.3}, \tag{6.10}$$

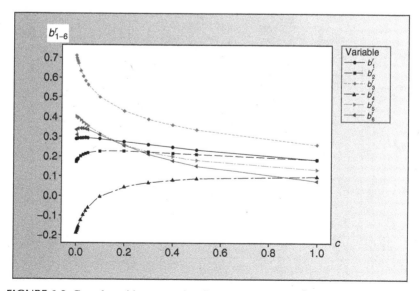

FIGURE 6.9 Complete ridge trace plot: Scatterplot of c vs. b^r values.

where

$$T = \frac{\text{trace}(X'X)^{-1}}{k} = \frac{\sum_{i=1}^{k} \frac{1}{\lambda_i}}{k}. \tag{6.11}$$

Let

$$c_i = \frac{k(\text{MS}_E)}{[b_0^r]'[b_0^r]}. \tag{6.12}$$

Note: k is the number of predictor b_i^r variables, less b_0 which equals 6 (b_1^r through b_6^r) in our example. MS_E is the mean square error, s^2, of the full regression on the correlation form of the x_i and y values, when the ridge regression computed sets $c = 0$. That is

$$[r_{xx} + cI]^{-1}r_{yx} = [r_{xx}]^{-1}r_{yx}.$$

$b_0^r =$ the beta coefficients of the ridge regression when $c = 0$.
The next iteration is

$$c_i = \frac{k(\text{MS}_E)}{[b_1^r]'[b_1^r]},$$

where k is the number of b_is, excluding b_0; MS_E is the mean square error, when $c = 0$; $b_1^r = [r_{xx} - c_1 I]^{-1}r_{yx}$, the matrix equation for ridge regression. The next iteration is

$$c_i = \frac{k(\text{MS}_E)}{[b_2^r]'[b_2^r]}, \text{ and so on.}$$

The iteration process is complete, when the first iteration results in

$$\frac{c_i - c_{i-1}}{c_{i-1}} \leq 20T^{-1.3}$$

To do that procedure, we run a regression on the transformed values, y and x, from Table 6.5 and Table 6.6, respectively. Table 6.12 combines those tables.

The researcher then regresses y on x_1, x_2, x_3, x_4, x_5, and x_6. Table 6.13 presents that regression. It gives us the b_i^r coefficients (notice $b_0 \approx 0$), as well as the MS_E value, using a standard procedure.*

---

*The analysis could also have been done using matrix form $b^r = [r_{xx}]^{-1} [r_{yx}]$, but the author has chosen to use a standard MiniTab routine to show that the regression can be done this way, too.

TABLE 6.12
Correlation Form Transformed y and x Values

Row	x_1	x_2	x_3	x_4	x_5	x_6	y
1	−0.301844	−0.169765	−0.227965	−0.154258	0.009667	0.117154	−0.218075
2	−0.268306	−0.186523	−0.227965	−0.160319	−0.038669	0.105114	−0.162642
3	−0.067077	−0.119489	−0.227965	−0.123952	0.170788	0.105114	−0.118295
4	−0.100615	−0.186523	−0.049169	−0.093646	−0.167566	0.237560	0.025832
5	−0.067077	−0.169765	−0.004470	−0.063340	−0.151454	0.321844	0.059092
6	0.000000	−0.052454	0.017880	−0.033034	−0.119230	0.333884	0.114525
7	0.268306	0.332994	0.375472	0.088191	0.315797	−0.015291	0.380606
8	0.268306	−0.186523	−0.227965	−0.366401	−0.522033	0.225519	−0.151555
9	0.536612	−0.354110	−0.339712	−0.381554	−0.409248	0.249600	−0.284595
10	−0.301844	0.098373	−0.004470	0.148803	−0.199790	−0.195900	−0.384375
11	−0.301844	0.165408	0.219025	0.451864	0.380246	−0.376508	−0.062862
12	−0.134153	−0.018937	0.174326	−0.033034	0.025779	−0.015291	0.103439
13	0.201230	0.534097	0.442520	0.451864	0.315797	−0.340386	0.436039
14	−0.100615	−0.169765	−0.317363	−0.154258	0.154676	−0.376508	−0.229162
15	0.368921	0.483821	0.397821	0.421558	0.235237	−0.376508	0.491473

TABLE 6.13
Regression on Transformed y, x Data

Predictor	Coef	St dev	t-ratio	P
b_0	−0.00005	0.02994	−0.00	0.999
b_1	0.2892	0.1612	1.79	0.111
b_2	0.1695	0.4577	0.37	0.721
b_3	0.7226	0.3932	1.84	0.103
b_4	−0.1956	0.3861	−0.51	0.626
b_5	0.4070	0.1937	2.10	0.069
b_6	0.3338	0.2317	1.44	0.188

$s = 0.115947$ R-sq $= 89.3\%$ R-sq(adj) $= 81.2\%$

Analysis of Variance

Source	DF	SS	MS	F	P
Regression	6	0.89314	0.14886	11.07	0.002
Error	8	0.10755	0.01344		
Total	14	1.00069			

The regression equation is $\hat{y} = -0.0001 + 0.289x_1 + 0.169x_2 + 0.723x_3 - 0.196x_4 + 0.407x_5 + 0.334x_6$.

Iteration 1, from Table 6.13,

$$b_0^r = \begin{bmatrix} 0.2892 \\ 0.1695 \\ 0.7226 \\ -0.1956 \\ 0.4070 \\ 0.3338 \end{bmatrix}.$$

So,

$$[b_0^r]'[b_0^r] = [0.2892 \; 0.1695 \; 0.7226 \; -0.1956 \; 0.407 \; 0.3338] \times \begin{bmatrix} 0.2892 \\ 0.1695 \\ 0.7226 \\ -0.1956 \\ 0.4070 \\ 0.3338 \end{bmatrix} = 0.949848,$$

$$c_1 = \frac{k(\mathrm{MS_E})}{[b_0^r]'[b_0^r]} = \frac{6(0.01344)}{0.949848} = 0.0849.$$

We use the c_1 value (0.0849) for the next iteration, Iteration 2.
Using matrix form of the correlation transformation:

$$b_1^r = (r_{xx} - c_1 I)^{-1} r_{yx},$$

where $c_1 = 0.0849$, $r_{xx} =$ Table 6.8, $I = 6 \times 6$ identity matrix, $r_{yx} =$ Table 6.9.

$$b_1^r = \begin{bmatrix} 0.292653 \\ 0.225860 \\ 0.516255 \\ -0.017225 \\ 0.325554 \\ 0.318406 \end{bmatrix},$$

$$[b_1^r]'[b_1^r] = 0.6108,$$

$$c_2 = \frac{6(0.01344)}{0.6108} = 0.1320.$$

Now we need to see if $(c_2 - c_1)/c_1 \leq T^{-1.3}$. $T = \sum_{i=1}^{k} \frac{1}{\lambda} i$, or the sum of the reciprocals of the eigenvalues of the $X'X$ matrix correlation form. Table 6.14 presents the eigenvalues.

$$\sum_{i=1}^{6} \left(\frac{1}{\lambda_i}\right) = \frac{1}{3.95581} + \frac{1}{1.17926} + \frac{1}{0.48270} + \frac{1}{0.28099} + \frac{1}{0.06124} + \frac{1}{0.04195} = 46.8984,$$

TABLE 6.14
Eigenvalues

Eigenvalue	3.95581	1.17926	0.48270	0.28099	0.06124	0.04195

$$T = \frac{\sum\limits_{i=1}^{n} \frac{1}{\lambda}}{k} = \frac{46.8984}{6} = 7.8164,$$

$$T = 7.8164,$$

$$20T^{-1.3} = 20\left(7.8164^{-1.3}\right) = 1.3808,$$

$$\frac{c_2 - c_1}{c_1} = \frac{0.1320 - 0.0849}{0.0849} = 0.5548.$$

Because $0.5548 < 1.3808$, the iteration is completed; the constant value $c_2 = 0.1320$.

Referring to Figure 6.9, $c = 0.1320$ looks reasonable enough.

In Step 6, we compute the regression using $b' = (r_{xx} + cI)^{-1} r_{yx}$, using $c = 0.1320$.

$$b' = \begin{bmatrix} 0.286503 \\ 0.228457 \\ 0.473742 \\ 0.016608 \\ 0.293828 \\ 0.291224 \end{bmatrix}.$$

The regression equation correlation form is

$$y^* = 0.287\left(x_1^*\right) + 0.228\left(x_2^*\right) + 0.474\left(x_3^*\right) + 0.017\left(x_4^*\right) + 0.294\left(x_5^*\right) + 0.291\left(x_6^*\right),$$

where y^*, x_i^* is the correlation form.

In Step 7, we convert the correlation form estimate back to the original scale by first finding $\bar{y}$, s_y, $\bar{x}$, and s_x in the original scale, from Table 6.1A (Table 6.15).

Find $b_0 = \bar{y} - (b_1\bar{x}_1 + b_2\bar{x}_2 + \ldots + b_6\bar{x}_6)$, and

$$b_i = \left(\frac{s_y}{s_{x_i}}\right)b_i^r,$$

TABLE 6.15
Calculations from Data in Table 6.1A

	$\bar{x}_i$	s_{x_i}
x_1	29.000	7.973
x_2	3.113	1.596
x_3	2.020	1.196
x_4	1.509	0.882
x_5	55.400	16.587
x_6	3.127	2.220
$\bar{y} = 75.667$		
$s_y = 24.115$		

where b_i^r was computed for $c = 0.1320$. This will convert the b_is to the original data scale. To find b_0, we need to compute the b_i values first, to bring them to the original scale:

$$b_1 = \frac{24.115}{7.973}(0.287) = 0.868,$$

$$b_2 = \frac{24.115}{1.596}(0.228) = 3.445,$$

$$b_3 = \frac{24.115}{1.196}(0.474) = 9.557,$$

$$b_4 = \frac{24.115}{0.882}(0.017) = 0.465,$$

$$b_5 = \frac{24.115}{16.587}(0.294) = 0.427,$$

$$b_6 = \frac{24.115}{2.220}(0.291) = 3.160.$$

Next, calculate b_0:

$$b_0 = 75.667 - [0.868(29) + 3.445(3.113) + 9.557(2.02) + 0.465(1.509) \\ + 0.427(55.4) + 3.16(3.127)],$$

$$b_0 = -13.773.$$

The final ridge regression equation, in original scale, is

$$\hat{y} = -13.773 + 0.0868(x_1) + 3.445(x_2) + 9.557(x_3) + 0.465(x_4)$$
$$+ 0.427(x_5) + 3.16(x_6).$$

CONCLUSION

The ridge regression analysis can be extremely useful with regressions that have correlated x_i predictor values. When the data are in correlation form, it is useful to run a variety of other tests, such as ANOVA, for the model; to be sure, it is adequate. In matrix form, the computations are

Source of Variance			
Regression	$SS_R = \dfrac{SS}{b^{r'}X'Y} - \left(\dfrac{1}{n}\right)Y'JY$	k	$MS_R = \dfrac{SS_R}{k}$
Error	$SS_E = Y'Y - b^{r'}X'Y$	$n - k - 1$	$MS_E = \dfrac{SS_E}{n - k - 1}$
Total	$SS_T = Y'Y - \left(\dfrac{1}{n}\right)Y'JY$	$n - 1$	

$J = n \times n$ square matrix of all 1s,
$$\begin{bmatrix} 1 & \cdots & \cdots & 1 \\ \vdots & \cdots & \cdots & \vdots \\ \vdots & \cdots & \cdots & \vdots \\ 1 & \cdots & \cdots & 1 \end{bmatrix}$$
, $1/n$ is scalar of the

reciprocal of the sample size, n; $\widehat{Y}$ predicted $= Xb^r$, all in correlation form; $e = $ residual $= Y - \widehat{Y}$.

In conclusion, it can be said that when x_i predictors are correlated, the variance often is so large that the regression is useless. Ridge regression offers a way to deal with this problem very effectively.

7 Polynomial Regression

Polynomial regression models are useful in situations in which the curvilinear response function is too complex to linearize by means of a transformation, and an estimated response function fits the data adequately. Generally, if the modeled polynomial is not too complex to be generalized to a wide variety of similar studies, it is useful. On the other hand, if a modeled polynomial "overfits" the data of one experiment, then, for each experiment, a new polynomial must be built. This is generally ineffective, as the same type of experiment must use the same model if any iterative comparisons are required. Figure 7.1 presents a dataset that can be modeled by a polynomial function, or that can be set up as a piecewise regression. It is impossible to linearize this function by a simple scale transformation.

For a dataset like this, it is important to follow two steps:

1. Collect sufficient data that are replicated at each x_i predictor variable.
2. Perform true replication, not just repeated measurements in the same experiment.

True replication requires actually repeating the experiment n times. Although this sounds like a lot of effort, it will save hours of frustration and interpretation in determining the true data pattern to be modeled.

Figure 7.2 shows another problem—that of inadequate sample points within the x_is. The large "gaps" between the x_is represent unknown data points. If the model were fit via a polynomial or piecewise regression with both replication and repeated measurements, the model would still be inadequate. This is because the need for sufficient data, specified in step 1, was ignored.

Another type of problem occurs when repeated measurements are taken, but the study was not replicated (Figure 7.3). The figure depicts a study that was replicated five times, and each average repeated measurement plotted. That a predicted model based on the data from any single replicate is inadequate and unreliable is depicted by the distribution of the "•" replicates.

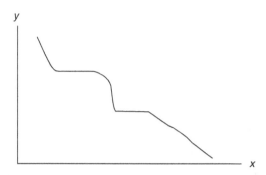

FIGURE 7.1 Polynomial function.

OTHER POINTS TO CONSIDER

1. It is important to keep the model's order as low as possible. Order is the value of the largest exponent.

$$\hat{y} = b_0 + b_1 x_1 + b_2 x_1^2 \qquad (7.1)$$

is a second-order (quadratic) model in one variable, x_1.

$$\hat{y} = b_0 + b_1 x_1^2 + b_2 x_2^2 \qquad (7.2)$$

is a second-order model in two x_i variables, x_1, x_2.

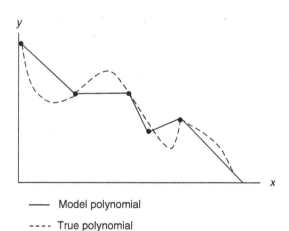

—— Model polynomial

---- True polynomial

FIGURE 7.2 Inadequate model of the actual data.

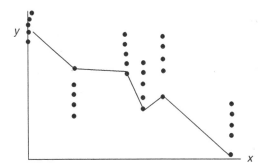

—— Represents one experiment with repeated measurements

• Represents each of five replicated experiments with
  repeated measurements

FIGURE 7.3 Modeling with no true replication.

A representation of the kth order polynomial is

$$\hat{y} = b_0 + b_1 x_1 + b_2 x^2 + \cdots + B_k x^k. \tag{7.3}$$

Because a small value is the key to robustness, k should never be greater than 2 or 3, unless one has extensive knowledge of the underlying function.

2. Whenever possible, linearize a function via a transformation. This will greatly simplify the statistical analysis. This author's view is that, usually, it is far better to linearize with a transformation than work in the original scale that is exponential. We discussed linearizing data in previous chapters.
3. Extrapolating is a problem, no matter what the model, but it is particularly risky with nonlinear polynomial functions.

For example, as shown in Figure 7.4, extrapolation occurs when someone wants to predict y at $x + 1$. There really is no way to know that value unless a measurement is taken at $x + 1$.

Interpolations can also be very problematic. Usually, only one or a few measurements are taken at each predictor value and gaps appear between predictor values as well, where no measured y response was taken. Interpolations, in these situations, are not data-driven, but function-driven. Figure 7.4 depicts the theoretical statistical function as a solid line, but the actual function may be as depicted by the dashed lines or any number of other possible

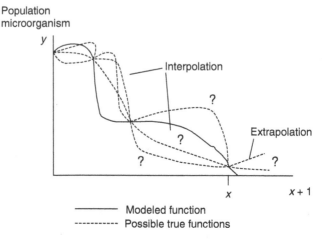

FIGURE 7.4 Modeling for extrapolation.

configurations. There is no way to know unless enough samples are replicated at enough predictor values in the range of data, as previously discussed.

4. Polynomial regression models often use data that are ill-conditioned, in that the matrix $[\mathbf{X}'\mathbf{X}]^{-1}$ is unstable and error-prone. This usually results in the variance (MS_E) that is huge. We discussed aspects of this situation in Chapter 6. When the model $\hat{y} = b_0 + b_1x_1 + b_2x_1^2$ is used, x_1^2 and x_1 will be highly correlated because x_1^2 is the square of x_1. If it is not serious due to excessive range spread, for example, in the selection of the x_i values, it may not be a problem, but it should be evaluated.

As seen in Chapter 6, ridge regression can be of use, as well as centering the x_i variable, $x' = x - \bar{x}$ or standardizing, $x' = (x - \bar{x})/s$, when certain x_i variables have extreme ranges relative to other x_i variables. Another solution could be to drop any x_i predictor variable not contributing to the regression function. We saw how to do this through partial regression analysis.

The basic model of polynomial regression is

$$Y = \beta_0 + \beta_1 X_1 + \beta_2 X_2^2 + \cdots + \beta_k X_k^k + \varepsilon \qquad (7.4)$$

estimated by

$$\hat{y} = b_0 + b_1 x_1 + b_2 x_2 + \cdots + b_k x_k^k + e \qquad (7.5)$$

or for centered data,

$$\hat{y} = b_0 + b_1 x_i^* + b_2 x_2^{*2} + \cdots + b_k x_k^* + e, \tag{7.6}$$

where $x_2^* = x_i - \bar{x}$ to center the data.

Therefore, $x_{1_i}^* = x_{1_i} - \bar{x}_1$, $x_{2_i}^* = x_{2_i} - \bar{x}_2$, and so on. Once the model's b_is have been computed, the data can be easily converted into the original noncentered scale (Chapter 6).

Polynomial regression is still considered a linear regression model in general because the b_i values remain linear, even though the x_is are not. Hence, the sum of squares computation is still employed. That is,

$$b = [\mathbf{X'X}]^{-1} \mathbf{X'Y}.$$

As previously discussed, some statisticians prefer to start with a larger model (backward elimination) and from that model, eliminate x_i predictor variables that do not contribute significantly to the increase in SS_R or decrease in SS_E. Others prefer to build a model using forward selection. The strategy is up to the researcher. A general rule is that the lower-order exponents appear first in the model. This ensures that the higher-order variables are removed first if they do not contribute. For example,

$$\hat{y} = b_0 + b_1 x_1 + b_2 x_2^2 + b_3 x_3^3.$$

Determining the significance of the variables would begin with comparing the higher-order to the lower-order model, sequentially:

First, x_3^3 is evaluated: $\quad SS_{R_{(x_3^3 | x_1, x_2^2)}} = SS_{R_{(x_1, x_2^2, x_3^3)}} - SS_{R_{(x_1, x_2^2)}}.$

Then, x_2^2 is evaluated: $\quad SS_{R_{(x_2^2 | x_1)}} = SS_{R_{(x_1, x_2^2)}} - SS_{R_{(x_1)}}.$

Finally, x_1 is evaluated: $\quad SS_{R_{(x_1)}} = SS_{R_{(x_1)}}.$

The basic procedure is the same as that covered in earlier chapters.

Example 7.1: In a wound-healing evaluation, days in the healing process (x_1) were compared with the number of epithelial cells cementing the wound (y). Table 7.1 presents these data. The researcher noted that the healing rate seemed to model a quadratic function. Hence, x_1^2 was also computed.

The model $\hat{y} = b_0 + b_1 x_1 + b_2 x_1^2$ was fit via least squares; Table 7.2 presents the computation. The researcher then plotted the actual y_i cell-count data against the day's sample; Figure 7.5 presents the results. Next, the predicted cell-count data (using the model $\hat{y} = b_0 + b_1 x_1 + b_2 x_1^2$) were plotted against x_i predictor values (days) (Figure 7.6). Then, the researcher superimposed the predicted and actual values. In Figure 7.7, one can see that the actual and predicted values fit fairly well. Next, the researcher decided to compute

TABLE 7.1
Wound-Healing Evaluation, Example 7.1

n	y_i	x_{1_i}	$x_{1_i}^2$
1	0	0	0
2	0	0	0
3	0	0	0
4	3	1	1
5	0	1	1
6	5	1	1
7	8	2	4
8	9	2	4
9	7	2	4
10	10	3	9
11	15	3	9
12	17	3	9
13	37	4	16
14	35	4	16
15	93	4	16
16	207	5	25
17	256	5	25
18	231	5	25
19	501	6	36
20	517	6	36
21	511	6	36
22	875	7	49
23	906	7	49
24	899	7	49
25	1356	8	64
26	1371	8	64
27	1223	8	64
28	3490	9	81
29	3673	9	81
30	3051	9	81
31	6756	10	100
32	6531	10	100
33	6892	10	100
34	6901	11	121
35	7012	11	121
36	7109	11	121
37	7193	12	144
38	6992	12	144
39	7009	12	144

Note: where y_i are the cells enumerated per grid over wound, $x_{1_i} = \text{day}$, $x_{1_i}^2 = \text{day}^2$.

TABLE 7.2
Least-Squares Computation, Example 7.1 Data

Predictor	Coef	St. Dev	t-Ratio	p
b_0	342.3	317.4	1.08	0.288
b_1	−513.1	122.9	−4.17	0.000
b_2	96.621	9.872	9.79	0.000
$s = 765.1$		$R^2 = 93.1\%$		$R^2_{(adj)} = 92.7\%$

The regression equation is $\hat{y} = b_0 + b_1 x_1 + b_2 x_i^2 = 342 - 513 x_1 + 96.6 x_1^2$.

the residuals to search for any patterns (Table 7.3). A definite pattern was found in the sequences of the "+" and "−" runs.

The researcher concluded that the days beyond 10 would be dropped for they held no benefit in interpreting the study. Also, because the range of y is so great, 0–7009, most statisticians would have performed a centering transformation on the data ($x_i^* = x_i - \bar{x}$) to reduce the range spread, but this researcher wanted to retain the data in the original scale. The researcher also removed days prior to day 2, hoping to make a better polynomial predictor. The statistical model that was iteratively fit was

$$\hat{y} = b_0 + b_1 x_1 + b_2 x_2,$$

where $x_1 = $ days, and $x_2 = x_1^2 = $ days^2. The regression analysis, presented in Table 7.4, looked promising, and the researcher thought the model was valid.

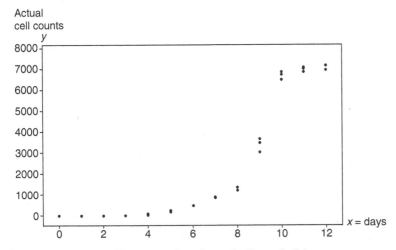

FIGURE 7.5 y vs. x_1, cell count vs. day of sample, Example 7.1.

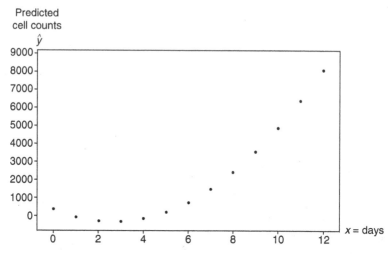

FIGURE 7.6 $\hat{y}$ vs. predicted x_1, Example 7.1.

As can be seen, the $R^2_{(adj)} = 0.905$, and the analysis of variance table portrays the model as highly significant in explaining the sum of squares, yet inadequate with all the data in the model. In Figure 7.8, we can see that the removal of $x_1 < 2$ and $x_1 > 10$ actually did not help.

Clearly, there is multicollinearity in this model, but we will not concern ourselves with this now (although we definitely would, in practice). The

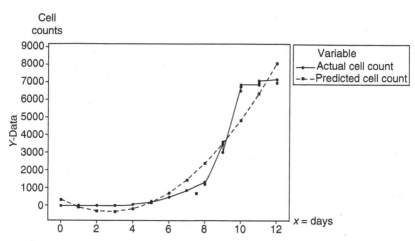

FIGURE 7.7 Actual (y) and predicted ($\hat{y}$) cell counts over days (x_1), Example 7.1.

TABLE 7.3
Computed Residuals, $e_i = y_i - \hat{y}_i$, Example 7.1

n	y	$\hat{y}$	$y - \hat{y} = e$
1	0	342.25	−342.25
2	0	342.25	−342.25
3	0	342.25	−342.25
4	3	−74.19	77.19
5	0	−74.19	74.19
6	5	−74.19	79.19
7	8	−297.40	305.40
8	9	−297.40	306.40
9	7	−297.40	304.40
10	10	−327.36	337.36
11	15	−327.36	342.36
12	17	−327.36	344.36
13	37	−164.08	201.08
14	35	−164.08	199.08
15	93	−164.08	257.08
16	207	192.44	14.56
17	256	192.44	63.56
18	231	192.44	38.56
19	501	742.20	−241.20
20	517	742.20	−225.20
21	511	742.20	−231.20
22	875	1485.21	−610.21
23	906	1485.21	−579.21
24	899	1485.21	−586.21
25	1356	2421.46	−1065.46
26	1371	2421.46	−1050.46
27	1223	2421.46	−1198.46
28	3490	3550.95	−60.95
29	3673	3550.95	122.05
30	3051	3550.95	−499.95
31	6756	4873.68	1882.32
32	6531	4873.68	1657.32
33	6892	4873.68	2018.32
34	6901	6389.65	511.35
35	7012	6389.65	622.35
36	7109	6389.65	719.35
37	7193	8098.87	−905.87
38	6992	8098.87	−1106.87
39	7009	8098.87	−1089.87

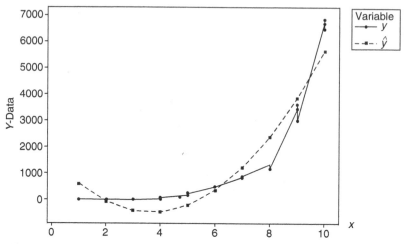

FIGURE 7.8 Scatter plot of y and $\hat{y}$ on $x - \hat{x} = x'$, with $x_1 < 2$ and $x_1 > 10$ removed, Example 7.1.

researcher decided to evaluate the model via a partial F test. Let us first examine the contribution of x_2:

$$SS_{R_{(x_2|x_1)}} = SS_{R_{(x_1,x_2)}} - SS_{R_{(x_1)}}.$$

The sum of squares regression, $SS_{R_{(x_1,x_2)}}$, is found in Table 7.4. Table 7.5 presents the regression model containing only x_1, $SS_{R_{(x_1)}}$.

TABLE 7.4
Full Model Regression with $x_1 < 2$ and $x_1 > 10$ Removed, Example 7.1

Predictor	Coef	SE Coef	t	P
b_0	1534.6	438.5	3.50	0.002
b_1	−1101.9	183.1	−6.02	0.000
b_2	151.74	16.23	9.35	0.000
$s = 645.753$		$R^2 = 91.2\%$		$R^2_{(adj)} = 90.5\%$

Analysis of Variance

Source	DF	SS	MS	F	P
Regression	2	16,111,053	58,055,527	139.22	0.000
Error	27	11,258,907	416,997		
Total	29	127,369,960			
Source	DF	SEQ SS			
x_1	1	79,638,851			
x_2	1	36,472,202			

The regression equation is $\hat{y} = 1535 + 1102x_1 - 152x_2$.

TABLE 7.5
Regression with x_1 in the Model and $x_1 < 2$ and $x_1 > 10$ Removed, Example 7.1

Predictor	Coef	St. Dev	t-Ratio	p
b_0	-1803.7	514.9	-3.50	0.002
b_1	567.25	82.99	6.84	0.000
$s = 1305.63$		$R^2 = 62.5\%$		$R^2_{(adj)} = 61.2\%$

Analysis of Variance

Source	DF	SS	MS	F	P
Regression	1	79,638,851	79,638,851	46.72	0.000
Error	28	47,731,109	1,704,682		
Total	29	127,369,960			

The regression equation is $\hat{y} = -1804 + 567x_1$.

So,

$$SS_{R_{(x_2|x_1)}} = SS_{R_{(x_1,x_2)}} - SS_{R_{(x_1)}} = 116,111,053 - 79,638,851 = 36,472,202$$

$$F_{c_{(x_2|x_1)}} = \frac{SS_{R_{(x_2|x_1)}}}{MS_{E_{(x_1,x_2)}}} = \frac{36,472,202}{416,997} = 87.4639$$

$$F_{T(\alpha,1,n-k-1)} = F_{T(0.05,1,30-2-1)} = F_{T(0.05,1,27)}$$
$$= 4.21 \text{ (from Table C, the F distribution table).}$$

Because $F_c = 87.4639 > F_T = 4.21$, we can conclude that the x_2 predictor variable is significant and should be retained in the model. Again, $F_{c_{(x_2|x_1)}}$ measures the contribution of x_2 to the sum of squares regression, given that x_1 is held constant.

The removal of $x < 2$ and $x > 10$ data points has not really helped the situation. The model and the data continue to be slightly biased. In fact, the $R^2_{(adj)}$ value for the latest model is less than the former. Often, in trying to fit polynomial functions, one just chases the data, sometimes endlessly. In addition, even if the model fits the data, in a follow-up experiment, the model is shown to be not robust and needing change. The problem with this, according to fellow scientists, is that one cannot easily distinguish between the study and the experimental results with confidence.

In this example, taking the $\log_{10}$ value of the colony-forming units would have greatly simplified the problem, by log-linearizing the data. This should have been done, particularly with $x < 2$ and $x > 10$ values of the model. Sometimes, linearizing the data will be impossible, but linearizing segments of the data function and performing a piecewise regression may be the best procedure. Using piecewise regression, the three obvious rate differences can

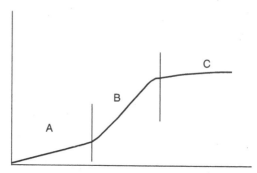

FIGURE 7.9 Original data for Example 7.1 in sigmoidal shape.

be partitioned into three linear components: A, B, and C (Figure 7.9). We discuss this later in this book, using dummy variables.

Example 7.2: Let us, however, continue with our discussion of polynomials. We need to be able to better assess the lack-of-fit model, using a more formal method. We will look at another example, that of biofilm grown on a catheter canula in a bioreactor. This study used two types of catheters, an antimicrobial-treated test and a nontreated control, and was replicated in triplicate, using the bacterial species, *Staphylococcus epidermidis*, a major cause of catheter-related infections. Because venous catheterization can be long-term without removing a canula, the biofilm was grown over the course of eight days. Table 7.6 presents the resultant data in exponential form.

In this experiment, the nontreated control and the treated test samples are clearly not linear, especially those for the nontreated canula. To better model these data, they were transformed by a $\log_{10}$ transformation of the microbial counts, the dependent variable. This is a common procedure in microbiology (Table 7.7).

The antimicrobially-treated and nontreated canulas' $\log_{10}$ microbial counts are plotted against days in Figure 7.10.

From Table 7.7, one can see that the $\log_{10}$ counts from the treated canulas were so low in some cases that the recommended minimum for reliable colony-count estimates (30 colonies per sample) was not reached in 14 of the 24 samples. Yet, these were the data and were used anyway, with the knowledge that the counts were below recommended detection limits. The data from the treated canulas appear to be approximately $\log_{10}$ linear. Hence, a simple regression analysis was first performed on those data (Table 7.8).

Figure 7.11 presents the predicted regression line superimposed over the data. Table 7.9 presents the actual, predicted, and residual values.

Notice that there is a definite pattern in the residual "+" and "−" values.

Instead of chasing data, presently, the model is "good enough." The b_0 intercept is negative (-0.6537) and should not be interpreted as the actual day

---

TABLE 7.6
Colony Counts of *Staphylococcus Epidermidis* from Treated and Nontreated Canulas, Example 7.2

n	Colony Counts ($y_{nontreated}$)	Colony Counts ($y_{treated}$)	Day
1	0	0	1
2	0	0	1
3	0	0	1
4	1×10^1	0	2
5	1.2×10^1	0	2
6	1.1×10^1	0	2
7	3.9×10^1	0	3
8	3.7×10^1	0	3
9	4.8×10^1	0	3
10	3.16×10^2	3.0×10^0	4
11	3.51×10^2	0	4
12	3.21×10^2	1.0×10^0	4
13	3.98×10^3	5.0×10^0	5
14	3.81×10^3	0	5
15	3.92×10^3	1.6×10^1	5
16	5.01×10^4	2.1×10^1	6
17	5.21×10^4	3.7×10^1	6
18	4.93×10^4	1.1×10^1	6
19	3.98×10^6	5.8×10^1	7
20	3.80×10^6	5.1×10^1	7
21	3.79×10^6	4.2×10^1	7
22	1.27×10^9	6.2×10^1	8
23	1.25×10^9	5.1×10^1	8
24	1.37×10^9	5.8×10^1	8

1 value. Instead, it merely points out the regression function that corresponds to the best estimate of the regression slope when $x = 0$. For each day, the microbial population increased 0.31 $\log_{10}$ times, which demonstrates the product that has good microbial inhibition. The adjusted coefficient of determination is $\approx 81.0\%$, meaning that about 81% of the variability in the data is explained by the regression equation.

Notice that the data for the nontreated canula were not linearized by a $\log_{10}$ transformation. Hence, we will add another x_i variable, x_2, into the regression equation, where $x_2 = x_1^2$, to see if this models the data better. Ideally, we did not want to do this, but we need to model the data. Hence, the equation becomes

$$\hat{y} = b_0 + b_1 x_1 + b_2 x_2,$$

TABLE 7.7
Log_{10} Transformation of the Dependent Variable, y, Example 7.2

n	$y_{nontreated}$	$y_{treated}$	x (Day)
1	0.00	0.00	1
2	0.00	0.00	1
3	0.00	0.00	1
4	1.00	0.00	2
5	1.07	0.00	2
6	1.04	0.00	2
7	1.59	0.00	3
8	1.57	0.00	3
9	1.68	0.00	3
10	2.50	0.48	4
11	2.55	0.00	4
12	2.51	0.00	4
13	3.60	0.70	5
14	3.58	0.00	5
15	3.59	1.20	5
16	4.70	1.32	6
17	4.72	1.57	6
18	4.69	1.04	6
19	6.60	1.76	7
20	6.58	1.71	7
21	6.58	1.62	7
22	9.10	1.79	8
23	9.10	1.71	8
24	9.14	1.76	8

where

$$x_2 = x_1^2.$$

Table 7.10 presents the nontreated canula regression analysis, and Figure 7.12 demonstrates that, although there is some bias in the model, it is adequate for the moment. Table 7.11 provides the values y_i, x_1, x_1^2, $\hat{y}_i$, and e_i.

The rate of growth is not constant in a polynomial function; therefore, the derivative (d/dx) must be determined. This can be accomplished using the power rule:

$$\frac{d}{dx}(x^n) = nx^{n-1},$$

$$\hat{y} = 0.1442 + 0.0388x_1 + 0.13046x^2$$

$$\text{slope of } \hat{y} = \frac{d}{dx}(0.1442 + 0.0388x_1 + 0.13046x^2) = 1(0.0388) + 2(0.13046)$$

$$(7.7)$$

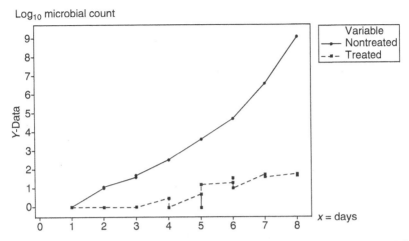

FIGURE 7.10 Log_{10} microbial counts from treated and nontreated canulas, Example 7.2.

The slope, or rate of population growth $= 0.0388 + 0.2609x$ for any day, x.
On day 1:
slope $= 0.0388 + 0.2609(1) = 0.2997 \approx 0.3$ $\log_{10}$, which is the same rate observed from the treated canula.
On day 3:
slope $= 0.0388 + 0.2609(3) = 0.82$, that is, an increase in microorganisms at day 3 of 0.82 $\log_{10}$.
On day 8:
slope $= 0.0388 + 0.2609(8) = 2.126$ $\log_{10}$ at day 8.

TABLE 7.8
Regression Analysis of Log_{10} Counts from Treated Canulas, Example 7.2

Predictor	Coef	St. Dev	t-Ratio	p
Constant b_0	−0.6537	0.1502	−4.35	0.000
b_1	0.29952	0.02974	10.07	0.000
$s = 0.3339$		$R^2 = 82.2\%$		$R^2_{(adj)} = 81.4\%$

Analysis of Variance

Source	DF	SS	MS	F	P
Regression	1	11.304	11.304	101.41	0.000
Error	22	2.452	0.111		
Total	23	13.756			

The regression equation is $\hat{y} = -0.654 + 0.300x_1$.

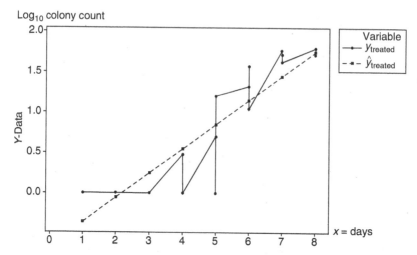

FIGURE 7.11 Scatter plot of y_{treated}, x, with predicted $\hat{y}_{\text{treated}}$, x.

Note also that the adjusted coefficient of determination, r^2, is about 99% (see Table 7.10). The fit is not perfect, but for preliminary work, it is all right. These data are also in easily understandable terms for presenting to management, a key consideration in statistical applications.

Let us compute the partial F test for this model, $\hat{y} = b_0 + b_1 x_1 + b_2 x_1^2$. The MiniTab regression routines, as well as those of many other software packages, provide the information in standard regression printouts. It can always be computed, as we have done previously, comparing the full and the reduced models.

The full regression model presented in Table 7.10 has a partial analysis of variance table, provided here:

Source	DF	SEQ SS
$SS_{R(x1)}$	1	185.361
$SS_{R(x2|x1)}$	1	8.578

The summed value, 193.939, approximates 193.938, which is the value of $SS_{R(x_1,x_2)}$.

The F_c value for

$$SS_{R(x_2|x_1)} = \frac{SS_{R(x_2|x_1)}}{MS_{E(x_1,x_2)}} = \frac{8.578}{0.074} = 115.92,$$

is obviously significant at $\alpha = 0.05$.

TABLE 7.9
Actual y_i Data, Fitted $\hat{y}$ Data, and Residuals, Treated Canulas,
Example 7.2

Row	x	y	$\hat{y}$	$y - \hat{y} = e$
1	1	0.00	−0.35417	0.354167
2	1	0.00	−0.35417	0.344167
3	1	0.00	−0.35417	0.354167
4	2	0.00	−0.05464	0.054643
5	2	0.00	−0.05464	0.054643
6	2	0.00	−0.05464	0.054643
7	3	0.00	0.24488	−0.244881
8	3	0.00	0.24488	−0.244881
9	3	0.00	0.24488	−0.244881
10	4	0.48	0.54440	−0.064405
11	4	0.00	0.54440	−0.544405
12	4	0.00	0.54440	−0.544405
13	5	0.00	0.84393	−0.143929
14	5	0.00	0.84393	−0.843929
15	5	1.20	0.84393	0.356071
16	6	1.32	1.14345	0.176548
17	6	1.57	1.14345	0.426548
18	6	1.04	1.14345	−0.103452
19	7	1.76	1.44298	0.317024
20	7	1.71	1.44298	0.267024
21	7	1.62	1.44298	0.177024
22	8	1.79	1.74250	0.047500
23	8	1.71	1.74250	−0.032500
24	8	1.76	1.74250	0.017500

Hence, the full model that includes x_1 and x_2 is the one to use.

$$\hat{y} = b_0 + b_1 x_1 + b_2 x_2,$$

where $x_2 = x_1^2$.

The partial F tests on other models are constructed exactly as presented in Chapter 4.

LACK OF FIT

Recall that the lack-of-fit test partitions the sum of squares error (SS_E) into two components: pure error, the actual random error component and lack of fit, a nonrandom component that detects discrepancies in the model. The lack-of-fit computation is a measure of the degree to which the model does not fit or represent the actual data.

TABLE 7.10
Nontreated Canula Regression Analysis, Example 7.2

Predictor	Coef	St. Dev	t-Ratio	p
b_0	0.1442	0.2195	0.66	0.518
b_1	0.0388	0.1119	0.35	0.732
b_2	0.13046	0.01214	10.75	0.000

$s = 0.2725$ $\qquad$ $R^2 = 99.2\%$ $\qquad$ $R^2_{(adj)} = 99.1\%$

Analysis of Variance

Source	DF	SS	MS	F	P
Regression	2	193.938	96.969	1305.41	0.000
Error	21	1.560	0.074		
Total	23	195.498			

Source	DF	SEQ SS
$SS_{R_{(x_1)}}$	1	185.361
$SS_{R_{(x_2, x_1)}}$	1	8.578

The regression equation is $\hat{y} = 0.144 + 0.039x_1 + 0.130x_1^2$

In Example 7.2, note that each x_i value was replicated three times ($j = 3$). That is, three separate y_{ij} values were documented for each x_i value. Those y_{ij} values were then averaged to provide a single $\bar{y}_i$ value for each x_i.

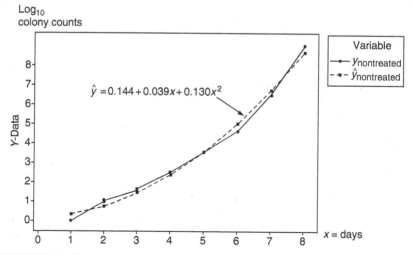

FIGURE 7.12 Scatter plot of $y_{\text{nontreated}}$, x, with predicted regression line, Example 7.2.

TABLE 7.11
The y_i, x_1, x_1^2, $\hat{y}_i$, and e_i Values, Nontreated Canulas, Example 7.2

n	y_i	x_1	$x_{1_i}^2 = x_{2_i}$	$\hat{y}_i$	$y_i - \hat{y}_i = e_i$
1	0.00	1	1	0.31347	−0.313472
2	0.00	1	1	0.31347	−0.313472
3	0.00	1	1	0.31347	−0.313472
4	1.00	2	4	0.74363	0.256369
5	1.07	2	4	0.74363	0.326369
6	1.04	2	4	0.74363	0.296369
7	1.59	3	9	1.43470	0.155298
8	1.57	3	9	1.43470	0.135298
9	1.68	3	9	1.43470	0.245298
10	2.50	4	16	2.38669	0.113314
11	2.55	4	16	2.38669	0.163314
12	2.51	4	16	2.38669	0.123314
13	3.60	5	25	3.59958	0.000417
14	3.58	5	25	3.59958	−0.019583
15	3.59	5	25	3.59958	−0.009583
16	4.70	6	36	5.07339	−0.373393
17	4.72	6	36	5.07339	−0.353393
18	4.69	6	36	5.07339	−0.383393
19	6.60	7	49	6.80812	−0.208115
20	6.58	7	49	6.80812	−0.228115
21	6.58	7	49	6.80812	−0.228115
22	9.10	8	64	8.80375	0.296250
23	9.10	8	64	8.80375	0.296250
24	9.14	8	64	8.80375	0.336250

x_i	y_{ij}	$\bar{y}_i$
1	0.00, 0.00, 0.00	0.00
2	1.00, 1.07, 1.04	1.04
3	1.59, 1.57, 1.68	1.61
4	2.50, 2.55, 2.51	2.52
5	3.60, 3.58, 3.59	3.59
6	4.70, 4.72, 4.69	4.70
7	6.60, 6.58, 6.58	6.59
8	9.10, 9.10, 9.14	9.11

c, the number of x_i values that were replicated is equal to 8. That is, all 8 x_i observations were replicated, so $n = 24$.

SS_{pe}, sum of squares pure error $= \sum_{j=1}^{n}(y_{ij} - \bar{y}_j)^2$, which reflects the variability of the y_{ij} replicate values about the mean of those values, $\bar{y}_j$.

From this

$$SS_{pe} = (0 - 0)^2 + (0 - 0)^2 + (0 - 0)^2 + \cdots + (9.10 - 9.11)^2 + (9.14 - 9.11)^2$$

$SS_{pe} = 0.0129$

$SS_{lack-of-fit} = SS_E - SS_{pe} = 1.560 - 0.013 = 1.547$

This is merely the pure "random" error subtracted from SS_E, providing an estimate of unaccounted for, nonrandom, lack-of-fit variability. Table 7.12, the lack-of-fit ANOVA table, presents these computations specifically.

Both F tests are highly significant ($F_c > F_T$); that is, the regression model and the lack of fit are significant. Note that degrees of freedom were calculated as $SS_{LF} = c - (k + 1) = 8 - 2 - 1 = 5$, and $SS_{pe} = n - c = 24 - 8 = 16$, where k, number of x_i independent variables $= 2$; c, number of replicated x_i values $= 8$; and n, sample size $= 24$.

Clearly, the regression is significant, but the lack- of- fit is also significant. This means that there is bias in the modeled regression equation, which we already knew. Therefore, what should be done? We can overfit the sample set to model these data very well, but in a follow-up study, the overfit model most likely will have to be changed. How will this serve the purposes of a researcher? If one is at liberty to fit each model differently, there is no problem. However, generally, the main goal of a researcher is to select a robust model that may not provide the best estimate for each experiment, but does so for the entire class of such studies.

TABLE 7.12
ANOVA Table with Analysis of Nontreated Canulas

Predictor	Coef	SE Coef	t	P	
b_0	0.1442	0.2195	0.66	0.518	
b_1	0.0388	0.1119	0.35	0.732	
b_2	0.13046	0.01214	10.75	0.000	
$s = 0.272548$		$R^2 = 99.2\%$		$R^2_{(adj)} = 99.1\%$	

Analysis of Variance

Source	DF	SS	MS	F	P
Regression	2	193.938	96.969	1305.41	0.000
Residual error	21	1.560	0.074		
Lack- of- fit	5	1.547	0.309	388.83	0.000
Pure error	16	0.013	0.001		
Total	23	195.498			

The regression equation is $\hat{y} = 0.144 + 0.039x_1 + 0.130x_2$.

Specifically, in this example, a practical problem is that the variability is relatively low. When the variability is low, the lack of fit of the model is magnified. Figure 7.12 shows the values $\hat{y}$ and y plotted on the same graph, and the slight difference in the actual data and the predicted data can be observed. This is the lack-of-fit component. The y_i values are initially overestimated and then are underestimated by $\hat{y}_i$ for the next three time points. The day 4 $\hat{y}$ predictor and the y value are the same, but the next two y values are over-predicted, and the last one is underpredicted. Notice that this phenomenon is also present in the last column as the value $y_i - \hat{y}_i = e$ in Table 7.11. Probably, the best thing to do is leave the model as it is and replicate the study to build a more robust general model based on the outcomes of multiple separate pilot studies. The consistent runs of negative and positive residuals represent "lack of fit." A problem with polynomial regression for the researcher, specifically for fitting the small pilot model, is that the data from the next experiment performed identically may not even closely fit that model.

SPLINES (PIECEWISE POLYNOMIAL REGRESSION)

Polynomial regression can often be made far more effective by breaking the regression into separate segments called "splines." The procedure is similar to the piecewise linear regression procedure, using dummy or indicator variables, which we discuss in Chapter 9. Spline procedures, although breaking the model into component parts, continue to use exponents. Sometimes a low-order polynomial model cannot be fit precisely to the data, and the researcher does not want to build a complex polynomial function to model the data. In such cases, the spline procedure is likely to be applicable.

In the spline procedure, the function is subdivided into several component sections such that it will be easier to model the data (Figure 7.13). Technically, the splines are polynomial functions of order k; and they connect at the

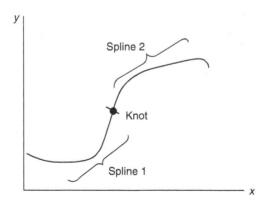

FIGURE 7.13 Splines.

"knot." The function values and the first $k-1$ derivatives must agree at the knot(s), so the spline is a continuous function with $k-1$ continuous derivatives. However, in practice, it is rarely this simple. To begin with, the true polynomial function is not known, so the derivatives tend to be rather artificial.

The position of the knots, for many practical purposes, can be determined intuitively. If the knot positions are known, a standard least-squares equation can be used to model them. If the knots are not known, they can be estimated via nonlinear regression techniques. Additionally, most polynomial splines are subject to serious multicollinearity in the x_i predictors, so the fewer splines, the better.

The general polynomial spline model is

$$y' = \sum_{j=0}^{d} \beta_{0j} x^j + \sum_{i=1}^{c} \sum_{j=0}^{d} \beta_i (x - t_i)^d, \qquad (7.8)$$

where

$$\left[\begin{matrix} x - t_i, & \text{if } x - t_i > 0 \\ 0, & \text{if } x - t_i \leq 0 \end{matrix} \right],$$

where

d is the order of splines 0, 1, 2, 3, and $j = 0, 1, \ldots, d$ (not recommended for greater than 3). The order is found by residual analysis and iteration. c is the number of knots.

For most practical situations, Montgomery et al. (2001) recommend using a cubic spline:

$$y' = \sum_{j=0}^{3} \beta_{0j} x^j + \sum_{i=1}^{c} \beta_i (x - t_i)^3, \qquad (7.9)$$

where c is the number of knots, $t_1 < t_2 < \cdots < t_c$; t_i is the knot value at x_i

$$(x - t_i) = \begin{cases} x - t_i, & \text{if } x - t_i > 0 \\ 0, & \text{if } x - t_i \leq 0 \end{cases}.$$

Therefore, if there are two knots, say $t_i = 5$, and $t_i = 10$, then, by Equation 7.9:

$$y' = \beta_{00} + \beta_{01} x + \beta_{02} x^2 + \beta_{03}^3 x^3 + \beta_1 (x - 5)^3 + \beta_2 (x - 10)^3 + \varepsilon. \qquad (7.10)$$

This model is useful, but often, a square spline is also useful. That is,

$$y' = \sum_{j=0}^{2} \beta_{0j} x^j + \sum_{i=1}^{c} \beta_i (x - t_i)^2. \qquad (7.11)$$

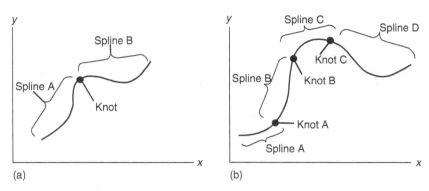

FIGURE 7.14 Polynomial splines with knots.

If there is one knot, for example,

$$y' = \beta_{00} + \beta_{01}x + \beta_{02}x^2 + \beta_1(x - t)^2 + \varepsilon$$

again, where

$$(x - t_i) = \begin{bmatrix} x - t_i, & \text{if } x - t_i > 0 \\ 0, & \text{if } x - t_i \leq 0 \end{bmatrix}.$$

Let us refer to data for Example 7.1, the wound-healing evaluation. With the polynomial spline-fitting process, the entire model can be modeled at once. Figure 7.5 shows the plot of the number of cells cementing the wound over days. As the curve is sigmoidal in shape, it is difficult to model without a complex polynomial, but is more easily modeled via a spline fit.

The first step is to select the knot(s) position(s) (Figure 7.14). Two possible knot configurations are provided for different functions. Figure 7.14a portrays one knot and two splines; Figure 7.14b portrays three knots and four splines. There is always one spline more than the number of total knots.

The fewer the knots, the better. Having some familiarity with data can be helpful in finding knot position(s), because both under- and overfitting the data pose problems. Besides, each spline should have only one extreme and one inflection point per section. For the data from Example 7.1, we use two knots because there appear to be three component functions. The proposed configuration is actually hand-drawn over the actual data (Figure 7.15).

The knots chosen were $t_1 =$ day 5 and $t_2 =$ day 9; Figure 7.5 shows that this appears to bring the inflection points near these knots. There is only one inflection point per segment. Other t_i values could probably be used, so it is not necessary to have an exact fit. Knot selection is not easy and is generally

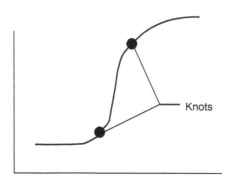

FIGURE 7.15 Proposed knots, Example 7.1.

an iterative exercise. If the function $f(x)$ is known, note that the inflection points of the tangent line $f(x)'$ or d/dx, can be quickly discovered by the second derivative, $f(x)''$. Although this process can be a valuable tool, it is generally not necessary in practice.

Recall from Example 7.1 that the y_i data were collected on cells per wound closure and x_i was the day of measurement—0 through 12. Because there is a nonlinear component that we will keep in that basic model, which is $\hat{y} = b_0 + b_1 x + b_2 x^2$, and adding the spline, the model we use is

$$\hat{y}' = b_{00} + b_{01}x + b_{02}x^2 + b_1(x - 5)^2 + b_2(x - 9)^2,$$

where

$$(x - 5) = \begin{cases} x - 5, & \text{if } x - 5 > 0 \\ 0, & \text{if } x - 5 \leq 0 \end{cases}$$

and

$$(x - 9) = \begin{cases} x - 9, & \text{if } x - 9 > 0 \\ 0, & \text{if } x - 9 \leq 0 \end{cases}.$$

Table 7.13 provides the input data points.

$$\hat{y}' = b_{00} + b_{01}x + b_{02}x^2 + b_1(x - 5)^2 + b_2(x - 9)^2.$$

Notice that when $x \leq 5$ (spline 1), the prediction equation is

$$\hat{y}' = b_{00} + b_{01}x + b_{02}x^2.$$

When $x > 5$ but $x \leq 9$ (spline 2), the equation is

$$\hat{y}' = b_{00} + b_{01}x + b_{02}x^2 + b_1(x - 5)^2.$$

TABLE 7.13
Input Data Points, Spline Model of Example 7.1

n	y	x_i	x_i^2	$(x_i - 5)^2$	$(x_i - 9)^2$
1	0	0	0	0	0
2	0	0	0	0	0
3	0	0	0	0	0
4	3	1	1	0	0
5	0	1	1	0	0
6	5	1	1	0	0
7	8	2	4	0	0
8	9	2	4	0	0
9	7	2	4	0	0
10	10	3	9	0	0
11	15	3	9	0	0
12	17	3	9	0	0
13	37	4	16	0	0
14	35	4	16	0	0
15	93	4	16	0	0
16	207	5	25	0	0
17	257	5	25	0	0
18	231	5	25	0	0
19	501	6	36	1	0
20	517	6	36	1	0
21	511	6	36	1	0
22	875	7	49	4	0
23	906	7	49	4	0
24	899	7	49	4	0
25	1356	8	64	9	0
26	1371	8	64	9	0
27	1223	8	64	9	0
28	3490	9	81	16	0
29	3673	9	81	16	0
30	3051	9	81	16	0
31	6756	10	100	25	1
32	6531	10	100	25	1
33	6892	10	100	25	1
34	6901	11	121	36	4
35	7012	11	121	36	4
36	7109	11	121	36	4
37	7193	12	144	49	9
38	6992	12	144	49	9
39	7009	12	144	49	9

When $x > 9$ (spline 3), the regression equation is

$$\hat{y}' = b_{00} + b_{01}x + b_{02}x^2 + b_1(x - 5)^2 + b_2(x - 9)^2.$$

Via the least-squares equation (Table 7.14), we create the following regression.
Notice that the $R^2_{(adj)}$ value is 97.6%, better than that provided by the model,
$\hat{y} = b_0 + b_1x + b_2x^2$. Table 7.15 presents the values $\hat{y}_i'$, x_{1i}, x_{1i}^2, $\hat{y}_i$, and e_i.

Figure 7.16 plots the y_i vs. x_i and the $\hat{y}_i'$ vs. x_i for a little better fit than that
portrayed in Figure 7.7, using the model, $\hat{y}' = b_0 + b_1x + b_2x^2$.

Although the polynomial spline model is slightly better than the original
polynomial model, there continues to be bias in the model. In this researcher's
view, the first knot should be moved to $x = 8$, and the second knot should be
moved to $x = 10$. Then, the procedure should be repeated. We also know that
it would have been far better to $\log_{10}$ linearize the y_i data points. Hence, it is
critical to use polynomial regression only when all other attempts fail.

SPLINE EXAMPLE DIAGNOSTIC

From Table 7.14, we see, however, that t tests (t-ratios) for b_{00}, b_{01}, and b_{02}
are not significantly different from 0 at $\alpha = 0.05$. $b_{00} = y$ intercept when $x = 0$
is not significantly different from 0, which is to be expected, because the

TABLE 7.14
Least-Squares Equation, Spline Model of Example 7.1

Predictor	Coef	St. Dev	t-Ratio	P
b_{00}	−140.4	222.3	−0.63	0.532
b_{01}	264.2	168.1	1.57	0.125
b_{02}	−50.61	25.71	−1.97	0.057
b_1	369.70	50.00	7.39	0.000
b_2	−743.53	87.78	−8.47	0.000

$s = 441.7$ $R^2 = 97.8\%$ $R^2_{(adj)} = 97.6\%$

Analysis of Variance

Source	DF	SS	MS	F	P
Regression	4	298,629,760	74,657,440	382.66	0.000
Error	34	6,633,366	195,099		
Total	38	305,263,136			

Source	DF	SEQ SS
x	1	228,124,640
x^2	1	56,067,260
$(x - 5)^2$	1	441,556
$(x - 9)^2$	1	13,996,303

The regression equation is $\hat{y}' = -140 + 264x - 50.6x^2 + 370(x - 5)^2 - 744(x - 9)^2$.

TABLE 7.15
Values $\hat{y}_i'$, x_{1_i}, $x_{1_i}^2$, $\hat{y}_i$, and e_i, Spline model of Example 7.1

n	y_i	x_i	$\hat{y}_i'$	$y_i - \hat{y}_i' = e_i$
1	0	0	−140.36	140.36
2	0	0	−140.36	140.36
3	0	0	−140.36	140.36
4	3	1	73.21	−70.21
5	0	1	73.21	−73.21
6	5	1	73.21	−68.21
7	8	2	185.56	−177.56
8	9	2	185.56	−176.56
9	7	2	185.56	−178.56
10	10	3	196.70	−186.70
11	15	3	196.70	−181.70
12	17	3	196.70	−179.70
13	37	4	106.62	−69.62
14	35	4	106.62	−71.62
15	93	4	106.62	−13.62
16	207	5	−84.68	291.68
17	257	5	−84.68	341.68
18	231	5	−84.68	315.68
19	501	6	−7.49	508.49
20	517	6	−7.49	524.49
21	511	6	−7.49	518.49
22	875	7	707.87	167.13
23	906	7	707.87	198.13
24	899	7	707.87	191.13
25	1356	8	2061.41	−705.41
26	1371	8	2061.41	−690.41
27	1223	8	2061.41	−838.41
28	3490	9	4053.12	−563.12
29	3673	9	4053.12	−380.12
30	3051	9	4053.12	−1002.12
31	6756	10	5939.49	816.51
32	6531	10	5939.49	591.51
33	6892	10	5939.49	952.51
34	6901	11	6976.97	−75.97
35	7012	11	6976.97	35.03
36	7109	11	6976.97	132.03
37	7193	12	7165.59	27.41
38	6992	12	7165.59	−173.59
39	7009	12	7165.59	−156.59

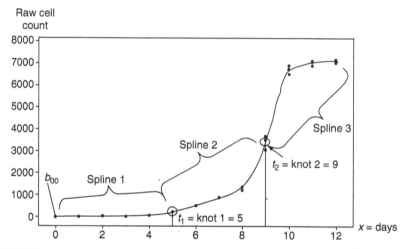

FIGURE 7.16 Proposed spline/knot configuration of data scatter plot, Example 7.1.

intercept of the data is $x = 0$ and $y = 0$. $b_{01} = x$ initially follows a straight line (no slope) at the low values of x, as expected. $b_{02} = x^2$ is hardly greater than 0, again at the initial values, but then increases in slope, making it borderline significant at $0.057 > \alpha$. However, as we learned, slopes should really be evaluated independently, so using a partial F test is a better strategy. Because the entire spline model is very significant, in terms of the F test, let us perform the partial F analysis.

For clarification, we recall

$$
\begin{aligned}
x_{01} &= x \\
x_{02} &= x^2 \\
x_1 &= (x - 5)^2 \\
x_2 &= (x - 9)^2.
\end{aligned}
$$

Let us determine the significance of x_2:

$$SS_{R(x_2 | x_{01}, x_{02}, x_1)} = SS_{R(x_{01}, x_{02}, x_1, x_2)} - SS_{R(x_{01}, x_{02}, x_1)}.$$

From Table 7.14, the full model is $SS_{R(x_{01}, x_{02}, x_1, x_2)} = 298,629,760$, and $MS_{E(x_{01}, x_{02}, x_1, x_2)} = 195,099$.

From Table 7.16, the partial model provides $SS_{R(x_{01}, x_{02}, x_1)} = 284,633,472$.

$$SS_{R(x_2 | x_{01}, x_{02}, x_1)} = 298,629,760 - 284,633472 = 13,996,288$$

$$F_{c(x_2 | x_{01}, x_{02}, x_1)} = \frac{SS_{R(x_2 | x_{01}, x_{02}, x_1)}}{MS_{E(x_{01}, x_{02}, x_1, x_2)}} = \frac{13,996,288}{195,099} = 71.74.$$

TABLE 7.16
Partial F Test of x_2, Spline Model of Example 7.1

Predictor	Coef	St. Dev	t-Ratio	P
b_{00}	160.7	381.4	0.42	0.676
b_{01}	−307.5	267.6	−1.15	0.258
b_{02}	64.99	37.86	1.72	0.095
b_1	49.16	56.80	0.87	0.393
$s = 767.7$		$R^2 = 93.2\%$		$R^2_{(adj)} = 92.7\%$

Analysis of Variance

Source	DF	SS	MS	F	P
Regression	3	284,633,472	94,877,824	160.97	0.000
Error	35	20,629,668	589,419		
Total	38	305,263,136			

The regression equation is $\hat{y} = 161 - 307x + 65.0x_2 + 492(x_1 - 5)^2$.

To test the significance of b_2, which corresponds to x_2 or $(x - 9)^2$, the hypothesis is

$$H_0: \beta_2 = 0,$$

$$H_A: \beta_2 \neq 0.$$

If $F_c > F_T$, reject H_0 at α.

Let us set $\alpha = 0.05$. $F_{T(\alpha;1,n-k-1)}$ (which is based on the full model) $= F_{T(0.05,1,39-4-1)} = F_{T(0.05,1,34)} \approx 4.17$ (from Table C). Because F_c (71.74) $> F_T$ (4.17), reject H_0 at $\alpha = 0.05$. Clearly, the $(x - 9)^2$ term associated with β_2 is significant.

The readers can test the other partial F test on their own. Notice, however, that the spline procedure provides a much better fit of the data than does the original polynomial. For work with splines, it is important first to model the curve and then scrutinize the modeled curve overlaid with the actual data. If the model has some areas that do not fit the data by a proposed knot, try moving the knot to a different x value and reevaluate the model. If this does not help, change the power of the exponent. As must be obvious by now, this is usually an iterative process requiring patience.

LINEAR SPLINES

In Chapter 9, we discuss piecewise multiple regressions with "dummy variables," but the use of linear splines can accomplish the same thing. Knots, again, are the points of the regression that link two separate linear splines (see Figure 7.17).

Cell count

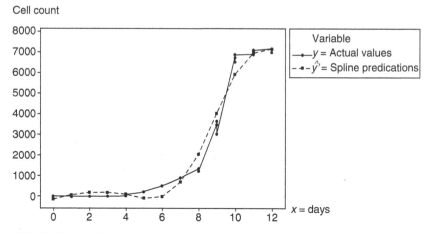

FIGURE 7.17 Spline vs. actual data.

Figure 7.18a is a regression with two splines and one knot, and Figure 7.18b is a regression with four splines and three knots. Note that these graphs are similar to those in Figure 7.14, but describe linear splines.

As with polynomial splines, the knots will be one count less than the number of splines. It is also important to keep the splines to a minimum. This author prefers to use a linear transformation of the original data and then, if required, use a knot to connect two spline functions.

The linear formula is

$$Y = \sum_{j=0}^{1} \beta_{0j} x^j + \sum_{i=1}^{c} \beta_i (x - t_i)^c, \qquad (7.12)$$

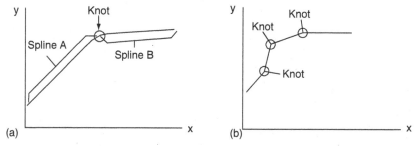

FIGURE 7.18 Linear splines.

where c is the number of knots. If there is one knot, c, the equation is

$$Y = \sum_{j=0}^{1} \beta_{0j} x^j + \sum_{i=1}^{1} \beta(x - t_i), \tag{7.13}$$

$$Y = \beta_{00} + \beta_{01} x + \beta_1 (x - t_i), \tag{7.14}$$

which is estimated by

$$\hat{y}' = b_{00} + b_{01} x + b_1 (x - t_i), \tag{7.15}$$

where t is the x value at the knot and $x - t = \begin{cases} x - t, & \text{if } x - t > 0 \\ 0, & \text{if } x - t \le 0 \end{cases}$.
If $x \le t$, then the equation reduces to

$$\hat{y}' = b_{00} + b_{01} x$$

because b_1 drops out of the equation.

For a two-knot ($c = 2$), three-spline (power 1, or linear) application, the equation is

$$Y = \sum_{j=0}^{1} \beta_{0j} x^j + \sum_{i=1}^{c} \beta_i (x - t_i) \tag{7.16}$$

$$Y = \sum_{j=0}^{1} \beta_{0j} x^j + \sum_{i=1}^{2} \beta_i (x - t_i) \tag{7.17}$$

$$Y = \beta_{00} + \beta_{01} x + \beta_1 (x - t_1) + \beta_2 (x - t_2),$$

which is estimated by

$$\hat{y}' = \sum_{j=0}^{1} b_{0j} x^j + \sum_{i=1}^{2} b_i (x - t_i), \tag{7.18a}$$

$$\hat{y}' = b_{00} + b_{01} x + b_1 (x - t_1) + b_2 (x - t_2).$$

For fitting data that are discontinuous, the formula must be modified. Use

$$Y = \sum_{j=0}^{p} \beta_{0j} x^j + \sum_{i=1}^{c} \sum_{j=0}^{p} \beta_{ij} (x - t_i)^j, \tag{7.18b}$$

where p is the power of the model, $j = 0, 1, 2, \ldots, p$, and c is the number of knots.

Suppose this is a linear spline ($p = 1$) with $c = 1$ or one knot. Then,

$$\hat{y}' = b_{00} + b_{01}x + b_1(x - t_i),$$

where

$$x - t_1 = \begin{cases} x - t, & \text{if } x - t > 0 \\ 0, & \text{if } x - t \leq 0 \end{cases}.$$

Let us consider Example 7.3.

Example 7.3: In product stability studies, it is known that certain products are highly sensitive to ultraviolet radiation. In a full-spectrum light study, a clear-glass configuration of product packaging was subjected to constant light for seven months to determine the effects. At the end of each month, HPLC analysis was conducted on two samples to detect any degradation of the product, in terms of percent potency.

Month	0	1	2	3	4	5	6	7
Sample 1%	100	90	81	72	15	12	4	1
Sample 2%	100	92	79	69	13	9	6	2

Figure 7.19 shows a scatter plot of the actual data points. Between months 3 and 4, the potency of the product declined drastically. Initially, it may seem wise to create three splines: the first spline covering months 0–3, a second spline covering months 3–4, and a third spline covering months 4–7.

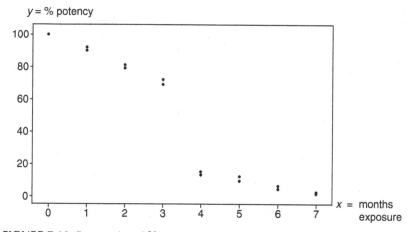

FIGURE 7.19 Scatter plot of % potency by months of exposure data.

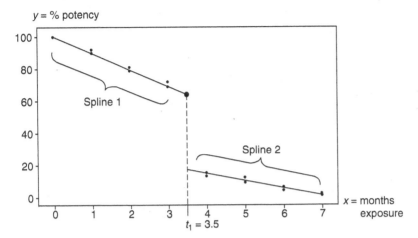

FIGURE 7.20 Proposed knot, % potency by months of exposure data, Example 7.3.

However, as there are no measurements in the period between months 3 and 4, the rate would be completely "unknown." So, only for simplifying the model, a knot was constructed between $x = 3$ and 4, specifically at 3.5, as shown in the scatter plot (Figure 7.20).

The model generally used is

$$\hat{y}' = \sum_{j=0}^{1} b_{0j}\, x^j + \sum_{i=1}^{1} b_i(x - t_1),$$

but this is a discontinuous fraction, so it must be modified to

$$\hat{y}' = \sum_{j=0}^{1} b_{0j}\, x^j + \sum_{i=1}^{1} \sum_{j=0}^{1} b_{ij}(x - t_i)^j$$

or

$$\hat{y}' = b_{00} + b_{01}x + b_{10}(x - t_1)^0 + b_{11}(x - t_1)^1,$$

where

$$t_1 = x = 3.5$$

$$(x - t)^0 = \begin{cases} 0, & \text{if } x - t_1 \le 0 \\ 1, & \text{if } x - t_1 \ge 0 \end{cases}$$

$$(x - t)^1 = \begin{cases} 0, & \text{if } x - t_1 \le 0 \\ x - t, & \text{if } x - t_1 > 0 \end{cases}.$$

Table 7.17 presents the input data.

TABLE 7.17
Input Data, One Knot and Two Splines, Example 7.3

Row	x	y	$(x-t)^0$	$(x-t)^1$
1	0	100	0	0.0
2	0	100	0	0.0
3	1	90	0	0.0
4	1	92	0	0.0
5	2	81	0	0.0
6	2	79	0	0.0
7	3	72	0	0.0
8	3	69	0	0.0
9	4	15	1	0.5
10	4	13	1	0.5
11	5	12	1	1.5
12	5	9	1	1.5
13	6	4	1	2.5
14	6	6	1	2.5
15	7	1	1	3.5
16	7	2	1	3.5

TABLE 7.18
Regression Analysis, One Knot and Two Splines, Example 7.3

Predictor	Coef	St. Dev	t-Ratio	p
b_{00}	100.300	0.772	129.87	0.000
b_{01}	−9.9500	0.4128	−24.10	0.000
b_1	−49.125	1.338	−36.72	0.000
b_2	5.6500	0.5838	9.68	0.000

$s = 1.305$ $\qquad R^2 = 99.9\%$ $\qquad R^2_{(adj)} = 99.9\%$

Analysis of Variance

Source	DF	SS	MS	F	P
Regression	3	25277.5	8425.8	4944.25	0.000
Error	12	20.5	1.7		
Total	15	25297.9			

Source	DF	SEQ SS
x	1	22819.5
$(x-t)^0$	1	2298.3
$(x-t)^1$	1	159.6

The regression equation is $\hat{y} = 100 - 9.95x - 49.1(x-t)^0 + 5.65(x-t)^1$.

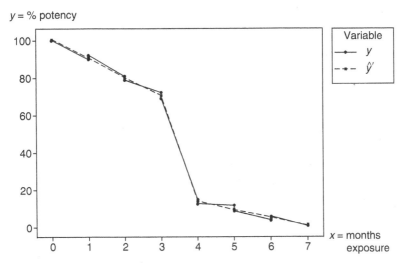

FIGURE 7.21 y, x and $\hat{y}'$, x, Example 7.3.

The regression analysis is presented in Table 7.18.

The graphic presentation of the overlaid actual and predicted $\hat{y}'$ values against x values are presented in Figure 7.21. Figure 7.22 breaks the regression into the actual components.

Finally, the data, x, y, $\hat{y}'$, and e are presented in Table 7.19. Clearly, this model fits the data extremely well.

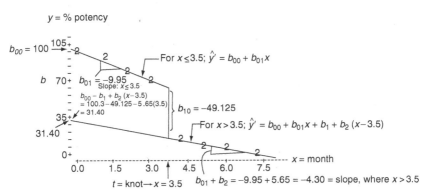

FIGURE 7.22 Breakdown of model components.

TABLE 7.19
x, y, $\hat{y}'$, and e for One Knot and Two Splines, Example 7.3

n	x	y	$\hat{y}'$	e
1	0	100	100.30	−0.30000
2	0	100	100.30	−0.30000
3	1	90	90.35	−0.35000
4	1	92	90.35	1.65000
5	2	81	80.40	0.60000
6	2	79	80.40	−1.40000
7	3	72	70.45	1.55000
8	3	69	70.45	−1.45000
9	4	15	14.20	0.80000
10	4	13	14.20	−1.20000
11	5	12	9.90	2.10000
12	5	9	9.90	−0.90000
13	6	4	5.60	−1.60000
14	6	6	5.60	0.40000
15	7	1	1.30	−0.30000
16	7	2	1.30	0.70000

8 Special Topics in Multiple Regression

INTERACTION BETWEEN THE x_i PREDICTOR VARIABLES

Interaction between x_i predictor variables is a common phenomenon in multiple regression practices. Technically, a regression model contains only independent x_i variables and is concerned with the predicted additive effects of each variable. For example, for the model, $\hat{y} = b_0 + b_1x_1 + b_2x_2 + b_3x_3 + b_4x_4$, the predictor x_i components that make up the SS_R are additive if one can add the SS_R values for the separate individual regression models ($\hat{y} = b_0 + b_1x_1$; $\hat{y} = b_0 + b_2x_2$; $\hat{y} = b_0 + b_3x_3$; $\hat{y} = b_0 + b_4x_4$), and their sum equals the SS_R of the full model. This condition rarely occurs in practice, so it is important to add interaction terms to "check" for significant interaction effects. Those interaction terms that are not significant can be removed.

For example, in the equation, $\hat{y} = b_0 + b_1x_1 + b_2x_2 + b_3x_1x_2$, the interaction term is

$$x_1x_2. \tag{8.1}$$

In practice, if the interaction term is not statistically significant at the chosen α, the SS_R contribution of that variable is added to the SS_E term, as well as its one degree of freedom lost in adding the interaction term.

The key point is, when interaction is significant, the b_i regression coefficients involved no longer have independent and individual meaning; instead, their meaning is conditional. Take the equation:

$$\hat{y} = b_0 + b_1x_1 + b_2x_2, \tag{8.2}$$

b_1, in this equation, represents the amount of change in the mean response, y, due to a unit change in x_1, given x_2 is held constant.

But in Equation 8.3, b_1 now is not the change in y for a unit change in x_1, holding x_2 constant:

$$y = b_0 + b_1x_1 + b_2x_2 + b_3x_1x_3. \tag{8.3}$$

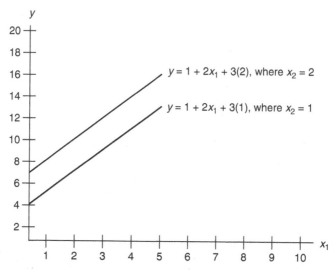

FIGURE 8.1 Additive model, no interaction.

Instead, $b_1 + b_3 x_2$ is the mean response change in y for a unit change in x_1, holding x_2 constant. Additionally, $b_2 + b_3 x_1$ is the change in the mean response of y for a unit change in x_2, holding x_1 constant. This, in essence, means that the effect of one x_i predictor variable depends in part on the level of the other predictor x_i variable, when interaction is present.

To illustrate this, suppose we have a function, $y = 1 + 2x_1 + 3x_2$. Suppose there are two levels of x_2: $x_2 = 1$ and $x_2 = 2$. The regression function with two values of x_2 is plotted in Figure 8.1. The model is said to be additive, for the y intercepts change but not the slopes; they are parallel. Hence, no interaction exists.

Now, suppose we use the same function with the interaction present. Let us assume that $b_3 = -0.50$, $y = 1 + 2x_1 + 3x_2 - 0.50x_1x_2$, and $x_2 = 1$ and 2 again. Note that both the intercepts and the slopes differ (Figure 8.2).

Neither the slopes are parallel, nor are the intercepts equal. In cases of interaction, the intercepts can be equal, but the slopes will always differ. That is, interaction is present because the slopes are not parallel. Figure 8.3 portrays the general patterns of interaction through scatterplots.

The practical aspect of interaction is that it does not make sense to discuss a regression in terms of one x_i without addressing the other x_is that are affected in the interaction. Conditional statements, not blanket statements, can be made. As previously mentioned, it is a good idea to check for interaction by including interaction terms. To do this, one just includes the possible combinations of the predicted variables, multiplying them to get their cross-products.

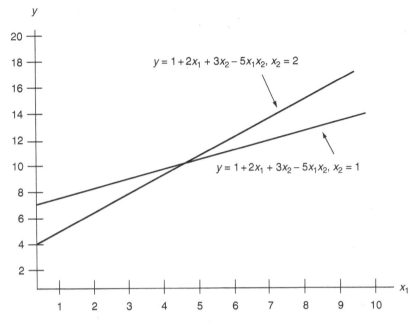

FIGURE 8.2 Nonadditive model, interaction present.

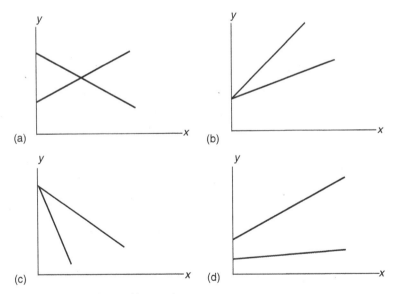

FIGURE 8.3 Other views of interaction.

For example, suppose there are two predictors, x_1 and x_2. The complete model, with interaction, is:

$$\hat{y} = b_0 + b_1 x_1 + b_2 x_2 + b_3 x_1 x_2.$$

Often the interaction term is portrayed as a separate predictor variable, say, x_3, where $x_3 = x_1 \cdot x_2$, or as a z term, where $z_1 = x_1 \cdot x_2$.

The use of the partial F-test is also an important tool in interaction determination. If $F(x_3 | x_1, x_2)$ is significant, for example, then significant interaction is present, and the x_1 and x_2 terms are conditional. That is, one cannot talk about the effects of x_1 without taking x_2 into account. Suppose there are three predictor variables, x_1, x_2, and x_3. Then, the model with all possible interactions is:

$$\hat{y} = b_0 + b_1 x_1 + b_2 x_2 + b_3 x_3 + b_4 x_4 + b_5 x_5 + b_6 x_6 + b_7 x_7$$

where $x_4 = x_1 x_2$, $x_5 = x_1 x_3$, $x_6 = x_2 x_3$, $x_7 = x_1 x_2 x_3$.

Each of the two-way interactions can be evaluated using partial F-tests, as can the three-way interaction.

If $F(x_7 | x_1, x_2, x_3, x_4, x_5, x_6)$ is significant, then there is significant three-way interaction. Testing two- and three-way interaction is so easy with current statistical software that it should be routinely done in all model-building.

CONFOUNDING

Confounding occurs when there are variables of importance that influence other measured predictor variables. Instead of the predictor variable measuring Effect X, for example, it also measures Effect Y. There is no way to determine to what degree Effects X and Y contribute independently as well as together, so they are said to be confounded, or mixed. For example, in surgically associated infection rates, suppose that, unknown to the researcher, 5% of all patients under 60 years of age, but otherwise healthy, develop nosocomial infections, 10% of patients of any age who suffer immune-compromising conditions do, and 20% of all individuals over 80 years old do. Confounding occurs when the under 60-year-old group, the immunocom-promised group, and the over 60-year-old group are lumped together in one category. This can be a very problematic situation, particularly if the researcher makes rather sweeping statements about nosocomial infections, as if no confounding occurred. However, at times, a researcher may identify confounding factors, but combines the variable into one model to provide a generalized statement, such as "all surgical patients" develop nosocomial infections.

Example 8.1: In a preoperative skin preparation evaluation, males and females are randomly assigned to test products and sampled before antimicrobial

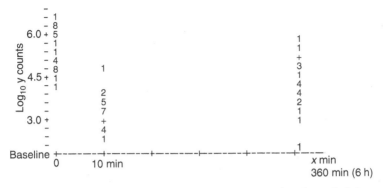

FIGURE 8.4 Plot of baseline and 10 min, 3 h, and 6 h samples, Example 8.1.

treatment (baseline), as well as 10 min and 6 h postantimicrobial treatment. Figure 8.4 provides the data collected in $\log_{10}$ colony count scale, with both sexes pooled in a scatter plot.

The baseline average is 5.52 $\log_{10}$. At 10 min posttreatment, the average is 3.24 $\log_{10}$, and at 360 min (6 h), the average is 4.55 $\log_{10}$. The actual $\log_{10}$ values separated between males and females are provided in Table 8.1.

Figure 8.5 and Figure 8.6 present the data from male and female subjects, respectively.

When the averages are plotted separately (see Figure 8.7), one can see that they provide a much different picture than that of the averages pooled. Sex of the subject was confounding in this evaluation. Also, note the interaction. The slopes of A and B are not the same at any point. We will return to this example when we discuss piecewise linear regression using dummy variables.

However, in practice, sometimes confounding is unimportant. What if it serves no purpose to separate the data on the basis of male and female? The important point is to be aware of confounding predictor variables.

UNEQUAL ERROR VARIANCES

We have discussed transforming y and x values to linearize them, as well as removing effects of serial correlation. But transformations can also be valuable in eliminating nonconstant error variances. Unequal error variances are often easily determined by a residual plot. For a simple linear regression, $\hat{y} = b_0 + b_1 x_1 + e$, the residual plot will appear similar to Figure 8.8, if a constant variance is present.

Because the e values are distributed relatively evenly around "0," there is no detected pattern of increase or decrease in the residual plot. Now view Figure 8.9a and Figure 8.9b. The residual errors get larger in Figure 8.9a and smaller in Figure 8.9b, as the x values increase.

TABLE 8.1
Log$_{10}$ Colony Counts, Example 8.1

n	Minute	Males	Females
1	0	6.5	4.9
2	0	6.2	4.3
3	0	6.0	4.8
4	0	5.9	5.2
5	0	6.4	4.7
6	0	6.1	4.8
7	0	6.2	5.1
8	0	6.0	5.2
9	0	5.8	4.8
10	0	6.2	4.9
11	0	6.2	5.3
12	0	6.1	4.8
13	0	6.2	4.9
14	0	6.3	5.0
15	0	6.4	4.5
16	10	3.2	4.7
17	10	3.5	3.2
18	10	3.0	3.5
19	10	3.8	3.6
20	10	2.5	3.1
21	10	2.9	2.7
22	10	3.1	3.1
23	10	2.8	3.1
24	10	3.5	3.5
25	10	3.1	3.8
26	10	2.8	3.4
27	10	3.4	3.4
28	10	3.1	3.4
29	10	3.3	2.6
30	10	3.1	2.9
31	360	5.2	3.5
32	360	4.8	3.8
33	360	5.2	4.0
34	360	4.7	3.8
35	360	5.1	4.1
36	360	5.3	4.1
37	360	5.7	4.3
38	360	4.5	5.0
39	360	5.1	5.1
40	360	5.2	4.1
41	360	5.1	4.0

(continued)

TABLE 8.1 (continued)
Log₁₀ Colony Counts, Example 8.1

n	Minute	Males	Females
42	360	5.2	3.3
43 .	360	5.1	4.8
44	360	5.0	2.9
45	360	5.1	3.5

0 = baseline prior to treatment.
10 = 10 min posttreatment sample.
360 = 360 min (6 h) posttreatment sample.

A simple transformation procedure can often remove the unequal scatter in e. But this is not the only procedure available; weighted least-squares regression can also be useful.

RESIDUAL PLOTS

Let us discuss more about residual plots. Important plots to generate in terms of residuals include:

1. The residual values, $y_i - \hat{y}_i = e_i$, plotted against the fitted values, $\hat{y}_i$. This residual scatter graph is useful in:
   a. portraying the differences between the predicted $\hat{y}$ and the actual y_i, which is the e_is, and the predicted $\hat{y}_i$ values,

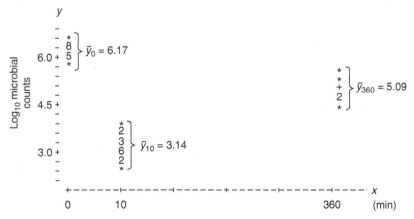

FIGURE 8.5 Log₁₀ colony counts with averages for males, Example 8.1.

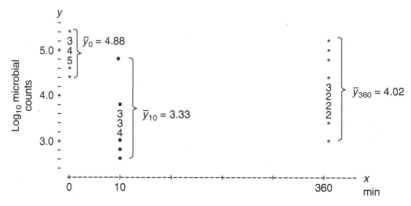

FIGURE 8.6 Log_{10} colony counts with averages for females, Example 8.1.

    b. the randomness of the error term, e_i, and
    c. outliers or large e_is.
2. Additionally, the e_i values should be plotted against each x_i predictor variable. This plot can often present patterns, such as seen in Plot a and Plot b of Figure 8.9. Also, the randomness of the error terms vs. the predictor variables and outliers can usually be visualized.
3. Residuals can be useful in model diagnostics in multiple regression by plotting interaction terms.
4. A plot of the absolute e_i, or $|e_i|$, as well as e_i^2 against $\hat{y}_i$ can also be useful for determining the consistency of the error variance. If non-uniformity is noted in the above plots, plot the $|e_i|$ and e_i^2 against each x_i predictor variable.

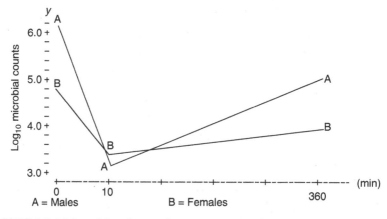

FIGURE 8.7 Male and female sample averages, Example 8.1.

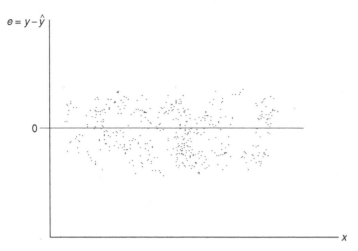

FIGURE 8.8 Residual plot of constant variance.

Several formal tests are available to evaluate whether the error variance is constant.

MODIFIED LEVENE TEST FOR CONSTANT VARIANCE

This test for constant variance does not depend on the error terms (e_i) being normally distributed. That is, the test is very robust, even if the error terms are not normal, and is based on the size of the $y_i - \hat{y}_i = e_i$ error terms. The larger the e_i^2, the larger the s_y^2. Because a large s_y^2 value may be due to a constant variance, the data set is divided into two groups, n_1 and n_2. If, say, the variance is increasing as the x_i values increase, then the $\sum e_i^2$ lower values of n_1 should be less than the $\sum e_i^2$ upper values of n_2.

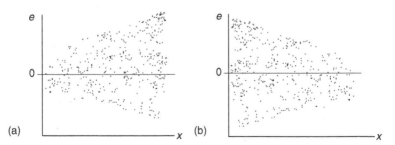

FIGURE 8.9 Residual plots of nonconstant variances.

PROCEDURE

To perform this test, the data are divided into two groups—one in which the x_i predictor variables are low, the other in which predictor variables are high (Figure 8.10).

Although the test can be conducted for multiple x_i predictor variables at once, it also generally works well using only one x_i predictor, given the predictor is significant through the partial F-test for being in the model. The goal is simple: to detect the increase or the decrease of e_i values with a magnitude increase of the x_i. To keep the test robust, the absolute or positive values of the e_is are used. The procedure involves a two-sample t-test to determine whether the mean of the absolute difference of one group is significantly different from the mean of the absolute difference of the other. The absolute deviations usually are not normally distributed, but they can be approximated by the t distribution when the sample size of each group is not too small, say, both $n_1 > 10$ and $n_2 > 10$.

Let $e_{i1} =$ the ith residual from the n_1 group of lower values of x_i, and $e_{i2} =$ the ith residual for the n_2 group of higher values of x_i.

$n_1 =$ sample size of the lower x_i group
$n_2 =$ sample size of the upper x_i group
$e'_1 =$ median of the lower e_i group
$e'_2 =$ median of the upper e_i group
$d_{i1} = |e_{i1} - e'_1| =$ absolute deviation of the lower x_i group
$d_{i2} = |e_{i2} - e'_2| =$ absolute deviation of the upper x_i group

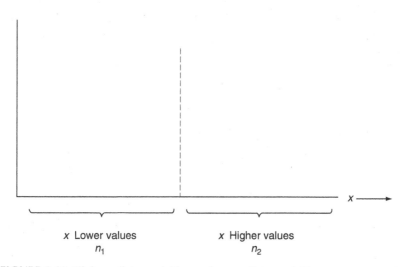

FIGURE 8.10 High predictor variables vs. low predictor variables.

The test statistic is

$$t_c = \frac{\bar{d}_1 - \bar{d}_2}{s\sqrt{(1/n_1) + (1/n_2)}},$$ (8.4)

where

$$s^2 = \frac{\sum_{i=1}^{n_1}(d_{i_1} - \bar{d}_1)^2 + \sum_{i=1}^{n_2}(d_{i_2} - \bar{d}_2)^2}{n_1 + n_2 - 2}.$$ (8.5)

If $t_c > t_{t(\alpha, n_1 + n_2 - 2)}$, reject H_0.

Let us work out an example (Example 8.2). In a drug stability evaluation, an antimicrobial product was held at ambient temperature (~68°F) for 12 months. The potency (%) through HPLC was measured, 10^6 colony-forming units (CFU) of *Staphylococcus aureus* (methicillin-resistant) were exposed to the product for 2 min, and the microbial reductions ($\log_{10}$ scale) were measured. Table 8.2 provides the data.

The proposed regression model is:

$$\hat{y} = b_0 + b_1 x_1 + b_2 x_2 + e$$

where $\hat{y}$ = % potency, x_1 = month of measurement, and x_2 = microbial $\log_{10}$ reduction value.

The regression model parameters are presented in Table 8.3. and the regression evaluation of the data in Table 8.2 are presented in Table 8.4.

We will consider x_1 (months) as the main predictor value with the greatest value range, 1 through 12. Note, by a t-test, each independent predictor variable is highly significant in the model ($p < 0.01$). A plot of the e_is vs. x_1, presented in Figure 8.11, demonstrates, by itself, a nonconstant variance. Often, this pattern is masked by extraneous outlier values. The data should be "cleaned" of these values to better see a nonconstant variance situation, but often the Modified Levene will identify a nonconstant variance, even in the presence of the "noise" of outlier values.

Without even doing a statistical test, it is obvious that, as months go by, the variability in the data increases. Nevertheless, let us perform the Modified Levene Test.

First, divide the data into two groups, n_1 and n_2, consisting of both y and x_i data points. One does not have to use all the data points; a group of the first and last will suffice. So, let us use the first three and the last three months (Table 8.5).

Group 1 = first three months
Group 2 = last three months

TABLE 8.2
Time-Kill Data, Example 8.2

y (Potency%)	x_1 (Month)	x_2 (Log$_{10}$ kill)
100	1	5.0
100	1	5.0
100	1	5.1
100	2	5.0
100	2	5.1
100	2	5.0
98	3	4.8
99	3	4.9
99	3	4.8
97	4	4.6
96	4	4.7
95	4	4.6
95	5	4.7
87	5	4.3
93	5	4.4
90	6	4.0
85	6	4.4
82	6	4.6
88	7	4.5
84	7	3.2
88	7	4.1
87	8	4.4
83	8	4.5
79	8	3.6
73	9	4.0
86	9	3.2
80	9	3.0
81	10	4.2
83	10	3.1
72	10	2.9
70	11	2.3
88	11	3.1
68	11	1.0
70	12	1.0
68	12	2.1
52	12	0.3

y = potency, the measure of the kill of *Staphylococcus aureus* following a 2 min exposure; 100% = fresh product ≈ 5 log$_{10}$ reduction.

x_1 = month of test = end of month.

x_2 = log$_{10}$ reduction in a 10^6 CFU population of *S. aureus* in 2 min.

TABLE 8.3
Time-Kill Data, Including Predicted y, x_1, x_2, $\hat{y}$, and $e_i = y - \hat{y}$,
Example 8.2

n	y	x_1	x_2	$\hat{y}$	e
1	100	1	5.0	101.009	−1.0089
2	100	1	5.0	101.009	−1.0089
3	100	1	5.1	101.009	−1.4390
4	100	2	5.0	99.261	0.7393
5	100	2	5.1	99.691	0.3092
6	100	2	5.0	99.261	0.7393
7	98	3	4.8	96.652	1.3476
8	99	3	4.9	97.083	1.9175
9	99	3	4.8	96.652	2.3476
10	97	4	4.6	94.044	2.9559
11	96	4	4.7	94.474	1.5258
12	95	4	4.6	94.044	0.9559
13	95	5	4.7	92.726	2.2739
14	87	5	4.3	91.006	−4.0057
15	93	5	4.4	91.436	1.5642
16	90	6	4.0	87.967	2.0328
17	85	6	4.4	89.688	−4.6876
18	82	6	4.6	90.548	−8.5478
19	88	7	4.5	88.370	−0.3696
20	84	7	3.2	82.778	1.2217
21	88	7	4.1	86.649	1.3508
22	87	8	4.4	86.191	0.8086
23	83	8	4.5	86.621	−3.6215
24	79	8	3.6	82.751	−3.7506
25	73	9	4.0	82.723	−9.7229
26	86	9	3.2	79.282	6.7179
27	80	9	3.0	78.422	1.5781
28	81	10	4.2	81.835	−0.8350
29	83	10	3.1	77.104	5.8962
30	72	10	2.9	76.244	−4.2436
31	70	11	2.3	71.915	−1.9149
32	88	11	3.1	75.356	12.6443
33	68	11	1.0	66.324	1.6764
34	70	12	1.0	64.575	5.4245
35	68	12	2.1	69.307	−1.3066
36	52	12	0.3	61.565	−9.5648

TABLE 8.4
Regression Evaluation, Example 8.2

Predictor	Coef	St. Dev	t-Ratio	p
b_0	81.252	6.891	11.79	0.000
b_1	−1.7481	0.4094	−4.27	0.000
b_2	4.301	1.148	3.75	0.001

$s = 4.496$　　　　$R^2 = 86.5\%$　　　　$R^2_{(adj)} = 85.7\%$

Source	DF	SS	MS	F	p
Regression	2	4271.9	2135.9	105.68	0.000
Error	33	667.0	20.2		
Total	35	4938.9			

The regression equation is $\hat{y} = 81.3 - 1.75x_1 + 4.30x_2$.

The $e'_1 =$ median of error in lower group $= 0.73927$, and $e'_2 =$ median of error in upper group $= -0.83495$.

---

n_1	$d_1 = \lvert e_{i_1} - e'_1 \rvert,\ e'_1 = 0.73927$	n_2	$d_2 = \lvert e_{i_2} - e'_2 \rvert,\ e'_2 = -0.83495$
1	1.74813	10	0.00000
1	1.74813	10	6.7311
1	2.17823	10	3.4087
2	0.00000	11	1.0800
2	0.43011	11	13.4792
2	0.00000	11	2.5113
3	0.60832	12	6.2595
3	1.17822	12	0.4716
3	1.60832·	12	8.7298
Sum the errors (absolute value)	$\sum \lvert e_{i_1} - e'_1 \rvert = 9.4995$		$\sum \lvert e_{i_1} - e'_2 \rvert = 42.671$

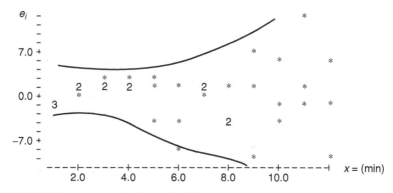

FIGURE 8.11　e_is vs. x_1 plot, Example 8.2.

TABLE 8.5
x_1 Data for First Three Months and Last Three Months, Example 8.2

Group 1 (first three months)			Group 2 (last three months)		
n_1	y	x_1	n_2	y	x_1
1	100	1	1	81	10
2	100	1	2	83	10
3	100	1	3	72	10
4	100	2	4	70	11
5	100	2	5	88	11
6	100	2	6	68	11
7	98	3	7	70	12
8	99	3	8	68	12
9	99	3	9	52	12

Error Group 1			Error Group 2		
n_1	x_{i_1}	e_{i_1}	n_2	x_{i_2}	e_{i_2}
1	1	−1.00886	1	10	−0.8350
2	1	−1.00886	2	10	5.8962
3	1	−1.43896	3	10	−4.2436
4	2	0.73927	4	11	−1.9149
5	2	0.30916	5	11	12.6443
6	2	0.73927	6	11	1.6764
7	3	1.34759	7	12	5.4245
8	3	1.91749	8	12	−1.3066
9	3	2.34759	9	12	−9.5648

Next, find the average error difference, $\bar{d}_i$:

$$\bar{d}_i = \frac{\sum \left| e_{ij} - e'_j \right|}{n_i}$$

$$\bar{d}_1 = \frac{9.4995}{9} = 1.0555$$

$$\bar{d}_2 = \frac{42.671}{9} = 4.7413$$

Next, we will perform the six-step procedure to test whether the two groups are different in error term magnitude.

Step 1: State the test hypothesis.

$H_0: \bar{d}_1 = \bar{d}_2$, the mean differences of the two groups are equal (constant variance)

$H_A: \bar{d}_1 \neq \bar{d}_2$, the above is not true (nonconstant variance)

Step 2: Determine the sample size and set the α level.
$n_1 = n_2 = 9$, and $\alpha = 0.05$

Step 3: State the test statistic to use (Equation 8.4).

$$t_c = \frac{\bar{d}_1 - \bar{d}_2}{s\sqrt{\frac{1}{n_1} + \frac{1}{n_2}}}.$$

Step 4: State the decision rule. This is a two-tail test, so if $|t_c| > |t_t|$, reject H_0 at $\alpha = 0.05$.

$t_t = t_{\text{tabled}} = t_{(\alpha/2;\ n_1 + n_2 - 2)} = t_{(0.05/2;\ 9 + 9 - 2)}$

$t_t = t_{(0.025;\ 16)} = 2.12$ (Table B).

Step 5: Compute the test statistic (Equation 8.5). First, we must find s, where

$$s^2 = \frac{\sum(d_{i_1} - \bar{d}_1)^2 + \sum(d_{i_2} - \bar{d}_2)^2}{n_1 + n_2 - 2}$$

In Tabular Form:

$(d_{i_1} - \bar{d}_1)^2$	$(d_{i_2} - \bar{d}_2)^2$
0.47973	22.4799
0.47973	3.9593
1.26053	1.7758
1.11407	13.4053
0.39111	76.3514
1.11407	4.9727
0.19997	2.3048
0.01506	18.2300
0.30561	15.9085
$\sum(d_{i_1} - \bar{d}_1)^2 = 5.3599$	$159.3877 = \sum(d_{i_2} - \bar{d}_2)^2$

$$s^2 = \frac{5.3599 + 159.3877}{9 + 9 - 2}$$

$s^2 = 10.2968$, and $s = 3.2089$ (Equation 8.4)

$$t_c = \frac{1.0555 - 4.7413}{3.2089\sqrt{\frac{1}{9} + \frac{1}{9}}}$$

$t_c = -2.4366$
$|t_c| = 2.4366$

Step 6: Draw the conclusion.
Because $|t_c| = 2.4366 > |t_t| = 2.12$, reject H_0. The variance is not constant at $\alpha = 0.05$. In practice, the researcher would probably not want to transform the data to make a constant variance. Instead, the spreading pattern exhibited in Figure 8.11 alerts the researcher that the stability of the product is deteriorating at a very uneven rate. Not only is the potency decreasing, it is also decreasing at an increasingly uneven rate. One can clearly see this from the following:

$$\sum (d_1 - \bar{d}_1)^2 < \sum (d_2 - \bar{d}_2)^2$$

BREUSCH–PAGAN TEST: ERROR CONSTANCY

This test is best employed when the error terms are not highly serially correlated, either by assuring this with the Durbin–Watson test or after the serial correlation has been corrected. It is best used when the sample size is large, assuring normality of the data.

The test is based on the relationship of the s_i^2 to the ith level of x in the following way:

$$\ell n \, s_i^2 = f_0 + f_1 x_i$$

The equation implies that s_i^2 increases or decreases with x_i, depending on the sign ("+" or "−") of f_1. If $f_1 = $ "−," the s_i^2 values decrease with x_i. If $f_1 = $ "+," the s_i^2 values increase with x_i. If $f_1 \approx 0$, then the variance is constant.

The hypothesis is:

$H_0: f_1 = 0$
$H_A: f_1 \neq 0$

The n must be relatively large, say, $n > 30$, and the e_i values normally distributed.

The test statistic, a Chi-Square statistic, is:

$$\chi_c^2 = \frac{SS_{R_M}}{2} \div \left(\frac{SS_E}{n}\right)^2. \tag{8.6}$$

For one x_i predictor variable, in cases of simple linear regression, e_i^2 equals the squared residual $(y_i - \hat{y})^2$, as always. Let SS_{RM} equal the sum of squares regression on the e_i^2 vs. the x_i. That is, the value, $(y_i - \hat{y})^2 = e_i^2$, is used as the y, or predictor value in this test. The e_i values are squared, and a simple linear regression is performed to provide the SS_{RM} term. The SS_E term is the sum of squares error of the original equation, where e_i^2 is not used as the dependent variable. The Chi-Square test statistic tabled value, χ_t^2, has one degree of freedom, $\chi_{t(\alpha,1)}^2$. If $\chi_c^2 > \chi_t^2$, reject H_0 at α.

We will use the data from Example 8.2 and do the test using x_i again, or y_i, where $x = $ month and $y = $ potency%.

Step 1: State the test hypothesis.

$H_0: f_1 = 0$ (variance is constant)
$H_A: f_1 \neq 0$ (variance is not constant)

Step 2: Set $\alpha = 0.05$, and $n = 36$.

Step 3: The test statistic is $\chi_c^2 = \frac{SS_{RM}}{2} \div \left(\frac{SS_E}{n}\right)^2$

Step 4: State the decision rule.
If $\chi_c^2 > \chi_{t(\alpha,1)} = \chi_{t(0.05,1)} = 3.841$ (Chi Square Table, Table L), reject H_0 at $\alpha = 0.05$.

Step 5: Compute the statistic (Table 8.6), $\hat{y} = b_0 + b_1 x_1$
The next step is to calculate the e_i values and square them (Table 8.7).
Table 8.8 presents the regression results, $e_i^2 = b_0 + b_1 x_1$.
We now have the data needed to compute χ_c^2

$$\chi_c^2 = \frac{SS_{RM}}{2} \div \left(\frac{SS_E}{n}\right)^2$$

TABLE 8.6
Regression Evaluation, $y = $ Potency % and $x_1 = $ Month, Example 8.2

Predictor	Coef	St. Dev	t-Ratio	p
b_0	106.374	1.879	56.61	0.000
b_1	−3.0490	0.2553	− 11.94	0.000
$s = 5.288$		$R^2 = 80.7\%$		$R_{(adj)}^2 = 80.2\%$

Source	DF	SS	MS	F	p
Regression	1	3988.0	3988.0	142.60	0.00
Error	34	950.9	28.0		
Total	35	4938.9			

The regression equation is $\hat{y} = 106 - 3.05x_1$.

TABLE 8.7
Values of e_i^2, Example 8.2

n	$e_i^2 = (y - \hat{y})^2$	x_i
1	11.054	1
2	11.054	1
3	11.054	1
4	0.076	2
5	0.076	2
6	0.076	2
7	0.598	3
8	3.144	3
9	3.144	3
10	7.964	4
11	3.320	4
12	0.676	4
13	14.985	5
14	17.048	5
15	3.501	5
16	3.686	6
17	9.487	6
18	36.967	6
19	8.814	7
20	1.063	7
21	8.814	7
22	25.179	8
23	1.036	8
24	8.893	8
25	35.203	9
26	49.940	9
27	1.138	9
28	26.171	10
29	50.634	10
30	15.087	10
31	8.039	11
32	229.969	11
33	23.380	11
34	0.046	12
35	3.191	12
36	316.353	12

SS_{R_M} is SS_R of the regression $e^2 = b_0 + b_1 x$ (Table 8.8).
$SS_{R_M} = 24132$
SS_E is the sum-squared error from the regression of $\hat{y} = b_0 + b_1 x_1$ (Table 8.6).

TABLE 8.8
Regression Analysis of $e_i^2 = b_0 + b_1 x_1$, Example 8.2

Predictor	Coef	St. Dev	t-Ratio	p
b_0	−22.34	20.65	−1.08	0.287
b_1	7.500	2.806	2.67	0.011

$s = 58.13$ $\qquad$ $R^2 = 17.4\%$ $\qquad$ $R_{(adj)}^2 = 14.9\%$

Source	DF	SS	MS	F	p
Regression	1	24132	24132	7.14	0.011
Error	34	114881	3379		
Total	35	139013			

The regression equation is $e^2 = 22.3 + 7.50x_1$.

$SS_E = 950.9$
$\quad n = 36$

$$\chi_c^2 = \frac{24132}{2} \div \left(\frac{950.9}{36}\right)^2 = 17.29$$

Step 6: Decision.
Because $\chi_c^2(17.29) > \chi_t^2 = (3.841)$, conclude that the f_1 value is not constant, so a significant nonconstant variance is present, at $\alpha = 0.05$.

FOR MULTIPLE x_i VARIABLES

The same basic formula is used (Equation 8.6). The $y_i - \hat{y} = e_i$ values are taken from the entire or full model, but the e_i^2 values are regressed only on the x_i predictor variables to be evaluated or, if the entire model is used, all are regressed.

$$e_i^2 \text{ vs. } (x_i, x_{i+1}, \ldots, x_k)$$

The SS_{R_M} is the sum of squares regression with the x_i values to be evaluated in the model, and the SS_E is from the full model, $x_i, x_{i+1}, \ldots, x_k$.

$\chi_t^2 = \chi_{t(\alpha, q)}^2$, where q is the number of x_i variables in the SS_{R_M} model.
The same hypothesis is used, and the null hypothesis is rejected if $\chi_c^2 > \chi_t^2$.

Using the data from Table 8.2 and all x_i values, the regression equation is:

$$\hat{y} = b_0 + b_1 x_1 + b_2 x_2,$$

where $y = $ potency%, $x_1 = $ month, and $x_2 = \log_{10}$ kill.

The six-step procedure follows.

Step 1: State the test hypothesis:

H_0: $f_1 = 0$ (variance is constant)
H_A: $f_1 \neq 0$ (variance is nonconstant)

Step 2: Set α and the sample size, n:
$\alpha = 0.05$, and $n = 36$

Step 3: Write out the test statistic (Equation 8.6):

$$\chi_c^2 = \frac{SS_{R_M}}{2} \div \left(\frac{SS_E}{n}\right)^2$$

Step 4: Decision rule:
If $\chi_c^2 > \chi_{t(\alpha, q)}^2 = \chi_{t(0.05, 2)}^2 = 5.991$ (Table L), reject H_0 at $\alpha = 0.05$.

Step 5: Compute the statistic:
Table 8.4 presents the regression, $\hat{y} = 81.3 - 1.75x_1 - 4.30x_2$, where y = potency %, x_1 = month, and x_2 = $\log_{10}$ kill.
Next, the regression, $\hat{e}_i^2 = b_0 + b_1x_1 + b_2x_2$ is computed using the data in Table 8.9.
The regression of $e^2 = b_0 + b_1x_1 + b_2x_2$ is presented in Table 8.10.

$$\chi_c^2 = \frac{SS_{R_M}}{2} \div \left(\frac{SS_E}{n}\right)^2$$

SS_{R_M} is the SS_R of the regression, $e^2 = b_0 + b_1x_1 + b_2x_2$ (Table 8.10).
$SS_{R_M} = 7902$
SS_E = from the regression of $\hat{y} = b_0 + b_1x_1 + b_2x_2$ (Table 8.4).
$SS_E = 667$
$n = 36$

$$\chi_c^2 = \left(\frac{7902}{2}\right) \div \left(\frac{667}{36}\right)^2 = 11.51$$

Step 6:
Because $\chi_c^2 = (11.51) > \chi_t^2(5.991)$, reject H_0 at $\alpha = 0.05$. The variance is nonconstant.

Again, the researcher probably would be very interested in the increasing variance in this example. The data suggest that, as time goes by, not only does the potency diminish, but also with increasing variability. This could flag the researcher to sense a very serious stability problem. In this case, transforming the data to stabilize the variance may not be useful. That is, there should be a

TABLE 8.9
Values of e_i^2, Example 8.2

Row	e_i^2	x_1	x_2
1	1.018	1	5.0
2	1.018	1	5.0
3	2.071	1	5.1
4	0.547	2	5.0
5	0.096	2	5.1
6	0.547	2	5.0
7	1.816	3	4.8
8	3.677	3	4.9
9	5.511	3	4.8
10	8.737	4	4.6
11	2.328	4	4.7
12	0.914	4	4.6
13	5.171	5	4.7
14	16.045	5	4.3
15	2.447	5	4.4
16	4.132	6	4.0
17	21.974	6	4.4
18	73.066	6	4.6
19	0.137	7	4.5
20	1.493	7	3.2
21	1.825	7	4.1
22	0.654	8	4.4
23	13.115	8	4.5
24	14.067	8	3.6
25	94.534	9	4.0
26	45.131	9	3.2
27	2.491	9	3.0
28	0.697	10	4.2
29	34.765	10	3.1
30	18.009	10	2.9
31	3.667	11	2.3
32	159.878	11	3.1
33	2.810	11	1.0
34	29.425	12	1.0
35	1.707	12	2.1
36	91.485	12	0.3

practical reason for transforming the variance to stabilize it, not just for statistical reasons.

Before proceeding to the weighted least squares method, we need to discuss a basic statistical procedure that will be used in weighted regression.

TABLE 8.10
Regression Analysis of $e_i^2 = b_0 + b_1 x_1 + b_2 x_2$, Example 8.2

Predictor	Coef	St. Dev	t-Ratio	p
b_0	−25.29	48.99	−0.52	0.609
b_1	5.095	2.911	1.75	0.089
b_2	2.762	8.160	0.34	0.737
$s = 31.96$		R-sq $= 19.0\%$		$R^2_{(adj)} = 14.1\%$

Source	DF	SS	MS	F	p
Regression	2	7902	3951	3.87	0.031
Error	33	33715	1022		
Total	35	41617			

The regression equation is $e^2 = -25.3 + 5.10x_1 + 2.76x_2$.

VARIANCE STABILIZATION PROCEDURES

There are many cases in which an investigator will want to make the variance constant. Recall, when a variance, σ^2, is not constant, the residual plot will look like Figure 8.12.

The transformation of the y values depends upon the amount of curvature the procedure induces. The Box–Cox transformation "automatically finds the correct transformation," but it requires an adequate statistical software package and should not only be used as the final answer, but also should be checked. The same strategy is used in *Applied Statistical Designs for the Researcher* (Paulson, 2003). But from an iterative perspective, Montgomery et al. also present a useful variance standardizing schema.

Relationship of σ^2 to $E(y)$	$y' = y$ Transformation
$\sigma^2 \approx$ constant	$y' = y$ (no transformation needed)
$\sigma^2 = E(y)$	$y' = \sqrt{y}$ (significant transformation as in Poisson data)
$\sigma^2 = E(y)[1 - E(y)]$	$y' = \sin^{-1}(\sqrt{y})$ where $0 \le y_i \le 1$ (binomial data)
$\sigma^2 = [E(y)]^2$	$y' = \ell n(y)$
$\sigma^2 = [E(y)]^3$	$y' = y^{-\frac{1}{2}}$ (reciprocal square root transformation)
$\sigma^2 = [E(y)]^4$	$y' = y^{-1}$ (reciprocal transformation)

Once a transformation is determined for the regression, substitute y' for y and plot the residuals. The process is an iterative one. It is particularly important to correct a nonconstant σ^2 when providing confidence intervals for prediction. The least squares estimator will still be unbiased, but no longer for a minimum variance probability.

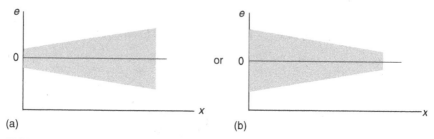

FIGURE 8.12 Residual plots: proportionally nonconstant variables.

WEIGHTED LEAST SQUARES

Recall that the general regression form is

$$Y_i = \beta_0 + \beta_1 x_1 + \cdots + \beta_k x_k + \varepsilon_i$$

The variance–covariance matrix is

$$\underset{n \times n}{\sigma^2(\varepsilon)} = \begin{bmatrix} \sigma_1^2 & 0 & \cdots & 0 \\ 0 & \sigma_2^2 & \cdots & 0 \\ \vdots & \vdots & \cdots & \vdots \\ 0 & 0 & \cdots & \sigma_n^2 \end{bmatrix}. \tag{8.7}$$

When the errors are not consistent, the b_i values are unbiased, but no longer portray the minimum variance. One must take into account that the different y_i observations for the n cases no longer have the same or constant reliability. The errors can be made constant by a weight assignment process, converting the σ_i^2 values by a $1/w_i$ term, where the largest σ_i^2 values—those with the most imprecision—are assigned the least weight.

The weighting process is merely an extension of the general variance–covariance matrix of the standard regression model, where $w =$ weight values, $1/w_i$, as diagonals and all other element values are 0, as in Equation 8.7.

Given that the errors are not correlated, but only unequal, the variance–covariance matrix can be made of the form:

$$\sigma^2 F = \sigma^2 \begin{bmatrix} \frac{1}{w_1} & 0 & \cdots & 0 \\ 0 & \frac{1}{w_2} & \cdots & 0 \\ \vdots & \vdots & \cdots & \vdots \\ 0 & 0 & \cdots & \frac{1}{w_n} \end{bmatrix}. \tag{8.8}$$

F is a diagonal matrix, and likewise is w, containing the weights, $w_1, w_2, \ldots,$ w_n. Similar to the normal least squares equation, the weighted least squares equation is of the form:

$$\hat{\beta}_w = (X'wX)^{-1}X'wY. \tag{8.9}$$

Fortunately, the weighted least squares estimators can easily be computed from standard software programs, where w is an $n \times n$ weight matrix

$$\underset{n \times n}{w} = \begin{bmatrix} w_1 & 0 & \cdots & 0 \\ 0 & w_2 & \cdots & 0 \\ \vdots & \vdots & \vdots & \vdots \\ 0 & 0 & \cdots & w_n \end{bmatrix}.$$

Otherwise, one can multiply each of the ith observed values, including the ones in the x_0 column, by the square root of the weight for that observation. This can be done for the x_is and the y_is. The standard least squares regression can then be performed. We will designate this standard data form of transformed values as S and Y:

$$S = \begin{bmatrix} 1 & x_{11} & \cdots & x_{1k} \\ 1 & x_{22} & \cdots & x_{2k} \\ \vdots & \vdots & \vdots & \vdots \\ 1 & x_{n1} & \cdots & x_{nk} \end{bmatrix} \quad Y = \begin{bmatrix} y_1 \\ y_2 \\ \vdots \\ y_n \end{bmatrix}. \tag{8.10}$$

Each x_i and y_i value in each row is multiplied by $\sqrt{w_i}$, the square root of the selected weight, to accomplish the transformation. The weighted transformation is

$$S_w = \begin{bmatrix} \overset{x_0}{1\sqrt{w_1}} & \overset{x_1}{x_{11}\sqrt{w_1}} & \overset{\cdots}{\cdots} & \overset{x_k}{x_k\sqrt{w_1}} \\ 1\sqrt{w_2} & x_{21}\sqrt{w_2} & \cdots & x_{2k}\sqrt{w_2} \\ \vdots & \vdots & \vdots & \vdots \\ 1\sqrt{w_n} & x_{n1}\sqrt{w_n} & \cdots & x_{nk}\sqrt{w_n} \end{bmatrix} \quad Y_w = \begin{bmatrix} \overset{y_i}{y_1\sqrt{w_1}} \\ y_2\sqrt{w_2} \\ \vdots \\ y_n\sqrt{w_n} \end{bmatrix}.$$

The final formula is

$$\hat{b}_w = (S'_w S_w)^{-1} S'_w Y_w = (X'wX)X'wY. \tag{8.11}$$

The weights follow the form, $w_i = 1/\sigma_i^2$, but the σ_i^2 values are unknown, as are the proper w_is. Recall that a large σ_i^2 is weighted less (by a smaller value) when compared with a smaller σ_i^2. This is reasonable, for the larger the variance, the less precise or certain one is.

ESTIMATION OF THE WEIGHTS

There are two general ways to estimate the weights:

1. when the e_is are increasing or decreasing by a proportional amount, and
2. regression of the e_i terms.

1. Proportionally increasing or decreasing e_i terms. Figure 8.12a is a pattern often observed in clinical trials of antimicrobial preoperative skin preparations and surgical handwash formulations. That is, the initial baseline population samples are very precise, but as the populations of bacteria residing on the skin decline posttreatment, the precision of the measurement decays. Hence, the error term ranges are small initially but increase over time. So, if σ_3^2 is three times larger than σ_1^2, and σ_2^2 is two times larger than σ_1^2, a possible weight choice would be: $w_1 = 1$, $w_2 = \frac{1}{2}$, and $w_3 = \frac{1}{3}$. Here, the weights can easily be assigned.

Figure 8.12b portrays the situation encountered, for example, when new methods of evaluation are employed, or new test teams work together. Initially, there is much variability but, over time, proficiency is gained, reducing the variability.

Although this is fine, one still does not know the σ_i^2 terms for each of the measurements. The σ_i^2 values are an estimate of σ^2 at the ith data point. The absolute value of e_i is an estimator of σ_i—that is, $|e_i| = \sigma_i$, or $\sqrt{\sigma_i^2}$.

The actual weight formula to use is

$$w_i = c\left(\frac{1}{\sigma_i^2}\right) = c\frac{1}{e_i^2},\tag{8.12}$$

where c = proportional constant and unknown, σ_i^2 = variance at a specific x_i, and e_i^2 = estimated variance at x_i.

Using this schema allows one to use Equation 8.9 in determining $\hat{b}_w$.

The weighted least squares variance–covariance matrix is

$$\sigma^2(\hat{b}_w) = \sigma^2(X'wX)^{-1}.\tag{8.13}$$

One does not know the actual value of c, so $\sigma^2(\hat{b}_w)$ is estimated by

$$s^2(\hat{b}_w) = MS_{E_w}(X'wX)^{-1},\tag{8.14}$$

where

$$MSE_w = \frac{\sum\limits_{i=1}^{n} w_i(y_i - \hat{y}_i)^2}{n-k} = \frac{\sum\limits_{i=1}^{n} w_i e_i^2}{n-k}, \tag{8.15}$$

where k = number of b_i values, excluding b_0.

Let us work out an example using the data from Example 8.2. We will use a flexible procedure with these data. As they are real data, the e_i terms bounce around, whereas they increase as x_1 increases. The predictor x_1 (month) has the most influence on the e_is, so it will be used as the sole x_i value. Table 8.11 provides the data, and in Figure 8.13, we see the error terms plotted against time, proportionately increasing in range.

We do not know what $1/\sigma^2$ is, but we can estimate the relative weights without knowing σ_i^2. We will focus on the $y - \hat{y}$ column in Table 8.12 and, for each of the three values per month, compute the absolute range, |high–low|. Some prefer to use only "near-neighbor" x_i values, but in pilot studies, this can lead to data-chasing. Above all, use a robust method. In this example, we will use near-neighbors of the x_1 predictor, the three replicates per month. The estimators do not have to be exact, and a three-value interval is arbitrary. The first range of $0.45 = |-1.2196 - (-1.6740)|$. Next, the relative weight (w_R) can be estimated. Because these data have a horn shape, we will call the lowest $|e_i|$ range 1, arbitrarily, even though the range is 0.45. This simplifies the process. It is wise to do the weighted regression iteratively, finding a weight system that is adequate, but not trying to make it "the weight system." Because $n = 36$, instead of grouping the like x_i values, we shall use them all. At this point, any x_i is considered as relevant as the rest.

Continuing with the example, Table 8.12 presents the regression with the weighted values in the equation, in which all x_i values are used. MiniTab computation, $\hat{b}_w = (X'wX)^{-1} X'wY$, automatically uses the weighted formula and the weights in a subroutine. If one does not have this option, one can compute $\hat{b}_w = (X'wX)^{-1} X'wY$.

Table 8.13 is the standard least squares model, and hence, contains exactly the same data as in Table 8.4. Notice that the MSE for the weighted values is $MSE = 1.05$, but for the unweighted values, is $MSE = 20.2$, which is a vast improvement of the model. Yet, if one plots the weighted residuals, one sees that they still show the same basic "form" of the unweighted residuals. This signals the need for another iteration. This time, the researcher may be better-off using a regression approach.

2. *Regression of the e_i terms to determine the weights.* The regression procedure rests on the assertion that $\sqrt{s_i^2} = \sqrt{e_i^2}$, or $s_i = |e_i|$ and $s_i^2 = e_i^2$. The s_i^2 values here are for each of the x_is in the multiple regression, with $e_i^2 = (y_i - \hat{y}_i)^2$. First, a standard regression is performed on the data; second, a separate regression with all the x_is in the model is performed on either e_i^2 or $|e_i|$. The weights are $w_i = 1/s_i^2 = 1/|e_i|^2$ with $c = 1$.

TABLE 8.11
Weight Computations, Example 8.2

n	y	x_1	x_2	$\hat{y}$	$y - \hat{y}$	|Range|	(w_R) Weight ratio to |e_i| in minutes	$w_i = \frac{1}{(w_R)}$
1	100	1	5.0	101.220	−1.2196			
2	100	1	5.0	101.220	−1.2196	0.45	1.00	1.00
3	100	1	5.1	101.674	−1.6740			
4	100	2	5.0	99.553	0.4665			
5	100	2	5.1	99.998	0.0121	0.45	1.00	1.00
6	100	2	5.0	99.533	0.4665			
7	98	3	4.8	96.938	1.0615			
8	99	3	4.9	97.393	1.6071	1.00	2.22	0.45
9	99	3	4.8	96.938	2.0615			
10	97	4	4.6	94.343	2.6566			
11	96	4	4.7	94.798	1.2021	2.00	4.44	0.23
12	95	4	4.6	94.343	0.6566			
13	95	5	4.7	93.112	1.8882			
14	87	5	4.3	91.294	−4.2939	6.18	13.73	0.07
15	93	5	4.4	91.748	1.2516			
16	90	6	4.0	88.244	1.7555			
17	85	6	4.4	90.062	4.9377	13.91	30.91	0.03
18	82	6	4.6	90.971	−8.9712			
19	88	7	4.5	88.831	−0.8306			
20	84	7	3.2	82.923	1.0773	1.91	4.24	0.24
21	88	7	4.1	87.013	0.9872			
22	87	8	4.4	86.690	0.3099			
23	83	8	4.5	87.145	−4.1445	4.45	9.89	0.10
24	79	8	3.6	83.054	−4.0544			
25	73	9	4.0	83.186	−10.1861			
26	86	9	3.2	79.550	6.4495	16.64	36.98	0.03
27	80	9	3.0	78.642	1.3584			
28	81	10	4.2	82.409	−1.4089			
29	83	10	3.1	77.410	5.5901	10.09	22.42	0.04
30	72	10	2.9	76.501	−4.5010			
31	70	11	2.3	72.088	−2.0881			
32	88	11	3.1	75.724	12.2762	14.36	31.91	0.03
33	68	11	1.0	66.180	1.8198			
34	70	12	1.0	64.494	5.5059			
35	68	12	2.1	69.493	−1.4931	14.82	32.93	0.03
36	52	12	0.3	61.313	−9.3128			

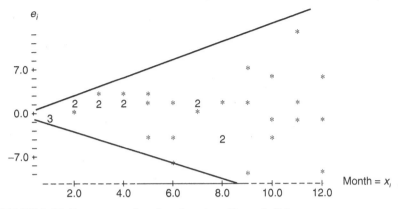

FIGURE 8.13 Error terms plotted against time, Example 8.2.

Some statisticians prefer to perform a regression analysis on the $|e_i|$ values to determine the weights to use without following the previous method (see Figure 8.14).

The $|e_i|$ values from the normal linear regression become the y_i values to determine the weights

$$|e_i| = y_i, \tag{8.16}$$
$$|e_i| = b_0 + b_1 x_1 + b_2 x_2.$$

The weights are computed as

$$\hat{w}_i = \frac{1}{|\hat{e}_i|^2}, \tag{8.17}$$

TABLE 8.12
Weighted Regression Analysis, Example 8.2

Predictor	Coef	SE Coef	t-Ratio	p
b_0	77.237	5.650	13.67	0.000
b_1	−1.4774	0.2640	−5.60	0.000
b_2	5.023	1.042	4.82	0.000

| $s = 1.02667$ | | $R^2 = 92.2\%$ | | $R^2_{(adj)} = 91.7\%$ |

Source	DF	SS	MS	F	p
Regression	2	411.9	205.96	195.39	0.000
Error	33	34.8	1.05		
Total	35	446.7			

The regression equation is $\hat{y} = 77.2 - 1.48x_1 + 5.02x_2$.

TABLE 8.13
Unweighted Regression Analysis

Predictor	Coef	St. Dev	t-Ratio	p
b_0	81.252	6.891	11.79	0.000
b_1	−1.7481	0.4094	−4.27	0.000
b_2	4.301	1.148	3.75	0.001

$s = 4.496$ $R^2 = 86.5\%$ $R^2_{(adj)} = 85.7\%$

Source	DF	SS	MS	F	p
Regression	2	4271.9	2135.9	105.68	0.000
Error	33	667.0	20.2		
Total	35	4938.9			

The regression equation is $\hat{y} = 81.3 − 1.75x_1 + 4.30x_2$.

for the standard deviation, or

$$\hat{w}_i = \frac{1}{e_i^2}$$

for the variance function.

The linear regression method, based on the computed $\hat{w}_i$, is presented in Table 8.14. The data used to compute the weights, $\hat{w}_i$, as well as the predicted $\hat{y}_w$, using the weights, and the error terms, $y_i − \hat{y}_{iw} = e_{iw}$, using the weights, are presented in Table 8.15.

Note the improvement of this model over the original and the proportional models. If the change in b_i parameters is great, it may be necessary to use the $|e_i|$ values of the weighted regression analysis as the y independent variable

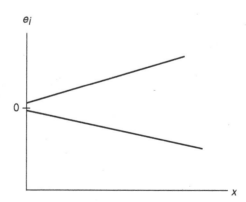

FIGURE 8.14 Slope of the expansion of the variance.

TABLE 8.14
Linear Regression to Determine Weights, Example 8.2

Predictor	Coef	SE Coef	t-Ratio	p
b_0	81.801	2.124	38.50	0.000
b_1	−1.69577	0.07883	−21.51	0.000
b_2	4.2337	0.3894	10.87	0.000

$s = 0.996302$ $\quad R^2 = 99.2\%$ $\quad R^2_{(adj)} = 99.1\%$

Source	DF	SS	MS	F	p
Regression	2	3987.2	1993.6	2008.45	0.000
Error	33	32.8	1.0		
Total	35	4020.0			

The regression equation is $\hat{y} = 81.8 - 1.70x_1 + 4.23x_2$.

and repeat the weight process iteratively a second or third time. In our case, the $R^2_{(adj)} \approx 0.99$, so another iteration will probably not be that useful.

In other situations, where there are multiple repeat readings for the x_i values, the e_i values at a specific x_i can provide the estimate for the weights. In this example, an s_i or s_i^2 would be calculated for each month, using the three replicates at each month. Because, at times, there was significant variability within each month, as well as between months (not in terms of proportionality), it probably would not have been as useful as the regression was. It is suggested that the reader make the determination by computing it.

RESIDUALS AND OUTLIERS, REVISITED

As was discussed in Chapter 3, outliers, or extreme values, pose a significant problem in that, potentially, they will bias the outcome of a regression analysis. When outliers are present, the questions always are "Are the outliers truly representative of the data that are extreme and must be considered in the analysis, or do they represent error in measurement, error in recording of data, influence of unexpected variables, and so on?" The standard procedure is to retain an outlier in an analysis, unless as assignable extraneous cause can be identified that proves the data point to be aberrant. If none can be found, or an explanation is not entirely satisfactory, one can present data analyses that include and omit one or more outliers, along with rationale explaining the implications, with and without.

In Chapter 3, it was noted that residual analysis is very useful for exploring the effects of outliers and nonnormal distributions of data, for how these relate to adequacy of the regression model, and for identifying and correcting for serially correlated data. At the end of the chapter, formulas for the process of

TABLE 8.15
Data for Linear Regression to Determine Weights, Example 8.2

Row	Nonweighted				e_i	$\hat{w}_i = \frac{1}{\|e_i\|^2}$	$\hat{y}_w$	$y - \hat{y}_w = e_{iw}$
	y	x_1	x_2	$\hat{y}$				
1	100	1	5.0	101.220	−1.2196	0.67	101.273	−1.2733
2	100	1	5.0	101.220	−1.2196	0.67	101.273	−1.2733
3	100	1	5.1	101.674	−1.6740	0.36	101.697	−1.6966
4	100	2	5.0	99.553	0.4665	4.59	99.578	0.4225
5	100	2	5.1	99.998	0.0121	6867.85	100.001	−0.0009
6	100	2	5.0	99.533	0.4665	4.59	99.578	0.4225
7	98	3	4.8	96.938	1.0615	0.89	97.035	0.9650
8	99	3	4.9	97.393	1.6071	0.39	97.458	1.5416
9	99	3	4.8	96.938	2.0615	0.24	97.035	1.9650
10	97	4	4.6	94.343	2.6566	0.14	94.492	2.5075
11	96	4	4.7	94.798	1.2021	0.69	94.916	1.0841
12	95	4	4.6	94.343	0.6566	2.32	94.492	0.5075
13	95	5	4.7	93.112	1.8882	0.28	93.220	1.7799
14	87	5	4.3	91.294	−4.2939	0.05	91.527	−4.5266
15	93	5	4.4	91.748	1.2516	0.64	91.950	1.0500
16	90	6	4.0	88.244	1.7555	0.32	88.561	1.4393
17	95	6	4.4	90.062	4.9377	0.04	90.254	4.7458
18	82	6	4.6	90.971	−8.9712	0.01	91.101	−9.1010
19	88	7	4.5	88.831	−0.8306	1.45	88.982	−0.9818
20	84	7	3.2	82.923	1.0773	0.86	83.478	0.5220
21	88	7	4.1	87.013	0.9872	1.03	87.288	0.7117
22	87	8	4.4	86.690	0.3099	10.41	86.863	0.1373
23	83	8	4.5	87.145	−4.1445	0.06	87.286	−4.2861
24	79	8	3.6	83.054	−4.0544	0.06	83.476	−4.4757
25	73	9	4.0	83.186	—	0.01	83.473	−10.4734
26	86	9	3.2	79.550	6.4495	0.02	80.086	5.9135
27	80	9	3.0	78.642	1.3584	0.54	79.240	0.7603
28	81	10	4.2	82.409	−1.4089	0.50	82.624	−1.6244
29	83	10	3.1	77.410	5.5901	0.03	77.967	5.0327
30	72	10	2.9	76.501	−4.5010	0.05	77.121	−5.1206
31	70	11	2.3	72.088	−2.0881	0.23	72.885	−2.8846
32	88	11	3.1	75.724	12.2762	0.01	76.272	11.7284
33	68	11	1.0	66.180	1.8198	0.30	67.381	0.6192
34	70	12	1.0	64.494	5.5059	0.03	65.685	4.3150
35	68	12	2.1	69.493	−1.4931	0.45	70.342	−2.3421
36	52	12	0.3	61.313	−9.3128	0.01	62.721	−10.7215

standardizing residual values were presented but the author did not expand that discussion for two reasons. First, the author and others [e.g., Kleinbaum et al. (1998)] prefer computing jackknife residuals, rather than standardized or Studentized ones. Secondly, for multiple regression, the rescaling of residuals by means of Studentizing and jackknifing procedures requires the use of matrix algebra to calculate hat matrices, explanations of which were deferred until we had explored models of multiple regression.

The reader is directed to Appendix II for a review of matrices and application of matrix algebra. Once that is completed, we will look at examples of Studentized and jackknifed residuals applied to data from simple linear regression models and then discuss rescaling of residuals as it applies to model leveraging due to outliers.

STANDARDIZED RESIDUALS

For sample sizes of 30 or more, the standardized residual is of value. The standardized residual just adjusts the residuals into a form where "0" is the mean, and a value of -1 or 1, represents 1 standard deviation, -2 or 2, represents 2 standard deviations, and so on.

The standardized residual is

$$S_{t_i} = \frac{e_i}{s_e},$$

where $e_i = y_i - \hat{y}_i$, and s_e is the standard deviation of the standard residual, where $k = $ number of b_is, excluding b_0

$$\sqrt{\frac{\sum e_i^2}{n - k - 1}}.$$

STUDENTIZED RESIDUALS

For smaller sample sizes ($n < 30$), the use of the Studentized approach is recommended, as it follows the Student's t-distribution with $n - k - 1$ df.

The Studentized residual (S_{r_i}) is computed as

$$S_{r_i} = \frac{e_i}{s\sqrt{1 - h_i}}. \tag{8.18}$$

The standard deviation of the Studentized residual is the divisor, $s\sqrt{1 - h_{ii}}$.

The h_{ii}, or leverage value measures the weight of the ith observation in terms of its importance in the model's fit. The value of h_{ii} will always be between 0 and 1, and, technically, represents the diagonal portion of a $(n \times n)$ hat matrix:

$$X(X'X)^{-1}X' = H. \qquad (8.19)$$

The standardized and Studentized residuals generally convey the same information, except when specific e_i residuals are large, the h_{ii} values are large, and/or the sample size is small. Then use the Studentized approach to the residuals.

JACKKNIFE RESIDUAL

The ith jackknife residual is computed by deleting the ith residual and, so, is based on $n - 1$ observations. The jackknife residual is calculated as

$$r_{(-i)} = S_{r_i}\sqrt{\frac{s^2}{s^2_{(-i)}}}, \qquad (8.20)$$

where

$s^2 = $ residual variance, $\frac{\sum e_i^2}{n-k-1}$,

$s^2_{(-i)} = $ residual variance with the ith residual removed,

$S_{r_i} = $ Studentized residual $= \frac{e_i}{s\sqrt{1-h_{ii}}}$,

$r_{(-i)} = $ jackknife residual.

The mean of the jackknife residual approximates 0, with a variance of

$$s^2 = \frac{\sum\limits_{i=1}^{n} r^2_{(-i)}}{n - k - 2}, \qquad (8.21)$$

which is slightly more than 1.

The degrees of freedom of $s^2_{(-i)}$ is $(n - k - 1) - 1$, where $k = $ number of b_is, not including b_0.

If the standard regression assumptions are met, and the same number of replicates is taken at each x_i value, the standardized, the Studentized, and jackknife residuals look the same. Outliers are often best identified by the jackknife residual, for it makes suspect data more obvious. For example, if the ith residual observation is extreme (lies outside the data pool), the $s_{(-i)}$ value will tend to be much smaller than s_i, which will make the $r_{(-i)}$ value larger in comparison to S_{r_i}, the Studentized residual. Hence, the $r_{(-i)}$ value will stand out for detection.

To Determine Outliers

In practice, Kleimbaum et al. (1998) and this author prefer computing the jackknife residuals over the standardized or Studentized ones, although the same strategy will be relevant to computing those.

Outlier Identification Strategy

1. Plot jackknife residuals $r_{(-i)}$ vs. x_i values (all the r_i corresponding to x_i values, except for the present $r_{(-i)}$ value).
2. Generate a Stem–Leaf display of $r_{(-i)}$ values.
3. Generate a Dotplot of the $r_{(-i)}$ values.
4. Generate a Boxplot of $r_{(-i)}$ values.
5. Once any extreme $r_{(-i)}$ values are noted, do not merely remove the corresponding x_i values from the data pool, but find out under what conditions they were collected, who collected them, where they were collected, and how they were input into the computer data record.

The jackknife procedure reflects an expectation $\varepsilon_i \sim N(0, \sigma^2)$, which is the basis for the Student's t-distribution at $\alpha/2$ and $n - k - 2$ degrees of freedom. The jackknife residual, however, must be adjusted, because there are, in fact, n tests performed, one for each observation. If $n = 20$, $\alpha = 0.05$, and a two-tail test is conducted, then the adjustment factor is

$$\frac{\frac{\alpha}{2}}{n} = \frac{0.025}{20} = 0.0013.$$

Table F presents corrected jackknife residual values, which essentially are Bonferroni corrections on the jackknife residuals. For example, let $\alpha = 0.05$, $k =$ the number of b_i values in the model, excluding b_0; say $k = 1$ and $n = 20$. In this case, Table F shows that a jackknife residual greater than 3.54 in absolute value, $|r_{(-i)}| > 3.54$, would be considered an outlier.

Leverage Value Diagnostics

In outlier data analysis, we are particularly concerned with also a specific x_i value's leverage and influence on the rest of the data. The leverage value, h_i, is equivalent to h_{ii}, the diagonal hat matrix, as previously discussed. We will use the term, h_i, as opposed to h_{ii}, when the computation is not derived from the hat matrix used extensively in multivariate regression. The leverage value measures the distance a specific x_{ij} value is from $\bar{\bar{x}}$, or the mean of all the x values. For, $Y_i = \beta_0 + \beta_1 x_1 + \varepsilon_i$, without correlation between any of the $x_{\cdot j}$ variables, the leverage value for the ith observation is of the form[*]:

---

[*]This requires that any correlation between the independent x variables is addressed prior to outlier data analysis. Also, all of the x_1 variables must be centered, $x_i - \bar{x}_1$ for a mean of 0 in order to use this procedure.

$$h_i = \frac{1}{n} + \sum_{j=1}^{k} \frac{x_{ij}^2}{(n-1)s_j^2}. \tag{8.22}$$

For linear regression in x_i, use

$$h_i = \frac{1}{n} + \frac{(x_i - \bar{x})^2}{(n-1)s_x^2},$$

where

$$s_j^2 = \frac{\sum\limits_{i=1}^{n} x_{ij}^2}{n-1} \tag{8.23}$$

for each x_j variable.

The h_i value lies between 0 and 1, that is, $0 \le h_i \le 1$, and is interpreted like a correlation coefficient. If $h_i = 1$, then $y_i = \hat{y}_i$. If a y intercept (b_0) is present, $h_i \ge 1/n$, and the average leverage is:

$$\bar{h}_i = \frac{k+1}{n}. \tag{8.24}$$

Also,

$$\sum_{i=1}^{n} h_i = k+1.$$

Hoaglin and Welsch (1978) recommend that the researcher closely evaluate any observation where $h_i > 2(k+1)/n$.

An F_i value can be computed for each value in a regression data set by means of

$$F_i = \frac{\frac{h_i - \frac{1}{n}}{k}}{\frac{1 - h_i}{n - k - 1}},$$

which follows an F distribution,

$$F_T \alpha'(k, n-k-1), \tag{8.25}$$

where

$$\alpha' = \frac{\alpha}{n}.$$

However, the critical value leverage table (Table H) will provide this value at $\alpha = 0.10$, 0.05, and 0.01; $n =$ sample size; and $k =$ number of b_i predictors, excluding b_0 ($k = 1$, for linear regression).

COOK'S DISTANCE

The Cook's distance (C_{d_i}) measures the influence of any one observation relative to the others. That is, it measures the change in b_1, the linear regression coefficient, when that observation, or an observation set, is removed from the aggregate set of observations. The calculation of C_i is:

$$C_{d_i} = \frac{e_i^2 h_i}{(k+1)s^2(1-h_i)^2}. \tag{8.26}$$

A Cook's distance value (C_{d_i}) may be large because an observation is large or because it has large Studentized residuals, Sr_i. The Sr_i value is not seen in Equation 8.26, but (C_{d_i}) can also be written as

$$C_{d_i} = \frac{Sr_i^2 h_i}{(k+1)(1-h_i)^2}.$$

A C_{d_i} value greater than 1 should be investigated.

Let us look at an example (Example 8.4). Suppose the baseline microbial average on the hands was 5.08 ($\log_{10}$ scale), and the average microbial count at time 0 following antimicrobial treatment was 2.17, for a 2.91 $\log_{10}$ reduction from the baseline value. The hands were gloved with surgeons' gloves for a period of 6 h. At the end of the 6-h period, the average microbial count was 4.56 $\log_{10}$, or 0.52 $\log_{10}$ less than the average baseline population. Table 8.16 provides these raw data, and Figure 8.15 presents a plot of the data.

In Figure 8.15, the baseline value (5.08), collected the week prior to product use, is represented as a horizontal.

A regression analysis is provided in Table 8.17.

Three observations have been flagged as unusual. Table 8.18 presents a table of values of x, y, e_i, $\hat{y}$, Sr_i, $r_{(-i)}$, and h_i.

Let us look at Table G, the Studentized table, where $k = 1$, $n = 30$, and $\alpha = 0.05$. Because there is no $n = 30$, we must interpolate using the formula:

value $=$ (lower tabled critical value)

$$+ \frac{([\text{upper tabled critical value}] - [\text{lower tabled critical value}])(\text{upper tabled } n - \text{actual } n)}{(\text{upper tabled } n) - (\text{lower tabled } n)}$$

value $= 2.87 + \dfrac{(3.16 - 2.87)(50 - 30)}{50 - 25} = 3.10.$

TABLE 8.16
Microbial Population Data, Example 8.4

n	Sample Time x	Log$_{10}$ Microbial Counts y
1	0	2.01
2	0	1.96
3	0	1.93
4	0	3.52
5	0	1.97
6	0	2.50
7	0	1.56
8	0	2.11
9	0	2.31
10	0	2.01
11	0	2.21
12	0	2.07
13	0	1.83
14	0	2.57
15	0	2.01
16	6	4.31
17	6	3.21
18	6	5.56
19	6	4.11
20	6	4.26
21	6	5.01
22	6	4.21
23	6	6.57
24	6	4.73
25	6	4.61
26	6	4.17
27	6	4.81
28	6	4.13
29	6	3.98
30	6	4.73

x = time; 0 = immediate sample, and 6 = 6 h sample.
y = log$_{10}$ microbial colony count averaged per two hands per subject.

Hence, any absolute value of S_{r_i} greater than 3.10, that is, $|S_{r_i}| > 3.10$, needs to be checked. We look down the column of S_{r_i} values and note 3.29388 at $n = 23$ is suspect. Looking also at the e_i values, we see 2.01, or a 2 log$_{10}$ deviation from 0, which is a relatively large deviation.

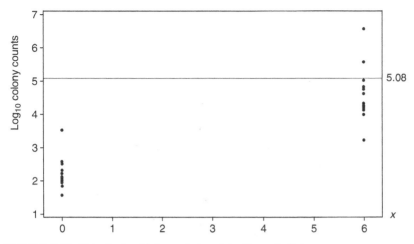

FIGURE 8.15 Plot of microbial population data, Example 8.4.

Let us now evaluate the jackknife residuals. The critical jackknife values are found in Table F, where $n = 30$, $k = 1$ (representing b_1), and $\alpha = 0.05$. We again need to interpolate.

TABLE 8.17
Regression Analysis, Example 8.4

Predictor	Coef	St. Dev	t-Ratio	p
b_0	2.1713	0.1631	13.31	0.000
b_1	0.39811	0.03844	10.36	0.000
$s = 0.6316$		$R^2 = 79.3\%$		$R^2(\text{adj}) = 78.6\%$

Analysis of Variance

Source	DF	SS	MS	F	p
Regression	1	42.793	42.793	107.26	0.000
Error	28	11.171	0.399		
Total	29	53.964			

Unusual Observations

Observations	C1	C2	Fit	St Dev Fit	Residual	St Residual
4	0.00	3.52	2.171	0.163	1.349	2.21 R
17	6.00	3.21	4.56	0.163	−1.350	−2.21 R
21	6.00	6.57	4.56	0.163	2.010	3.29 R

R denotes an observation with a large standardized residual (St Residual).
The regression equation is $\hat{y} = 2.17 + 0.398x$.

TABLE 8.18
Data Table, Example 8.4

Row	x	y	e_i	$\hat{y}$	Sr_i	$r_{(-i)}$	h_i
1	0	2.01	−0.16133	2.17133	−0.26438	−0.25994	0.0666667
2	0	1.96	−0.21133	2.17133	−0.34632	−0.34081	0.0666667
3	0	1.93	−0.24133	2.17133	−0.39548	−0.38945	0.0666667
4	0	3.52	1.34867	2.17133	2.21012	2.38862	0.0666667
5	0	1.97	−0.20133	2.17133	−0.32993	−0.32462	0.0666667
6	0	2.50	0.32867	2.17133	0.53860	0.53166	0.0666667
7	0	1.56	−0.61133	2.17133	−1.00182	−1.00189	0.0666667
8	0	2.11	−0.06133	2.17133	−0.10051	−0.09872	0.0666667
9	0	2.31	0.13867	2.17133	0.22724	0.22335	0.0666667
10	0	2.01	−0.16133	2.17133	−0.26438	−0.25944	0.0666667
11	0	2.21	0.03867	2.17133	0.06336	0.06223	0.0666667
12	0	2.07	−0.10133	2.17133	−0.16606	−0.16315	0.0666667
13	0	1.83	−0.34133	2.17133	−0.55936	−0.55237	0.0666667
14	0	2.57	0.39867	2.17133	0.65331	0.64649	0.0666667
15	0	2.01	−0.16133	2.17133	−0.26438	−0.25994	0.0666667
16	6	4.31	−0.25000	4.56000	−0.40969	−0.40351	0.0666667
17	6	3.21	−1.35000	4.56000	−2.21230	−2.39148	0.0666667
18	6	5.56	1.00000	4.56000	1.63874	1.69242	0.0666667
19	6	4.11	−0.45000	4.56000	−0.73743	−0.73128	0.0666667
20	6	4.26	−0.30000	4.56000	−0.49162	−0.48486	0.0666667
21	6	5.01	0.45000	4.56000	0.73744	0.73128	0.0666667
22	6	4.21	−0.35000	4.56000	−0.57356	−0.56656	0.0666667
23	6	6.57	2.01000	4.56000	3.29388	4.13288	0.0666667
24	6	4.73	0.17000	4.56000	0.27859	0.27395	0.0666667
25	6	4.61	0.05000	4.56000	0.08194	0.08047	0.0666667
26	6	4.17	−0.39000	4.56000	−0.63911	−0.63222	0.0666667
27	6	4.81	0.25000	4.56000	0.40969	0.40351	0.0666667
28	6	4.13	−0.43000	4.56000	−0.70466	−0.69818	0.0666667
29	6	3.98	−0.58000	4.56000	−0.95047	−0.94878	0.0666667
30	6	4.73	0.17000	4.56000	0.27859	0.27395	0.0666667

Studentized residual $= S_{r_i}$.
Jackknife residual $= r_{(-i)}$.
Leverage value $= h_i$.

$$3.5 + \frac{(3.51 - 3.50)(50 - 30)}{50 - 25} = 3.51.$$

So, any jackknife residual greater than 3.51, or $r_{(-i)} > |3.51|$, is suspect. Looking down the jackknife residual $r_{(-i)}$ column, we note that the value 4.13288 > 3.51, again at $n = 23$. Our next question is "what happened?"

TABLE 8.19
Stem–Leaf Display of Jackknife Residuals, Example 8.4

1	−2	3
1	−1	
2	−1	0
8	−0	976655
(10)	−0	443332210
12	0	002224
6	0	567
3	1	
3	1	6
2	2	3
1	2	
1	3	
1	3	
1	4	1

Going back to the study, after looking at the technicians' reports, we learn that a subject biased the study. Upon questioning the subject, technicians learned that the subject was embarrassed about wearing the glove and removed it before the authorized time; hence, the large colony counts.

Because this author prefers the jackknife procedure, we will use it for an example of a complete analysis. The same procedure would be done for calculating standardized and Studentized residuals. First, a Stem–Leaf display was computed of the $r_{(-i)}$ values (Table 8.19).

From the Stem–Leaf jackknife display, we see the 4.1 value, that is, $(r_{(-i)} = 4.1)$. There are some other extreme values, but not that unusual for this type of study.

Next, a Boxplot of the $r_{(-i)}$ values was printed, which showed the "0," depicting "outlier." There are three other extreme values that may be of concern, flagged by solid dots (Figure 8.16).

Finally, a Dotplot of the $r_{(-i)}$ values is presented, showing the data in a slightly different format (Figure 8.17).

Before continuing, let us also look at a Stem–Leaf display of the e_is, that is, the $y - \hat{y}$ values (Figure 8.18).

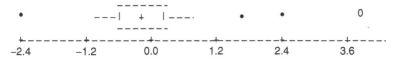

FIGURE 8.16 Boxplot display of jackknife residuals, Example 8.4.

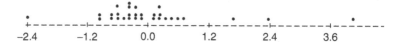

FIGURE 8.17 Dotplot display of jackknife residuals.

Note that the display does not accentuate the more extreme values, so they are more difficult to identify. Figure 8.19 shows the same data, but as a Studentized residual display.

Continuing with the data evaluation, the researcher determined that the data need to be separated into two groups. If a particularly low $\log_{10}$ reduction at time 0 was present, and a particularly high $\log_{10}$ reduction was observed at time 6, the effects would be masked.

The data were sorted by time of sample (0, 6). The time 0, or immediate residuals are provided in Table 8.20.

Table 8.20 did not portray any other values more extreme than were already apparent; it is just that we want to be more thorough. The critical value for Sr_i at $\alpha = 0.05 = |2.61|$ and $r_{(-i)} = |3.65|$, and none of the values in Table 8.21 exceed the critical values for Sr_i or $r_{(-i)}$ at $\alpha = 0.05$.

It is always a good idea to look at all the values on the upper or lower ends of a Stem–Leaf display, Boxplot or Dotplot. Figure 8.20 presents a Stem–Leaf display of the e_is at time 0.

We note that two residual values, -0.6 (Subject #7, 0.61133) and 1.3 (Subject #4, 1.34867) stand out. Let us see how they look on Boxplots and Dotplots.

The Boxplot (Figure 8.21) portrays the 1.3486 value as an outlier relative to the other e_i residual data points. Although we know that it is not that uncommon to see a value such as this, we will have to check.

Figure 8.22 portrays the same e_i data in Dotplot format. Because this author prefers the Stem–Leaf and Boxplots, we will use them exclusively in the future. The Dotplots have been presented only for reader interest.

1	−1	3
3	−0	65
(15)	−0	443333222211110
12	0	001112334
3	0	
3	1	03
1	1	
1	2	0

FIGURE 8.18 Stem–Leaf display of e_i values, Example 8.4.

1	-2	2
1	-1	
2	-1	0
8	-0	977655
(10)	-0	4433322211
12	0	002224
6	0	567
3	1	
3	1	6
2	2	2
1	2	
1	3	1

FIGURE 8.19 Studentized residuals, Example 8.4.

The Studentized residuals, S_{r_i}, at time 0 were next printed in a Stem–Leaf format (Figure 8.23). The lower value (Subject #7) now does not look so extreme, but the value for Subject #4 does. It does appear unique from the data pool, but even so, it is not that extreme.

The Boxplot (Figure 8.24) of the Studentized residuals, S_{r_i}, shows the Subject #4 datum as an outlier. We will cross check.

TABLE 8.20
Time 0 Residuals, Example 8.4

Row	Residuals	Studentized Residuals	Jackknife Residuals
n	e_i	S_{r_i}	$r_{(-i)}$
1	−0.16133	−0.26438	−0.25994
2	−0.21133	−0.34632	−0.34081
3	−0.24133	−0.39548	−0.38945
4	1.34867	2.21012	2.38862
5	−0.20133	−0.32993	−0.32462
6	0.32867	0.53860	0.53166
7	−0.61133	−1.00182	−1.00189
8	−0.06133	−0.10051	−0.09872
9	0.13867	0.22724	0.22335
10	−0.16133	−0.26438	−0.25994
11	0.03867	0.06336	0.06223
12	−0.10133	−0.16606	−0.16315
13	−0.34133	−0.55936	−0.55237
14	0.39867	0.685331	0.64649
15	−0.16133	−0.26438	−0.25994

TABLE 8.21
Residual Data 6 h after Surgical Wash, Example 8.4

Row	Residuals e_i	Studentized Residuals Sr_i	Jackknife Residuals $r_{(-i)}$
1	−0.25000	−0.40969	−0.40351
2	−1.35000	−2.21230	−2.39148
3	1.00000	1.63874	1.69242
4	−0.45000	−0.73743	−0.73128
5	−0.30000	−0.49162	−0.48486
6	0.45000	0.73744	0.73128
7	−0.35000	−0.57356	−0.56656
8	2.01000	3.29388	4.13288
9	0.17000	0.27859	0.27395
10	0.05000	0.08194	0.08047
11	−0.39000	0.63911	−0.63222
12	0.25000	0.40969	0.40351
13	−0.43000	−0.70466	−0.69818
14	−0.58000	−0.95047	−0.94878
15	0.17000	0.27859	0.27395

The jackknife residuals at time 0 are portrayed in the Stem–Leaf display (Figure 8.25). Again, the Subject #4 datum is portrayed as extreme, but not that extreme.

Figure 8.26 shows the $r_{(-i)}$ jackknife residuals plotted on the Boxplot display and indicates a single outlier.

1	−0	6
1	−0	
5	−0	3222
(5)	−0	11110
5	0	01
3	0	33
1	0	
1	0	
1	0	
1	1	
1	1	3

FIGURE 8.20 Stem–Leaf display of e_i values at time zero, Example 8.4.

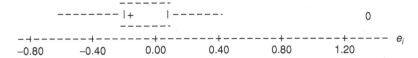

FIGURE 8.21 Boxplot of e_i, Example 8.4.

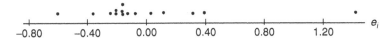

FIGURE 8.22 Dotplot display of e_i values at time 0, Example 8.4.

1	−1	0
2	−0	5
(8)	−0	33322211
5	0	02
3	0	56
1	1	
1	1	
1	2	2

FIGURE 8.23 Stem–Leaf display of Studentized residuals at time zero, Example 8.4.

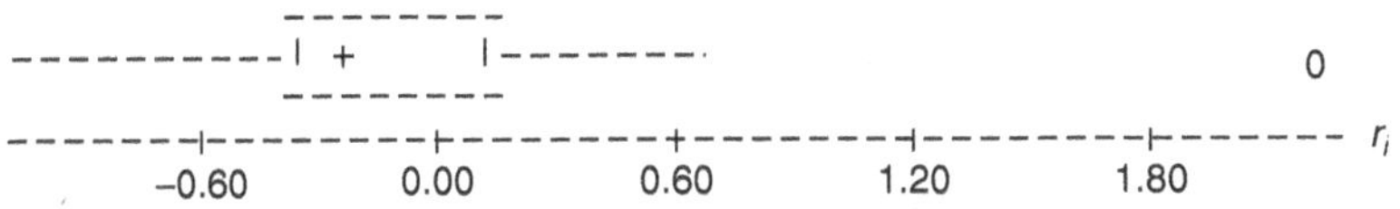

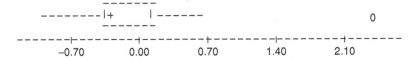

FIGURE 8.24 Boxplot of Studentized residuals at time 0, Example 8.4.

1	−1	0
2	−0	5
(8)	−0	33322210
5	0	02
3	0	56
1	1	
1	1	
1	2	3

FIGURE 8.25 Stem–Leaf display of jackknife residuals $r_{(-i)}$ at time zero, Example 8.4.

FIGURE 8.26 Boxplot display of jackknife residuals $r_{(-i)}$ at time 0, Example 8.4.

1	-2	3
1	-1	
(7)	-0	9766544
7	0	02247
2	1	6
1	2	
1	3	
1	4	1

FIGURE 8.27 Stem–Leaf display of jackknife residuals $r_{(-i)}$ at 6 h, Example 8.4.

Note that, whether one uses the e_i, Sr_i, or $r_{(-i)}$ residuals, in general, the same information results. It is really up to the investigator to choose which one to use. Before choosing the appropriate one, we suggest running all three until the researcher achieves a "feel" for the data. It is also a good idea to check out the lower and upper 5% of the values, just to be sure nothing is overlooked. "Check out" actually means to go back to the original data.

As it turned out, the 3.52 value at time zero was erroneous. The value could not be reconciled with the plate count data, so it was removed, and its place was labeled as "missing value." The other values were traceable and reconciled.

The 6 h data were evaluated next (Table 8.21).

Because we prefer using the jackknife residual, we will look only at the Stem–Leaf and Boxplot displays of these. Note that $Sr_i = 3.29388$ and $r_{(-i)} = 4.13288$, both exceed their critical values of 2.61 and 3.65, respectively.

Figure 8.27 is a Stem–Leaf display of the time 6 h data. We earlier identified the 6.57 value, with a 4.1 jackknife residual, as a spurious data point due to noncompliance by a subject.

The Boxplot of the jackknife residuals, 6 h, is presented in Figure 8.28.

The -2.39 jackknife value at 6 h is extreme, but is not found to be suspect after reviewing the data records. Hence, in the process of our analysis and validation, two values were eliminated: 6.57 at 6 h, and 3.52 at the immediate sample time. All other suspicious values were "checked out" and not removed. A new regression conducted on the amended data set increased R^2, as well as reducing the b_0 and b_1 values. The new regression is considered

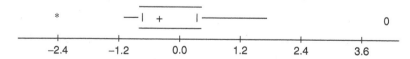

FIGURE 8.28 Boxplot display of jackknife residuals $r_{(-i)}$ at 6 h, Example 8.4.

TABLE 8.22
Regression Analysis, Outliers Removed, Example 8.4

Predictor	Coef	St. Dev	t-Ratio	p
Constant (b_0)	2.0750	0.1159	17.90	0.000
b_1	0.39024	0.02733	14.28	0.000
$s = 0.4338$		$R^2 = 88.7\%$		$R^2_{(adj)} = 88.3\%$

Analysis of Variance

Source	DF	SS	MS	F	p
Regression	1	38.376	38.376	203.89	0.000
Error	26	4.894	0.188		
Total	27	43.270			

Unusual Observations

Observations	C1	C2	Fit	St Dev Fit	Residual	St Resid
17	6.00	3.2100	4.4164	0.1159	-1.2064	-2.89 R
18	6.00	5.5600	4.4164	0.1159	1.1436	2.74 R

R denotes an observation with a large st. resid.
The regression equation is $\hat{y} = 2.08 + 0.390x$.

more "real." We know it is possible to get a three $\log_{10}$ immediate reduction, and the rebound effect is just over $1/3 \log_{10}$ per hour. The microbial counts do not exceed the baseline counts 6 h postwash.

The new analysis is presented in Table 8.22.

Table 8.23 presents the new residual indices. We see there are still extreme values relative to the general data pool, but these are not worth pursuing in this pilot study.

The mean of the y_i values at time 0 is 2.0750 $\log_{10}$, which computes to a 3.01 $\log_{10}$ reduction immediately postwash. It barely achieves the FDA requirement for a 3 $\log_{10}$ reduction, so another pilot study will be suggested to look at changing the product's application procedure. The y_i mean value at 6 h is 4.4164, which is lower than the mean baseline value, assuring the adequacy of the product's antimicrobial persistence.

Given that this study was a pilot study, the researcher decided not to "over" evaluate the data, but to move onto a new study. The product would be considered for further development as a new surgical handwash.

LEVERAGES AND COOK'S DISTANCE

Because MiniTab and other software packages also can provide values for leverage (h_i) and Cook's distance, let us look at them relative to the previous analysis with the two data points (#4 and #23) in the analysis.

TABLE 8.23
Residual Indices

Row	x_i	y_i	e_i	$\hat{y}_i$	Sr_i	$r_{(-i)}$
1	0	2.01	−0.06500	2.07500	−0.15548	−0.15253
2	0	1.96	−0.11500	2.07500	−0.27508	−0.27013
3	0	1.93	−0.14500	2.07500	−0.34684	−0.34089
4	0	*	*	*	*	*
5	0	1.97	−0.10500	2.07500	−0.25116	−0.24658
6	0	2.50	0.42500	2.07500	1.01660	1.01728
7	0	1.56	−0.51500	2.07500	−1.23188	−1.24483
8	0	2.11	0.03500	2.07500	0.08372	0.08211
9	0	2.31	0.23500	2.07500	0.56212	0.55458
10	0	2.01	−0.06500	2.07500	−0.15548	−0.15253
11	0	2.21	0.13500	2.07500	0.32292	0.31729
12	0	2.07	−0.00500	2.07500	−0.01196	−0.01173
13	0	1.83	−0.24500	2.07500	−0.58604	−0.57849
14	0	2.57	0.49500	2.07500	1.18404	1.19368
15	0	2.01	−0.06500	2.07500	−0.15548	−0.15253
16	6	4.31	−0.10643	4.41643	−0.25458	−0.24995
17	6	3.21	−1.20643	4.41643	−2.88578	−3.43231
18	6	5.56	1.14357	4.41643	2.73543	3.17837
19	6	4.11	−0.30643	4.41643	−0.73298	−0.72629
20	6	4.26	−0.15643	4.41643	−0.37418	−0.36790
21	6	5.01	0.59357	4.41643	1.41982	1.44958
22	6	4.21	−0.20643	4.41643	−0.49378	−0.48648
23	6	*	*	*	*	*
24	6	4.73	0.31357	4.41643	0.75006	0.74359
25	6	4.61	0.19357	4.41643	0.46302	0.45592
26	6	4.17	−0.24643	4.41643	−0.58946	−0.58191
27	6	4.81	0.39357	4.41643	0.94142	0.93929
28	6	4.13	−0.28643	4.41643	−0.68514	−0.67798
29	6	3.98	−0.43643	4.41643	−1.04394	−1.04582
30	6	4.73	0.31357	4.41643	0.75006	0.74359

Recall that the h_i value measures the distance for the $\bar{x}$ value. The formula is:

$$h_i = \frac{1}{n} + \frac{(x_i - \bar{x})^2}{(n-1)s_x^2},$$

where

$$s_x^2 = \frac{\sum(x_i - \bar{x})^2}{n-1}.$$

The x_i values are either 0 or 6, and $\bar{x} = 3$.

So, $0 - 3 = -3$, and $6 - 3 = 3$

The square of 3 is 9, so all the $(x_i - \bar{x})^2 = 9$, whether $x_i = 0$ or 6; hence, the associated hat matrix would be constant. That is, $\sum(x_i - \bar{x})^2$ is a summation of 30 observations of x_i each of which equals 9. Hence, $\sum(x_i - \bar{x})^2 = 270$.

$$s = \frac{\sum(x_i - \bar{x})^2}{n - 1} = \frac{270}{29} = 9.3103$$

$$h_0 = \frac{1}{30} + \frac{(0 - 3)^2}{29(9.3103)} = 0.0667, \text{ and}$$

$$h_6 = \frac{1}{30} + \frac{(6 - 3)^2}{29(9.3103)} = 0.0667.$$

The leverage values, h_i, in Table 8.24 are the same for all 30 values of x_i.

To see if the 30 h_i values are significant at $\alpha = 0.05$, we turn to Table H, the Leverage Table for $n = 30$, $k = 1$, and $\alpha = 0.05$, and find that $h_{\text{tabled}} = 0.325$. If any of the h_i values is >0.325, this would indicate an extreme observation in the x value. This, of course, is not applicable here, for all x_is are set at 0 or 6, and none of the h_i values >0.325.

The Cooks Distance, C_{d_i}, is the measure of the influence, or weight a single paired observation (x, y) has on the regression coefficients (b_0, b_1). Recall from Equation 8.26, $C_{d_i} = \frac{e_i^2 h_i}{(k+1)s^2(1-h_i)^2}$, or, from text, $= \frac{Sr_i h_i}{(k+1)(1-h_i)^2}$. Each value of C_{d_i} in Table 8.24 is multiplied by $n - k - 1$, or $30 - 2 = 28$, for comparison with tabled values.

The tabled value of C_{d_i} in Table I for $n = 25$ (without interpolating from $N = 30$), $\alpha = 0.05$, and $k = 1$ is 17.18, so any C_{d_i} value times 28 that is greater than 16.37 is significant. Observation #23 $(x = 6, y = 6.51)$ with a C_{d_i} of 0.374162, is the most extreme. Because $n - k - 1 = 28 \times 0.374162 = 10.4765 < 17.18$, we know that none of the C_{d_i} values is significant. In fact, a C_{d_i} value of at least 0.61 would have to be obtained to indicate a significant influence on b_0 or b_1.

Now that we have explored residuals and the various construances of them relative to simple linear regression, we will expand these into applications for multiple regression. Once again, review of matrix algebra (Appendix II) will be necessary.

LEVERAGE AND INFLUENCE

LEVERAGE: HAT MATRIX (x VALUES)

Certain values can have more "weight" in the determination of a regression curve than do other values. We covered this in linear regression (Chapter 3), and the application to multiple linear regression is straightforward. In Chapter 3,

TABLE 8.24
Leverage h_i and Cook's Distance

Row	x	y	h_i	C_{d_i}
1	0	2.01	0.0666667	0.002551
2	0	1.96	0.0666667	0.004377
3	0	1.93	0.0666667	0.005707
4	0	3.52	0.0666667	0.178246
5	0	1.97	0.0666667	0.003972
6	0	2.50	0.0666667	0.010586
7	0	1.56	0.0666667	0.036624
8	0	2.11	0.0666667	0.000369
9	0	2.31	0.0666667	0.001884
10	0	2.01	0.0666667	0.002551
11	0	2.21	0.0666667	0.000147
12	0	2.07	0.0666667	0.001006
13	0	1.83	0.0666667	0.011417
14	0	2.57	0.0666667	0.015575
15	0	2.01	0.0666667	0.002551
16	6	4.31	0.0666667	0.005930
17	6	3.21	0.0666667	0.177542
18	6	5.56	0.0666667	0.098782
19	6	4.11	0.0666667	0.019493
20	6	4.26	0.0666667	0.008586
21	6	5.01	0.0666667	0.020199
22	6	4.21	0.0666667	0.011732
23	6	6.51	0.0666667	0.374162
24	6	4.73	0.0666667	0.002967
25	6	4.61	0.0666667	0.000286
26	6	4.17	0.0666667	0.014601
27	6	4.81	0.0666667	0.006322
28	6	4.13	0.0666667	0.017784
29	6	3.98	0.0666667	0.032513
30	6	4.73	0.0666667	0.002967

simple linear regression, we saw the major leverage in regression occurs in the tails, or endpoints. Figure 8.29 portrays the situation where extreme values have leverage. Both regions A and B have far more influence on regression coefficients than does region C. In this case, however, it will not really matter, because regions A, B, and C are in a reasonably straight alignment.

In other cases of leverage, as shown in Figures 8.30a and b, extreme values at either end of the regression curve can pull or push the b_i estimates away from the main trend. In 8.30a, an extreme low value pulls the regression estimate down. In 8.30b, the extreme low value pushes the regression estimate

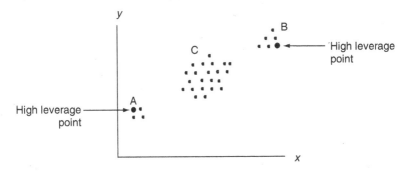

FIGURE 8.29 Extreme values with leverage.

up. Hence, it is important to detect these extreme influential data points. In multiple regression, they are not as obvious as they are in the simple linear regression condition, where one can simply look at a data scatterplot. In multiple linear regression, residual plots often will not reveal leverage value(s).

The hat matrix, a common matrix form used in regression analysis, can be applied effectively to uncovering points of "leverage," by detecting data points that are large or small, by comparison with near-neighbor values. Because parameter estimates, standard errors, predicted values ($\hat{y}_i$) and summary statistics are so strongly influenced by leverage values, if these are erroneous, they must be identified. As noted in Equation 8.19 earlier, the hat matrix is of the form:

$$\underset{n \times n}{\mathbf{H}} = \mathbf{X}(\mathbf{X'X})^{-1}\mathbf{X'}$$

$\mathbf{H}$ can be used to express the fitted values in vector $\hat{\mathbf{Y}}$.

$$\hat{\mathbf{Y}} = \mathbf{HY}. \tag{8.27}$$

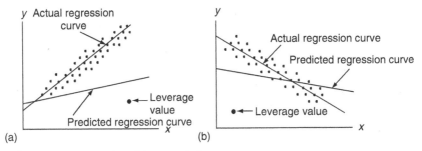

(a)   (b)

FIGURE 8.30 Examples of leverage influence.

H also can be used to provide the error term vector, **e**, where $\mathbf{e} = (\mathbf{I} - \mathbf{H})\mathbf{Y}$, and **I** is an $n \times n$ identity matrix, or the variance–covariance matrix, $\sigma^2(\mathbf{e})$, where

$$\sigma^2(\mathbf{e}) = \sigma^2(\mathbf{I} - \mathbf{H}). \tag{8.28}$$

The elements of h_{ii} of the hat matrix, "**H**," also provide an estimate of the leverage exerted by the ith row and the ith column value. By further manipulation, the actual leverage of any particular value set can be known.

Our general focus will be on the diagonal elements, h_{ii}, of the hat matrix, where

$$\boldsymbol{h_{ii} = x_i'(X'X)^{-1}x_i} \tag{8.29}$$

and $\boldsymbol{x_i'}$ is the transposed ith row of the **X** matrix.

The diagonal values of the hat matrix, the h_{ii}s, are standardized measures of the distance of the ith observation from the center of x_i value's space. Large h_{ii} values often give warning of observations that are extreme, in terms of leverage exerted on the main data set. The average value of the hat matrix diagonal is $\bar{h} = (k + 1)/n$, where $k =$ the number of b_i values, excluding b_0, and $n =$ number of observations. By convention, any observation for which the hat diagonal exceeds $2(\bar{h})$ or $2((k + 1)/n)$ is remote enough from the main data to be considered a "leverage point" and should be further evaluated. Basically, the researcher must continually ask "can this value be this extreme and be real?" Perhaps there is an explanation, and it leads the investigator to view the data set in a different light. Or, perhaps the value was misrecorded. In situations where $2(\bar{h}) > 1$, the rule, "greater than $2(\bar{h})$ initiates a leverage value," does not apply. This author suggests using $3(\bar{h})$ as a rule-of-thumb cut-off value for pilot studies, and $2(\bar{h})$ for larger, more definitive studies. If $h_{ii} > 2$ or $3(\bar{h})$, recomputed the regression with the set of x_i values removed from the analysis to see what happens.

Because the hat matrix is relevant only for the location of observations in x_i space, many researchers will use Studentized residual values, S_{r_i}, in relation to h_{ii} values, looking for observations with both large S_{r_i} values and large h_{ii} values. These will be values likely to be strong leverage points.

Studentized residuals usually are provided by standard statistical computer programs. As discussed earlier, these are termed Studentized residuals, because they approximate the Student's t distribution with $n - k - 1$ degrees of freedom, where k is the number of b_is in the data set, excluding b_0. As noted in Equation 8.18 earlier, the Studentized residual value, S_{r_i}, for multiple regression is:

$$S_{r_i} = \frac{e_i}{s\sqrt{1 - h_i}},$$

where $s\sqrt{1 - h_i}$ = standard deviation of the e_i values.
The mean of S_{r_i} is approximately 0, and the variance is:

$$\frac{\sum_{i=1}^{n} S_{r_i}^2}{n - k - 1}.$$

If any of the $|S_{r_i}|$ values is $> t_{(\alpha/2, \, n-k-1)}$, that value is considered a significant leverage value at α.

Let us look at an example (Example 8.5). Dental water lines have long been a concern for microbial contamination, in that microbial biofilms can attach to the lines and grow within them. As the biofilm grows, it can slough off into the line and a patient's mouth, potentially to cause an infection. A study was conducted to measure the amount of biofilm that could potentially grow in untreated lines over the course of six months. The researcher measured the microbial counts in $\log_{10}$ scale of microorganisms attached to the interior of the water line, the month (every 30 days), the water temperature, and the amount of calcium (Ca) in the water (Table 8.25). This information was necessary to the researcher in order to design a formal study of biocides for prevention of biofilms.

In this example, there is a three-month gap in the data (three to six months). The researcher is concerned that the six-month data points may be

TABLE 8.25
Dental Water Line Biofilm Growth Data, Example 8.5

n	$\log_{10}$ Colony–Forming Units Per mm^2 of Line (y)	Month (x_1)	Water Temperature, °C (x_2)	Calcium Levels of Water (x_3)
1	0.0	0	25	0.03
2	0.0	0	24	0.03
3	0.0	0	25	0.04
4	1.3	1	25	0.30
5	1.3	1	24	0.50
6	1.1	1	28	0.20
7	2.1	2	31	0.50
8	2.0	2	32	0.70
9	2.3	2	30	0.70
10	2.9	3	33	0.80
11	3.1	3	32	0.80
12	3.0	3	33	0.90
13	5.9	6	38	1.20
14	5.8	6	39	1.50
15	6.1	6	37	1.20

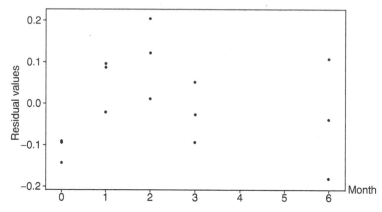

FIGURE 8.31 Residuals plotted against month of sampling, Example 8.5.

extremely influencing on a regression analysis. Figure 8.31 displays the residual plotted vs. month of sampling.

The regression model is presented in Table 8.26.

Looking at the regression model, one can see that x_3 (Ca level) probably serves no use in the model. That variable should be further evaluated using a partial F test.

Most statistical software packages (SAS, SPSS, and MiniTab) will print the diagonals of the hat matrix, $\mathbf{H} = \mathbf{X}(\mathbf{X}'\mathbf{X})^{-1}\mathbf{X}'$. Below is the MiniTab version. Table 8.27 presents the actual data, the h_{ii} values, and the S_{r_i} values.

TABLE 8.26
Regression Model of Data, Example 8.5

Predictor	Coef	St. Dev	t-Ratio	p
b_0	1.4007	0.5613	2.50	0.030
b_1	1.02615	0.06875	14.93	0.000
b_2	−0.05278	0.02277	−2.32	0.041
b_3	0.3207	0.2684	1.19	0.257*
$s = 0.1247$		$R^2 = 99.7\%$		$R^2_{(adj)} = 99.6\%$

$y = \log_{10}$ colony forming units.
b_1 = month.
b_2 = water temperature in lines.
b_3 = Ca level.
The regression equation is $\hat{y} = 1.40 + 1.03x_1 - 0.0528x_2 + 0.321x_3$.

TABLE 8.27
Actual Data with h_{ii} and S_{r_i} Values, Example 8.5

n	y	x_1	x_2	x_3	h_{ii}	S_{r_i}
1	0.0	0	25	0.03	0.207348	−0.80568
2	0.0	0	24	0.03	0.213543	−1.34661
3	0.0	0	25	0.04	0.198225	−0.83096
4	1.3	1	25	0.30	0.246645	0.88160
5	1.3	1	24	0.50	0.649604	−0.26627
6	1.1	1	28	0.20	0.228504	0.77810
7	2.1	2	31	0.50	0.167612	1.08816
8	2.0	2	32	0.70	0.322484	0.10584
9	2.3	2	30	0.70	0.176214	2.07424
10	2.9	3	33	0.80	0.122084	−0.79142
11	3.1	3	32	0.80	0.083246	0.42855
12	3.0	3	33	0.90	0.192055	−0.22285
13	5.9	6	38	1.20	0.399687	−0.36670
14	5.8	6	39	1.50	0.344164	−2.02117
15	6.1	6	37	1.20	0.448586	1.21754

$$2(\bar{h}) = \frac{2k+1}{n} = \frac{2(4)}{15} = 0.533.$$

So, if any $h_{ii} > 0.533$, that data point needs to be evaluated.

Observing the h_{ii} column, none of the six-month data is greater than 0.533. However, the h_{ii} value at $n = 5$ is 0.649604, which is greater. Further scrutiny shows that the value is "lowish" at the x_2 and "highish" at x_3, relative to the adjacent x_i values, leading one to surmise that it is not a "typo" or data input error, and should probably be left in the data set. Notice that the Studentized residual value, S_{r_i}, for $n = 5$ is not excessive, nor is any other $|S_{r_i}|$ value $> |2.201|.$[2] It is useful to use both the h_{ii} and the S_{r_i} values in measuring the leverage. If both are excessive, then one can be reasonably sure that excessive leverage exists.

Let us look at this process in detail. What if x_2 is changed, say a typographical input error at $n = 7$, where $x_2 = 31$ was actually mistakenly input as 3.1. How is this flagged? Table 8.28 provides a new regression that accommodates the change at $n = 7/x_2$.

Note that neither b_2 or b_3 are significant, nor is the constant significantly different from 0. The entire regression can be explained as a linear one, $\hat{y} = b_0 + b_1 x_1$, with the possibility of b_0 also canceling out.

Table 8.29 provides the actual data with h_{ii} and Studentized residuals.

---

[2]Referencing Table B; $t_{(a/2,\ n-k-1)} = t_{(0.025,11)} = 2.021$

TABLE 8.28
Regression Model with Error at $n = 7$, Example 8.5

Predictor	Coef	St. Dev	t-Ratio	p
b_0	0.1920	0.1443	1.33	0.210
b_1	0.93742	0.06730	13.93	0.000
b_2	−0.003945	0.005817	−0.68	0.512
b_3	0.2087	0.3157	0.66	0.522
$s = 0.1490$		$R^2 = 99.6\%$		$R^2_{(adj)} = 99.5\%$

The regression equation is $\hat{y} = 0.192 + 0.937x_1 − 0.00395x_2 + 0.209x_3$.

As can be seen at $n = 7$, $x_2 = 3.1$, and $h_{77} = 0.961969 > 3(\bar{h}) = \frac{3(4)}{15} = 0.8$. Clearly, the x_i values at 7 would need to be evaluated. Notice that S_{r7}, −2.4453, is a value that stands away from the group, but is not, by itself, excessive. Together, h_{77} and S_{r7} certainly point to one x_i series of values with high leverage. Notice how just one change in x_2 at $n = 7$ influenced the entire regression (Table 8.26 vs. Table 8.28). Also, note that x_2 (temperature) increases progressively over the course of the six months. Why this has occurred should be investigated further.

TABLE 8.29
Data for Table 8.28 with h_{ii} and Studentized Residuals, Example 8.5

Row	y	b_1	b_2	b_3	h_{ii}	S_{r_i}
1	0.0	0	25.0	0.03	0.217732	−0.74017
2	0.0	0	24.0	0.03	0.209408	−0.76688
3	0.0	0	25.0	0.04	0.208536	−0.75190
4	1.3	1	25.0	0.30	0.103712	1.55621
5	1.3	1	24.0	0.50	0.222114	1.25603
6	1.1	1	28.0	0.20	0.205295	0.28328
7	2.1	2	3.1	0.50	0.961969	−2.44530
8	2.0	2	32.0	0.70	0.191373	−0.62890
9	2.3	2	30.0	0.70	0.178048	1.63123
10	2.9	3	33.0	0.80	0.093091	−0.99320
11	3.1	3	32.0	0.80	0.086780	0.37091
12	3.0	3	33.0	0.90	0.174919	−0.44028
13	5.9	6	38.0	1.20	0.403454	−0.14137
14	5.8	6	39.0	1.50	0.344424	−1.54560
15	6.1	6	37.0	1.20	0.399146	1.67122

INFLUENCE: COOK'S DISTANCE

Previously in this chapter, we discussed Cook's distance for simple linear regression, a regression diagnostic that is used to detect an extreme value and its influence by removing it from the analysis and then observing the results. In multiple linear regression, the same approach is used, except that a data set is removed. Cook's distance lets the researcher determine just how influential the ith value set is.

The distance is measured in matrix terms as

$$D_i = \frac{\left(\hat{b}_{(-i)} - \hat{b}\right)' X'X \left(\hat{b}_{(-i)} - \hat{b}\right)}{pMS_E}, \tag{8.30}$$

where $\hat{b}_{(-i)}$ = estimate of $\hat{b}$, when the ith point is removed from the regression; p = number of b_i values, including b_0; $k + 1$; and MS_E = mean square error of the full model.

D_i can also be solved as

$$D_i = \frac{\left(\hat{Y} - \hat{Y}_{(-i)}\right)' \left(\hat{Y} - \hat{Y}_{(-i)}\right)}{pMS_E}, \tag{8.31}$$

where $\hat{Y} = HY$ (all n values fitted in a regression) and $\hat{Y}_{(-i)}$ = all values but the ith set fitted for predicting this vector

Instead of calculating a new regression for each i omitted, a simpler formula exists, if one must do the work by hand, without the use of a computer.

$$D_i = \frac{e_i^2}{pMS_E} \left[\frac{h_{ii}}{(1 - h_{ii})^2}\right]. \tag{8.32}$$

This formula stands alone and does not require a new computation of h_{ii} each time.

Another approach, too, that is often valuable uses the F table (Table C), even though the D_i value is not formally an F test statistic.

Step 1: H_0: $D_i = 0$ (Cook's distance parameter is 0)

H_A: $D_i \neq 0$ (Cook's distance parameter is influential)

Step 2: Set α.

Step 3: If $D_i > F_{T, \alpha, (p, n - p)}$, reject H_0 at α.

Generally, however, when $D_i > 1$, the removed point set is considered significantly influential and should be evaluated. In this case, y and the x_i set need to be checked out, not just the x_i set.

Let us again look at Example 8.5. The Cook's distance values are provided in Table 8.30. The critical value is $F_{T(0.05; \, 4, 15 - 4)} = 3.36$ (Table C). If $D_i > 3.36$, it needs to be flagged.

TABLE 8.30
Cook's Distance Values, Example 8.5

n	y	x_1	x_2	x_3	D_i
1	0.0	0	25	0.03	0.043850
2	0.0	0	24	0.03	0.114618
3	0.0	0	25	0.04	0.043914
4	1.3	1	25	0.30	0.064930
5	1.3	21	24	0.50	0.035893
6	1.1	1	28	0.20	0.046498
7	2.1	2	31	0.50	0.058626
8	2.0	2	32	0.70	0.001465
9	2.3	2	30	0.70	0.176956
10	2.9	3	33	0.80	0.022541
11	3.1	3	32	0.80	0.004503
12	3.0	3	33	0.90	0.003230
13	5.9	6	38	1.20	0.024294
14	5.8	6	39	1.50	0.418550
15	6.1	6	37	1.20	0.288825

Because no D_i value > 3.36, there is no reason to suspect undue influence of any of the value sets. Let us see what happens when we change $n = 7$ from 31 to a value of 3.1. Table 8.31 provides the y, x_i, and D_i values. One now

TABLE 8.31
y, x_i, and D_i Values with Error at x_2/n_7,
Example 8.5

n	y	x_1	x_2	x_3	D_i
1	0.0	0	25.0	0.03	0.0398
2	0.0	0	24.0	0.03	0.0405
3	0.0	0	25.0	0.04	0.0388
4	1.3	1	25.0	0.30	0.0620
5	1.3	1	24.0	0.50	0.1070
6	1.1	1	28.0	0.20	0.0057
7	2.1	2	3.1	0.50	26.0286
8	2.0	2	32.0	0.70	0.0248
9	2.3	2	30.0	0.70	0.1252
10	2.9	3	33.0	0.80	0.0253
11	3.1	3	32.0	0.80	0.0035
12	3.0	3	33.0	0.90	0.0111
13	5.9	6	38.0	1.20	0.0037
14	5.8	6	39.0	1.50	0.2786
15	6.1	6	37.0	1.20	0.3988

TABLE 8.32
Regression Analysis with Error at x_2/n_7, Example 8.5

Predictor	Coef	SE Coef	t-Ratio	p
b_0	0.1920	0.1443	1.33	0.210
b_1	0.93742	0.06730	13.93	0.000
b_2	−0.003945	0.005817	−0.68	0.512
b_3	0.2087	0.3157	0.66	0.522
$s = 0.149018$		R-sq = 99.6%		R-sq(adj) = 99.5%

The regression equation is $\hat{y} = 0.192 + 0.937x_1 - 0.00395x_2 + 0.209x_3$.

observes a D value of 26.0286, much larger than 3.36; 3.1 is, of course, an outlier, as well as an influential value.

Again, Table 8.32 portrays a different regression equation from that presented in Table 8.26, because we have created the same error that produced Table 8.28. While $R^2_{(adj)}$ continues to be high, the substitution of 3.1 for 31 at x_2/n_7 does change the regression.

OUTLYING RESPONSE VARIABLE OBSERVATIONS, y_i

Sometimes, a set of normal-looking x_i values may be associated with an extreme y_i value. The residual value, $e_i = y_i - \hat{y}$, often is useful for evaluating y_i values. It is important with multiple linear regression to know where the influential values of the regression model are. Generally, they are at the extreme ends, but not always.

We have discussed residual e_i analysis in other chapters, so we will not spend a lot of time revisiting this. Two forms of residual analyses are particularly valuable for use in multiple regression: semi-Studentized and Studentized residuals. A semi-Studentized residual, e'_i, is the ith residual value divided by the square root of the mean square error.

$$e'_i = \frac{e_i}{\sqrt{MS_E}} \tag{8.33}$$

The hat matrix can be of use in another aspect of residual analysis, the Studentized residual. Recall that $H = X(X'X)^{-1} X'$ is the hat matrix. $\hat{Y} = HY$ is the predicted vector, $\hat{Y}$, the product of the $n \times n$ H matrix times the Y value vector. $e = (I - H)Y$, the error of the residual vector can be determined by subtracting the $n \times n$ H matrix from an $n \times n$ identity matrix, I, and multiplying that result by the Y vector.

The variance–covariance of the residuals can be determined by

$$\sigma^2_{(e)} = \sigma^2(I - H). \tag{8.34}$$

So, the estimate of $\sigma^2_{(e)} = x^2_{(e_i)} = MS_E(1 - h_{ii})$, where

$$h_{ii} \text{ is the } i\text{th diagonal of the hat matrix.} \qquad (8.35)$$

We are interested in the Studentized residual, which is the ratio of e_i to $s_{(e_i)}$, where

$$s_{(e_i)} = \sqrt{MS_E(1 - h_{ii})} \qquad (8.36)$$

$$\text{Studentized residual} = S_{r_i} = \frac{e_i}{s_{(e_i)}}, \qquad (8.37)$$

which is the residual divided by the standard deviation of the residual.

Large Studentized residual values are suspect, and they follow the Student's t distribution with $n - k - 1$ degrees of freedom. Extreme residuals are directly related to the y_i values, in that $e_i = y_i - \hat{y}_i$.

However, it is more effective to use the same type of schema as the Cook's distance—that is, providing S_{r_i} values with the ith value set deleted. This tends to flag outlying y_i values very quickly. The fitted regression is computed based on all values but the ith one. That is, each of the $e_i = y_i - \hat{y}_i$s is omitted from the regression. The $n - 1$ values are refit via the least squares method. The x_i values of the omitted value are then plugged back into the regression equation to obtain $\hat{y}_{i(i)}$, the estimated i value of the equation not using the y, x_i data of that spot to produce the regression equation. The value, d_i (difference between the original y_i and the new $\hat{y}_{i(i)}$ value), is computed, providing a deleted residual.

$$d_i = y_i - \hat{y}_{i(i)}. \qquad (8.38)$$

Recall that, in practice, the method used does not require refitting the regression equation:

$$d_i = \frac{e_i}{1 - h_{ii}} \qquad (8.39)$$

where $e_i = y_i - \hat{y}_i$, an ordinary residual containing all the data and h_{ii} = diagonal of hat matrix

Of course, the larger h_{ii} is, the greater the deleted residual value will be. This is valuable—the deleted residual—for it helps identify large "y" influences where the ordinary residual would not.

STUDENTIZED DELETED RESIDUALS

The deleted residual and Studentized residual approaches can be combined for a more powerful test in a process of dividing the deleted residual, d_i, by the standard deviation of the deleted residual.

$$t_i = \frac{d_i}{s_{d_i}},$$ (8.40)

where

$$d_i = y_i - \hat{y}_{i(-i)} = \frac{e_i}{1 - h_{ii}}$$

$$s_{d_i} = \sqrt{\frac{MSE_i}{1 - h_{ii}}},$$ (8.41)

MSE_i = mean square error of the regression without the ith value in the regression equation.

The test can also be written in the form:

$$t_{c_i} = \frac{e_i}{\sqrt{MSE_i(1 - h_{ii})}}.$$ (8.42)

But, in practice, the t_{c_i} formula is cumbersome, because MSE_i must be repeatedly calculated for each new t_i.

Hence, if the statistical software package one is using does not have the ability to perform the test, it can easily be adapted to do so. Just use the form:

$$t_{c_i} = e_i \sqrt{\frac{n - k - 2}{SS_E(1 - h_{ii}) - e_i^2}}.$$ (8.43)

Those values high in absolute terms are potential problems in the y_i values— perhaps even outliers. A formal test—a Bonferroni procedure—can be used to determine not the influence of the y_i values, but whether the largest absolute values of a set of y_i values may be outliers.

If $|t_{c_i}| > |t_t|$, conclude that t_{c_i} values greater than $|t_t|$ are "outliers" at α. $t_t = t_{(\alpha/2c;\ n-k-2)}$, k = number of b_i values, excluding b_0, and c = contrasts.

Let us return to data in Example 8.5. In this example, in Table 8.27, y_6 will be changed to 4, and y_{13} to 7.9. Table 8.33 provides the statistical model.

The actual values, fitted values, residuals, and h_{ii} diagonals, are provided in Table 8.34.

$$e_i \times \left(\sqrt{\left(\frac{10}{8.479} \times (1 - h_i) - e_i^2 \right)} \right)$$

$$C22 = C16 \times \left(\sqrt{\left(\frac{10}{8.479} \times (1 - C21) - C19 \right)} \right).$$

TABLE 8.33
Statistical Model of Data from Table 8.27, with Changes at y_6 and y_{13}

Predictor	Coef	St. Dev	t-Ratio	p
b_0	−0.435	3.953	−0.11	0.914
b_1	1.5703	0.4841	3.24	0.008
b_2	0.0479	0.1603	0.30	0.771
b_3	−3.198	1.890	−1.69	0.119

$s = 0.8779$ $\qquad$ $R^2 = 89.0\%$ $\qquad$ $R^2_{(adj)} = 86.0\%$

Source	DF	SS	MS	F	p
Regression	3	68.399	22.800	29.58	0.000
Error	11	8.479	0.771		
Total	14	76.8778			

The regression equation is $\hat{y} = -0.43 + 1.57x_1 + 0.048x_2 - 3.20x_3$.

As can be seen, the e_i values for $y_6 = 2.16247$ and $y_{13} = 0.92934$. We can craft the t_{c_i} values by manipulating the statistical software, if the package does not have t_{c_i} calculating capability, using the formula:

$$t_{c_i} = e_i \sqrt{\frac{n - k - 2}{SS_E(1 - h_{ii}) - e_i^2}},$$

where $n - k - 2 = 15 - 3 - 2 = 10$, and $SS_E = 8.479$ (Table 8.34)

TABLE 8.34
Example 8.5 Data, with Changes at y_6 and y_{13}

n	y	x_1	x_2	x_3	e_i	$\hat{y}_i$	h_{ii}
1	0.0	0	25.0	0.03	−0.66706	0.66706	0.047630
2	0.0	0	24.0	0.03	−0.61915	0.61915	0.042927
3	0.0	0	25.0	0.04	−0.63509	0.63509	0.040339
4	1.3	1	25.0	0.30	−0.07403	1.37403	0.000772
5	1.3	1	24.0	0.50	0.61340	0.68660	0.645692
6	4.0	1	28.0	0.20	2.16247	1.83753	0.582281
7	2.1	2	31.0	0.50	−0.49232	2.59232	0.019017
8	2.0	2	32.0	0.70	−0.00072	2.00072	0.000000
9	2.3	2	30.0	0.70	0.39511	1.90489	0.013148
10	2.9	3	33.0	0.80	−0.39919	3.29919	0.008187
11	3.1	3	32.0	0.80	−0.15127	3.25127	0.000735
12	3.0	3	33.0	0.90	0.02057	2.97943	0.000040
13	7.9	6	38.0	1.20	0.92934	6.97066	0.310683
14	5.8	6	39.0	1.50	−0.25931	6.05931	0.017451
15	6.1	6	37.0	1.20	−0.82275	6.92275	0.323916

TABLE 8.35
Table 8.34, with e_i^2 and t_{c_i} Values

	C1	C2	C3	C4	C5	C7	C8	C9
Row	y	x_1	x_2	x_3	e_i	h_{ii}	e_i^2	t_{c_i}
1	0.0	0	25.0	0.03	−0.66706	0.207348	0.44498	−0.84203
2	0.0	0	24.0	0.03	−0.61915	0.213543	0.38335	−0.78098
3	0.0	0	25.0	0.04	−0.63509	0.198225	0.40334	−0.79418
4	1.3	1	25.0	0.30	−0.07403	0.246645	0.00548	−0.09267
5	1.3	1	24.0	0.50	0.61340	0.649604	0.37626	1.20417
6	4.0	1	28.0	0.20	2.16247	0.228504	4.67626	5.00703
7	2.1	2	31.0	0.50	−0.49232	0.167612	0.24238	−0.59635
8	2.0	2	32.0	0.70	−0.00072	0.322484	0.00000	−0.00095
9	2.3	2	30.0	0.70	0.39511	0.176214	0.15611	0.47813
10	2.9	3	33.0	0.80	−0.39919	0.122084	0.15935	−0.46771
11	3.1	3	32.0	0.80	−0.15127	0.083246	0.02288	−0.17183
12	3.0	3	33.0	0.90	0.02057	0.192055	0.00042	0.02485
13	7.9	6	38.0	1.20	0.92934	0.399687	0.86367	1.42951
14	5.8	6	39.0	1.50	−0.25931	0.344164	0.06724	−0.34985
15	6.1	6	37.0	1.20	−0.82275	0.448586	0.67691	−1.30112

We will add new columns to Table 8.34 ($C8$) for e_i^2 and t_{c_i} (Table 8.35). So the MiniTab procedure for computing t_{c_i} is:

Let

$$C9 = C5 \times \left(\sqrt{\left(\tfrac{10}{8.479} \times (1 - C7) - C8\right)} \right), C9 = t_{c_i}, C7 = h_i, C5 = e_i, C8 = e_i^2$$

Note that the really large t_{c_i} value is 5.00703, where $y_i = 4.0$, and a $t_{c_i} = 1.49951$ at $y_{13} = 7.9$. To determine the t_t value, set $\alpha = 0.05$. We will perform two contrasts, so $c = 2$. $t_{t(\alpha/2c; n-k-2)} = t_{t(0.05/4, 5-5)} = t_{t(0.0125, 10)} = 2.764$, from the Student's t Table (Table B). So, if $|t_i| > 2.764$, reject H_0. Only 5.00703 > 2.764, so it is an outlier with influence on the regression. We see that 1.42951 (y_{13}) is relatively large, but not enough to be significant.

INFLUENCE: BETA INFLUENCE

Additionally, one often is very interested as to how various values of y_i or x_i influence the estimated b_i coefficients in terms of standard deviation shifts. It is one thing to be influenced as a value, but a real effect is in the beta (b_i) coefficients. Belsey et al. (1980) have provided a useful method to do this, termed the DFBETAS.

$$\text{DFBETAS}_{j(-i)} = \frac{b_j - b_{j(-i)}}{\sqrt{s_{(-i)}^2 C_{ji}}},$$

where $b_j = j$th regression coefficient with data point, $b_{j(i)} = j$th regression coefficient without ith data point, $s^2_{(-i)} =$ variance error term of the $t_{j(-i)}$ coefficient, and $C_{jj} =$ diagonal element of the matrix $= (X'X)^{-1}$

A large DFBETAS$_{j(-i)} > 2\sqrt{n}$ means that the ith observation needs to be checked. The only problem is that, with small samples, the $2\sqrt{n}$ may not be useful. For large samples, $n \geq 30$, it works fine. In smaller samples, use Cook's distance in preference to DFBETAS$_{j(-i)}$.

SUMMARY

What is one to do if influence or leverage is great? Ideally, one can evaluate the data and find leverage and influence values to be mistakes in data collection or typographical errors. If they are not, then the researcher must make some decisions:

1. One can refer to the results of similar studies. For example, if one has done a number of surgical scrub evaluations using a standard method, has experience with that evaluative method, has used a reference product (and the reference product's results are consistent with those from similar studies), and if one has experience with the active antimicrobial, then an influential or leveraged, unexpected value may be removed.
2. Instead of removing a specific value, an analogy to a trim mean might be employed. Say 10% of the most extreme absolute residual values, Cook's distance values, or deleted Studentized values are simply removed; this is 5% of the extreme positive residuals and 5% of the negative ones. This sort of determination helps prevent "distorting" the data for one's gain.
3. One can perform the analysis with and without the extreme leverage/influential values and let the reader determine how they want to interpret the data.
4. Finally, the use of nonparametric regression is sometimes valuable.

9 Indicator (Dummy) Variable Regression

Indicator, or dummy variable regression, as it is often known, employs qualitative or categorical variables as all or some of its predictor variables, x_is. In the regression models discussed in the previous chapters, the x_i predictor variables were quantitative measurements, such as time, temperature, chemical level, or days of exposure. Indicator regression uses categorical variables, such as sex, machine, process, anatomical site (e.g., forearm, abdomen, inguinal region), or geographical location, and these categories are coded, which allows them to be ranked. For example, female may be represented as "0," and male as "1." Neither sex is rankable or distinguishable, except by the code "0" or "1."

Indicator regression, many times, employs both quantitative and qualitative x_i variables. For example, if one wished to measure the microorganisms normally found on the skin of men and women, relative to their age, the following regression model might be used

$$\hat{y} = b_0 + b_1 x_1 + b_2 x_2,$$

where
$\hat{y}$ is the $\log_{10}$ microbial counts per cm^2,
x_i the age of the subject, and
x_2 is 0 if male and 1 if female.

This model is composed of two linear regressions, one for males and the other for females.

For the males, the regression would reduce to

$$\hat{y} = b_0 + b_1 x_1 + b_2(0),$$
$$\hat{y} = b_0 + b_1 x_1.$$

For the females, the regression would be

$$\hat{y} = b_0 + b_1 x_1 + b_2(1),$$
$$\hat{y} = (b_0 + b_2) + b_1 x_1.$$

The plotted regression functions would be parallel—same slopes, but different y-intercepts. Neither 0 nor 1 is the required representative value to use—any will do—but they are the simplest to use.

In general, if there are c levels of a specific quantitative variable, they must be expressed in terms of $c - 1$ levels to avoid collinearity. For example, suppose multiple anatomical sites, such as the abdominal, forearm, subclavian, and inguinal, are to be evaluated in an antimicrobial evaluation. There are $c = 4$ sites, so there will be $c - 1 = 4 - 1 = 3$ dummy x variables. The model can be written as

$$\hat{y} = b_0 + b_1 x_1 + b_2 x_2 + b_3 x_3,$$

where

$$x_1 = \begin{cases} 1 = \text{if abdomen site,} \\ 0 = \text{if otherwise,} \end{cases}$$

$$x_2 = \begin{cases} 1 = \text{if forearm site,} \\ 0 = \text{if otherwise,} \end{cases}$$

$$x_3 = \begin{cases} 1 = \text{if subclavian site,} \\ 0 = \text{if otherwise.} \end{cases}$$

When $x_1 = x_2 = x_3 = 0$, the model represents the inguinal region. Let us write out the equations to better comprehend what is happening. The full model is

$$\hat{y} = b_0 + b_1 x_1 + b_2 x_2 + b_3 x_3. \tag{9.1}$$

The abdominal site model reduces to

$$\hat{y} = b_0 + b_1 x_1 = b_0 + b_1, \tag{9.2}$$

where $x_1 = 1$, $x_2 = 0$, and $x_3 = 0$.

The forearm site model reduces to

$$\hat{y} = b_0 + b_2 x_2 = b_0 + b_2, \tag{9.3}$$

where $x_1 = 0$, $x_2 = 1$, and $x_3 = 0$.

The subclavian site model reduces to

$$\hat{y} = b_0 + b_3 x_3 = b_0 + b_3, \tag{9.4}$$

where $x_1 = 0$, $x_2 = 0$, and $x_3 = 1$.

In addition, the inguinal site model reduces to

$$\hat{y} = b_0, \qquad (9.5)$$

where $x_1 = 0$, $x_2 = 0$, and $x_3 = 0$.

Let us now look at an example while describing the statistical process.

Example 9.1: In a precatheter-insertion skin preparation evaluation, four anatomical skin sites were used to evaluate two test products, a 70% isopropyl alcohol (IPA) and 70% IPA with 2% chlorhexidine gluconate (CHG). The investigator compared the products at four anatomical sites (abdomen, inguinal, subclavian, and forearm), replicated three times, and sampled for $\log_{10}$ microbial reductions both immediately and after a 24 h postpreparation period. The y values are $\log_{10}$ reductions from baseline (pretreatment) microbial populations at each of the sites.

There are four test sites, so there are $c - 1$, or $4 - 1 = 3$, dummy variables for which one must account. There are two test products, so $c - 1 = 2 - 1 = 1$ dummy variable per product. So, let

$$x_1 = \text{time of sample} = \begin{cases} 0 = \text{if immediate,} \\ 24 = \text{if 24 h,} \end{cases}$$

$$x_2 = \text{product} = \begin{cases} 1 = \text{if IPA,} \\ 0 = \text{if other,} \end{cases}$$

$$x_3 = \begin{cases} 1 = \text{if inguinal,} \\ 0 = \text{if other,} \end{cases}$$

$$x_4 = \begin{cases} 1 = \text{if forearm,} \\ 0 = \text{if other,} \end{cases}$$

$$x_5 = \begin{cases} 1 = \text{if subclavian,} \\ 0 = \text{if other.} \end{cases}$$

Recall that the abdominal site is represented by $b_0 + b_1 + b_2$, when $x_3 = x_4 = x_5 = 0$.

The full model is

$$\hat{y} = b_0 + b_1 x_1 + b_2 x_2 + b_3 x_3 + b_4 x_4 + b_5 x_5.$$

The actual data are presented in Table 9.1.

Table 9.2 presents the regression model derived from the data in Table 9.1. The reader will undoubtedly see that the output is the same as that previously observed.

TABLE 9.1
Actual Data, Example 9.1

Microbial Counts	Time	Product	Inguinal	Forearm	Subclavian
y	x_1	x_2	x_3	x_4	x_5
3.1	0	1	1	0	0
3.5	0	1	1	0	0
3.3	0	1	1	0	0
3.3	0	0	1	0	0
3.4	0	0	1	0	0
3.6	0	0	1	0	0
0.9	24	1	1	0	0
1.0	24	1	1	0	0
0.8	24	1	1	0	0
3.0	24	0	1	0	0
3.1	24	0	1	0	0
3.2	24	0	1	0	0
1.2	0	1	0	1	0
1.0	0	1	0	1	0
1.3	0	1	0	1	0
1.3	0	0	0	1	0
1.2	0	0	0	1	0
1.1	0	0	0	1	0
0.0	24	1	0	1	0
0.1	24	1	0	1	0
0.2	24	1	0	1	0
1.4	24	0	0	1	0
1.5	24	0	0	1	0
1.2	24	0	0	1	0
1.5	0	1	0	0	1
1.3	0	1	0	0	1
1.4	0	1	0	0	1
1.6	0	0	0	0	1
1.2	0	0	0	0	1
1.4	0	0	0	0	1
0.1	24	1	0	0	1
0.2	24	1	0	0	1
0.1	24	1	0	0	1
1.7	24	0	0	0	1
1.8	24	0	0	0	1
1.5	24	0	0	0	1
2.3	0	1	0	0	0
2.5	0	1	0	0	0
2.1	0	1	0	0	0
2.4	0	0	0	0	0

TABLE 9.1 (continued)
Actual Data, Example 9.1

Microbial Counts	Time	Product	Inguinal	Forearm	Subclavian
2.1	0	0	0	0	0
2.2	0	0	0	0	0
0.3	24	1	0	0	0
0.2	24	1	0	0	0
0.3	24	1	0	0	0
2.3	24	0	0	0	0
2.5	24	0	0	0	0
2.2	24	0	0	0	0

In order to fully understand the regression, it is necessary to deconstruct its meaning. There are two products evaluated, two time points, and four anatomical sites. From the regression model (Table 9.2), this is not readily apparent. So we will evaluate it now.

INGUINAL SITE, IPA PRODUCT, IMMEDIATE

Full model: $\hat{y} = b_0 + b_1x_1 + b_2x_2 + b_3x_3 + b_4x_4 + b_5x_5$.
The x_4 (forearm) and x_5 (subclavian) values are 0.

TABLE 9.2
Regression Model, Example 9.1

Predictor	Coef	St. Dev	t-Ratio	p
b_0	2.6417	0.1915	13.80	0.000
b_1	−0.034201	0.006514	−5.25	0.000
b_2	−0.8958	0.1563	−5.73	0.000
b_3	0.9000	0.2211	4.07	0.000
b_4	−0.8250	0.2211	−3.73	0.001
b_5	−0.6333	0.2211	−2.86	0.006
$s = 0.541538$		R-sq $= 76.2\%$		R-sq(adj) $= 73.4\%$

Analysis of Variance

Source	DF	SS	MS	F	P
Regression	5	39.4810	7.8962	26.93	0.000
Error	42	12.3171	0.2933		
Total	47	51.7981			

The regression equation is $\hat{y} = 2.64 - 0.034x_1 - 0.896x_2 + 0.900x_3 - 0.825x_4 - 0.633x_5$.

Hence, the model reduces to $\hat{y} = b_0 + b_1x_1 + b_2x_2 + b_3x_3$.
Time $= 0 = x_1$, product 1 is IPA $= 1$ for x_2, and the inguinal site is 1 for x_3.

$$\hat{y}_0 = b_0 + b_1(0) + b_2(1) + b_3(1),$$
$$\hat{y}_0 = b_0 + b_2 + b_3,$$
$$\hat{y}_0 = 2.6417 + (-0.8958) + 0.9000.$$

$\hat{y}_0 = 2.6459 \log_{10}$ reduction in microorganisms by the IPA product.

INGUINAL SITE, IPA $\pm$ CHG PRODUCT, IMMEDIATE

Full model: $\hat{y} = b_0 + b_1x_1 + b_2x_2 + b_3x_3 + b_4x_4 + b_5x_5$.
Time $= 0 = x_1$, and product is IPA $+$ CHG $= 0$ for x_2.

$$\hat{y} = b_0 + b_1(0) + b_2(0) + b_3(1) + b_4(0) + b_5(0),$$
$$\hat{y}_0 = b_0 + b_3,$$
$$\hat{y}_0 = 2.6417 + 0.9000.$$

$\hat{y}_0 = 3.5417 \log_{10}$ reduction in microorganisms by the IPA $+$ CHG product.

INGUINAL SITE, IPA PRODUCT, 24 H

$$x_1 = 24, \ x_2 = 1, \text{ and } x_3 = 1.$$
$$\hat{y}_{24} = 2.6417 + (-0.0342[24]) + (-0.8958[1]) + (0.9000[1]).$$

$\hat{y}_{24} = 1.8251 \log_{10}$ reduction in microorganisms by the IPA product at 24 h.

INGUINAL SITE, IPA $\pm$ CHG PRODUCT, 24 H

$$x_1 = 24, \ x_2 = 0, \text{ and } x_3 = 1.$$
$$\hat{y}_{24} = 2.6417 + (-0.0342[24]) + (0.9000[1]).$$

$\hat{y}_{24} = 2.7209 \log_{10}$ reduction in microorganisms by the IPA $+$ CHG product at 24 h.

Plotting these two products, the result is shown in Figure 9.1.

Note that there may be a big problem. The regression fits the same slope for both products, just different at the y-intercepts. This may not be adequate for what we are trying to do. The actual data for both at time 0 are nearly equivalent in this study, differing only at the 24 h period. Hence, the predicted values do not make sense.

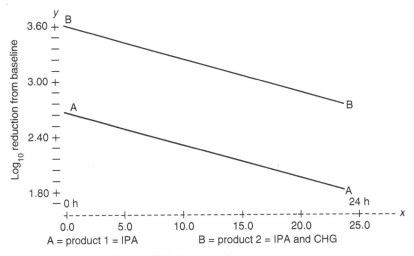

FIGURE 9.1 IPA and IPA + CHG, Example 9.1.

There may be an interaction effect. Therefore, we need to look at the data in Table 9.3, providing the actual data, fitted data, and residual data for the model. We see a $+/-$ pattern, depending on the x_i variable, so we check out the possible interaction, particularly because $R^2_{(adj)}$ for the regression is only 73.4% (Table 9.2).

The positive interactions that can occur are x_1x_2, x_1x_3, x_1x_4, x_1x_5, x_2x_3, x_2x_4, x_2x_5, $x_1x_2x_3$, $x_1x_2x_4$, and $x_1x_2x_5$. Note that we have limited the analysis to three-way interactions.

We code the interactions as $x_6 - x_{15}$. Specifically, they are

$$x_1x_2 = x_6,$$
$$x_1x_3 = x_7,$$
$$x_1x_4 = x_8,$$
$$x_1x_5 = x_9,$$
$$x_2x_3 = x_{10},$$
$$x_2x_4 = x_{11},$$
$$x_2x_5 = x_{12},$$
$$x_1x_2x_3 = x_{13},$$
$$x_1x_2x_4 = x_{14},$$
$$x_1x_2x_5 = x_{15}.$$

Table 9.4 provides the complete new set of data to fit the full model with interactions.

TABLE 9.3
Actual Data, Fitted Data, and Residual Data, Example 9.1

Row	y	x_1	x_2	x_3	x_4	x_5	$\hat{y}$	$y - \hat{y} = e$
1	3.1	0	1	1	0	0	2.64583	0.45417
2	3.5	0	1	1	0	0	2.64583	0.85417
3	3.3	0	1	1	0	0	2.64583	0.65417
4	3.3	0	0	1	0	0	3.54167	−0.24167
5	3.4	0	0	1	0	0	3.54167	−0.14167
6	3.6	0	0	1	0	0	3.54167	0.05833
7	0.9	24	1	1	0	0	1.82500	−0.92500
8	1.0	24	1	1	0	0	1.82500	−0.82500
9	0.8	24	1	1	0	0	1.82500	−1.02500
10	3.0	24	0	1	0	0	2.72083	0.27917
11	3.1	24	0	1	0	0	2.72083	0.37917
12	3.2	24	0	1	0	0	2.72083	0.47917
13	1.2	0	1	0	1	0	0.92083	0.27917
14	1.0	0	1	0	1	0	0.92083	0.07917
15	1.3	0	1	0	1	0	0.92083	0.37917
16	1.3	0	0	0	1	0	1.81667	−0.51667
17	1.2	0	0	0	1	0	1.81667	−0.61667
18	1.1	0	0	0	1	0	1.81667	−0.71667
19	0.0	24	1	0	1	0	0.10000	−0.10000
20	0.1	24	1	0	1	0	0.10000	−0.00000
21	0.2	24	1	0	1	0	0.10000	0.10000
22	1.4	24	0	0	1	0	0.99583	0.40417
23	1.5	24	0	0	1	0	0.99583	0.50417
24	1.2	24	0	0	1	0	0.99583	0.20417
25	1.5	0	1	0	0	1	1.11250	0.38750
26	1.3	0	1	0	0	1	1.11250	0.18750
27	1.4	0	1	0	0	1	1.11250	0.28750
28	1.6	0	0	0	0	1	2.00833	−0.40833
29	1.2	0	0	0	0	1	2.00833	−0.80833
30	1.4	0	0	0	0	1	2.00833	−0.60833
31	0.1	24	1	0	0	1	0.29167	−0.19167
32	0.2	24	1	0	0	1	0.29167	−0.09167
33	0.1	24	1	0	0	1	0.29167	−0.19167
34	1.7	24	0	0	0	1	1.18750	0.51250
35	1.8	24	0	0	0	1	1.18750	0.61250
36	1.5	24	0	0	0	1	1.18750	0.31250
37	2.3	0	1	0	0	0	1.74583	0.55417
38	2.5	0	1	0	0	0	1.74583	0.75417
39	2.1	0	1	0	0	0	1.74583	0.35417
40	2.4	0	0	0	0	0	2.64167	−0.24167
41	2.1	0	0	0	0	0	2.64167	−0.54167

TABLE 9.3 (continued)
Actual Data, Fitted Data, and Residual Data, Example 9.1

Row	y	x_1	x_2	x_3	x_4	x_5	$\hat{y}$	$y - \hat{y} = e$
42	2.2	0	0	0	0	0	2.64167	−0.44167
43	0.3	24	1	0	0	0	0.92500	−0.92500
44	0.2	24	1	0	0	0	0.92500	−0.72500
45	0.3	24	1	0	0	0	0.92500	−0.62500
46	2.3	24	0	0	0	0	1.82083	0.47917
47	2.5	24	0	0	0	0	1.82083	0.67917
48	2.2	24	0	0	0	0	1.82083	0.37917

Other interactions could have been evaluated, but the main candidates are presented here. Interactions between inguinal and abdominal were not used, because they will not interact.

The new model is

$$\hat{y} = b_0 + b_1 x_1 + \cdots + b_{15} x_{15}, \qquad (9.6)$$

or as presented in Table 9.5.

This model appears rather ungainly, and some of the x_i values could be removed. We will not do that at this point, but the procedures in Chapter 3 and Chapter 10 (backward, forward, or stepwise) would be used for this. Note that $R^2_{(adj)} = 98.2\%$, a much better fit.

By printing the y, $\hat{y}$, and e values, we can evaluate the configuration (Table 9.6). Let us compare product 1 and product 2 at the inguinal sites time 0 and time 24.

Figure 9.2 shows the new results.

Note that IPA, alone, and IPA + CHG initially produce about the same $\log_{10}$ microbial reductions (approximately a $3.3 \log_{10}$ reduction at time 0). However, over the 24 h period, the IPA, with no persistent antimicrobial effects, drifted toward the baseline level. The IPA + CHG, at the 24 h mark, remains at over a $3 \log_{10}$ reduction.

This graph shows the effects the way they really are. Note, however, that as the variables increase, the number of interaction terms skyrockets, eating valuable degrees of freedom. Perhaps, a better way to perform this study would be to separate the anatomical sites, because their results are not compared directly anyway, and use a separate statistical analysis for each. However, by the use of dummy variables, the evaluation can be made all at once. There is also a strong argument to do the study as it is, because the testing is performed on the same unit—a patient—just at different anatomical sites. Multiple analysis of variance could also be used where multiple dependent variables would be employed, but many readers would have trouble

TABLE 9.4
New Data Set to Account for Interaction, Example 9.1

Row	y	x_1	x_2	x_3	x_4	x_5	x_6	x_7	x_8	x_9	x_{10}	x_{11}	x_{12}	x_{13}	x_{14}	x_{15}
1	3.10	0	1	1	0	0	0	0	0	0	1	0	0	0	0	0
2	3.50	0	1	1	0	0	0	0	0	0	1	0	0	0	0	0
3	3.30	0	1	1	0	0	0	0	0	0	1	0	0	0	0	0
4	3.30	0	0	1	0	0	0	0	0	0	0	0	0	0	0	0
5	3.40	0	0	1	0	0	0	0	0	0	0	0	0	0	0	0
6	3.60	0	0	1	0	0	0	0	0	0	0	0	0	0	0	0
7	0.90	24	1	1	0	0	24	24	0	0	1	0	0	24	0	0
8	1.00	24	1	1	0	0	24	24	0	0	1	0	0	24	0	0
9	0.80	24	1	1	0	0	24	24	0	0	1	0	0	24	0	0
10	3.00	24	0	1	0	0	0	24	0	0	0	0	0	0	0	0
11	3.10	24	0	1	0	0	0	24	0	0	0	0	0	0	0	0
12	3.20	24	0	1	0	0	0	24	0	0	0	0	0	0	0	0
13	1.20	0	1	0	1	0	0	0	0	0	0	1	0	0	0	0
14	1.00	0	1	0	1	0	0	0	0	0	0	1	0	0	0	0
15	1.30	0	1	0	1	0	0	0	0	0	0	1	0	0	0	0
16	1.30	0	0	0	1	0	0	0	0	0	0	0	0	0	0	0
17	1.20	0	0	0	1	0	0	0	0	0	0	0	0	0	0	0
18	1.10	0	0	0	1	0	0	0	0	0	0	0	0	0	0	0
19	0.00	24	1	0	1	0	24	0	24	0	0	1	0	0	24	0
20	0.10	24	1	0	1	0	24	0	24	0	0	1	0	0	24	0
21	0.20	24	1	0	1	0	24	0	24	0	0	1	0	0	24	0
22	1.40	24	0	0	1	0	0	0	24	0	0	0	0	0	0	0
23	1.50	24	0	0	1	0	0	0	24	0	0	0	0	0	0	0
24	1.20	24	0	0	1	0	0	0	24	0	0	0	0	0	0	0
25	1.50	0	1	0	0	1	0	0	0	0	0	0	1	0	0	0
26	1.30	0	1	0	0	1	0	0	0	0	0	0	1	0	0	0
27	1.40	0	1	0	0	1	0	0	0	0	0	0	1	0	0	0
28	1.60	0	0	0	0	1	0	0	0	0	0	0	0	0	0	0
29	1.20	0	0	0	0	1	0	0	0	0	0	0	0	0	0	0
30	1.40	0	0	0	0	1	0	0	0	0	0	0	0	0	0	0
31	0.10	24	1	0	0	1	24	0	0	24	0	0	1	0	0	24
32	0.20	24	1	0	0	1	24	0	0	24	0	0	1	0	0	24
33	0.10	24	1	0	0	1	24	0	0	24	0	0	1	0	0	24
34	1.70	24	0	0	0	1	0	0	0	24	0	0	0	0	0	0
35	1.80	24	0	0	0	1	0	0	0	24	0	0	0	0	0	0
36	1.50	24	0	0	0	1	0	0	0	24	0	0	0	0	0	0
37	2.30	0	1	0	0	0	0	0	0	0	0	0	0	0	0	0
38	2.50	0	1	0	0	0	0	0	0	0	0	0	0	0	0	0
39	2.10	0	1	0	0	0	0	0	0	0	0	0	0	0	0	0
40	2.40	0	0	0	0	0	0	0	0	0	0	0	0	0	0	0

(continued)

TABLE 9.4 (continued)
New Data Set to Account for Interaction, Example 9.1

Row	y	x_1	x_2	x_3	x_4	x_5	x_6	x_7	x_8	x_9	x_{10}	x_{11}	x_{12}	x_{13}	x_{14}	x_{15}
41	2.10	0	0	0	0	0	0	0	0	0	0	0	0	0	0	0
42	2.20	0	0	0	0	0	0	0	0	0	0	0	0	0	0	0
43	0.30	24	1	0	0	0	24	0	0	0	0	0	0	0	0	0
44	0.20	24	1	0	0	0	24	0	0	0	0	0	0	0	0	0
45	0.30	24	1	0	0	0	24	0	0	0	0	0	0	0	0	0
46	2.30	24	0	0	0	0	0	0	0	0	0	0	0	0	0	0
47	2.50	24	0	0	0	0	0	0	0	0	0	0	0	0	0	0
48	2.20	24	0	0	0	0	0	0	0	0	0	0	0	0	0	0

TABLE 9.5
Revised Regression Model, Example 9.1

Predictor	Coef	St. Dev	t-Ratio	p
b_0	2.23333	0.08122	27.50	0.000
b_1	0.004167	0.004786	0.87	0.390
b_2	0.0667	0.1149	0.58	0.566
b_3	1.2000	0.1149	10.45	0.000
b_4	−1.0333	0.1149	−9.00	0.000
b_5	−0.8333	0.1149	−7.25	0.000
b_6	−0.088889	0.006769	−13.13	0.000
b_7	−0.018056	0.006769	−2.67	0.012
b_8	0.002778	0.006769	0.41	0.684
b_9	0.006944	0.006769	1.03	0.313
b_{10}	−0.2000	0.1624	−1.23	0.227
b_{11}	−0.1000	0.1624	−0.62	0.543
b_{12}	−0.0667	0.1624	−0.41	0.684
b_{13}	0.002778	0.009572	0.29	0.774
b_{14}	0.037500	0.009572	3.92	0.000
b_{15}	0.025000	0.009572	2.61	0.014

$s = 0.140683$ $R\text{-sq} = 98.8\%$ $R\text{-sq(adj)} = 98.2\%$

Analysis of Variance

Source	DF	SS	MS	F	p
Regression	15	51.1648	3.4110	172.34	0.000
Error	32	0.6333	0.0198		
Total	47	51.7981			

The regression equation is $\hat{y} = 2.23 + 0.00417x_1 + 0.067x_2 + 1.20x_3 - 1.03x_4 - 0.833x_5 - 0.0889x_6 - 0.0181x_7 + 0.00278x_8 + 0.0694x_9 - 0.200x_{10} - 0.100x_{11} - 0.067x_{12} + 0.00278x_{13} + 0.0375x_{14} + 0.0250x_{15}$.

TABLE 9.6
y, $\hat{y}$, and e Values, Revised Regression, Example 9.1

Row	y	$\hat{y}$	e
1	3.10	3.30000	−0.200000
2	3.50	3.30000	0.200000
3	3.30	3.30000	−0.000000
4	3.30	3.43333	−0.133333
5	3.40	3.43333	−0.033333
6	3.60	3.43333	0.166667
7	0.90	0.90000	−0.000000
8	1.00	0.90000	0.100000
9	0.80	0.90000	−0.100000
10	3.00	3.10000	−0.100000
11	3.10	3.10000	−0.000000
12	3.20	3.10000	0.100000
13	1.20	1.16667	0.033333
14	1.00	1.16667	−0.166667
15	1.30	1.16667	0.133333
16	1.30	1.20000	0.100000
17	1.20	1.20000	0.000000
18	1.10	1.20000	−0.100000
19	0.00	0.10000	−0.100000
20	0.10	0.10000	−0.000000
21	0.20	0.10000	0.100000
22	1.40	1.36667	0.033333
23	1.50	1.36667	0.133333
24	1.20	1.36667	−0.166667
25	1.50	1.40000	0.100000
26	1.30	1.40000	−0.100000
27	1.40	1.40000	0.000000
28	1.60	1.40000	0.200000
29	1.20	1.40000	−0.200000
30	1.40	1.40000	0.000000
31	0.10	0.13333	−0.033333
32	0.20	0.13333	0.066667
33	0.10	0.13333	−0.033333
34	1.70	1.66667	0.033333
35	1.80	1.66667	0.133333
36	1.50	1.66667	−0.166667
37	2.30	2.30000	0.000000
38	2.50	2.30000	0.200000
39	2.10	2.30000	−0.200000
40	2.40	2.23333	0.166667
41	2.10	2.23333	−0.133333

(*continued*)

TABLE 9.6 (continued)
y, $\hat{y}$, and e Values, Revised Regression, Example 9.1

Row	y	$\hat{y}$	e
42	2.20	2.23333	−0.033333
43	0.30	0.20667	0.033333
44	0.20	0.20667	−0.066667
45	0.30	0.20667	0.033333
46	2.30	2.33333	−0.033333
47	2.50	2.33333	0.166667
48	2.20	2.33333	−0.133333

comprehending a more complex design and, because a time element is present, the use of this dummy regression is certainly appropriate.

COMPARING TWO REGRESSION FUNCTIONS

When using dummy variable regression, one can directly compare the two or more regression lines. There are three basic questions:

1. Are the two or more intercepts different?
2. Are the two or more slopes different?
3. Are the two or more regression functions coincidental—the same at the intercept and in the slopes?

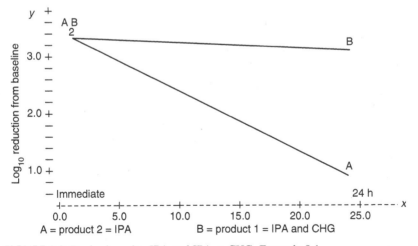

FIGURE 9.2 Revised results, IPA and IPA + CHG, Example 9.1.

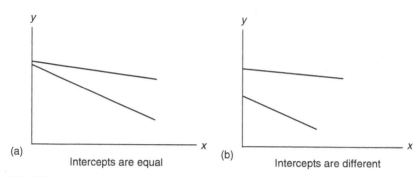

(a) Intercepts are equal   (b) Intercepts are different

FIGURE 9.3 Comparing two intercepts.

Figure 9.3a presents a case where the intercepts are the same, and Figure 9.3b presents a case where they differ.

Figure 9.4a presents a case where the slopes are different, and Figure 9.4b a case where they are the same.

Figure 9.5 presents a case where intercepts and slopes are identical.

Let us work an example beginning with two separate regression equations. We will use the data in Example 9.1.

The first set of data is for the IPA + CHG product (Table 9.7).

Figure 9.6 provides the data from the IPA + CHG product in $\log_{10}$ reductions at all sites.

Table 9.8 provides the linear regression analysis for the IPA + CHG product.

For the IPA alone, Table 9.9 provides the microbial, reduction data from all sites.

Figure 9.7 provides the plot of the IPA $\log_{10}$ reduction.

Table 9.10 provides the linear regression data.

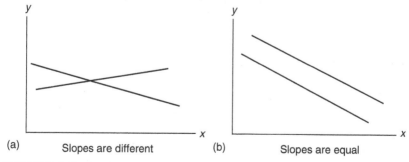

(a)   Slopes are different   (b)   Slopes are equal

FIGURE 9.4 Comparing two slopes.

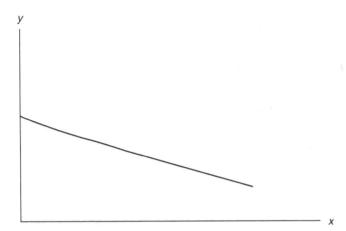

FIGURE 9.5 Identical slopes and intercepts.

TABLE 9.7
IPA + CHG Data, All Sites, Example 9.1

Row	y	x	
1	3.3	0	$y = \log_{10}$ reductions from baseline
2	3.4	0	
3	3.6	0	$x =$ time of sample
4	3.0	24	$0 =$ immediate
5	3.1	24	$24 = 24$ h
6	3.2	24	
7	1.3	0	
8	1.2	0	
9	1.1	0	
10	1.4	24	
11	1.5	24	
12	1.2	24	
13	1.6	0	
14	1.2	0	
15	1.4	0	
16	1.7	24	
17	1.8	24	
18	1.5	24	
19	2.4	0	
20	2.1	0	
21	2.2	0	
22	2.3	24	
23	2.5	24	
24	2.2	24	

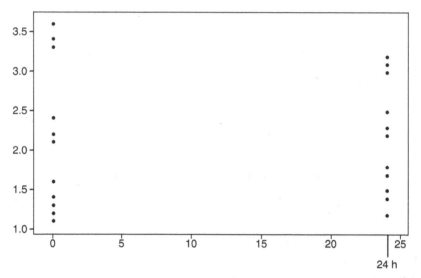

FIGURE 9.6 IPA + CHG product $\log_{10}$ reductions, all sites, Example 9.1.

COMPARING THE y-INTERCEPTS

When performing an indicator variable regression, it is often useful to compare two separate regressions for y-intercepts. This can be done using the six-step procedure.

TABLE 9.8
Linear Regression Analysis for IPA + CHG Product at All Sites,
Example 9.1

Predictor	Coef	St. Dev	t-Ratio	p
b_0	2.0667	0.2381	8.68	0.000
b_1	0.00208	0.01403	0.15	0.883

$s = 0.824713$ $R\text{-sq} = 0.1\%$ $R\text{-sq(adj)} = 0.0\%$

Analysis of Variance

Source	DF	SS	MS	F	p
Regression	1	0.0150	0.0150	0.02	0.883
Error	22	14.9633	0.6802		
Total	23	14.9783			

The regression equation is $\hat{y} = 2.07 + 0.0021x$.

TABLE 9.9
IPA Data, All Sites, Example 9.1

n	y	x
1	3.10	0
2	3.50	0
3	3.30	0
4	0.90	24
5	1.00	24
6	0.80	24
7	1.20	0
8	1.00	0
9	1.30	0
10	0.00	24
11	0.10	24
12	0.20	24
13	1.50	0
14	1.30	0
15	1.40	0
16	0.10	24
17	0.20	24
18	0.10	24
19	2.30	0
20	2.50	0
21	2.10	0
22	0.30	24
23	0.20	24
24	0.30	24

Step 1: Hypothesis.
There are three hypotheses available.

Upper Tail	Lower Tail	Two Tail
$H_0: \beta_{0A} \leq \beta_{0B}$	$H_0: \beta_{0A} \geq \beta_{0B}$	$H_0: \beta_{0A} = \beta_{0B}$
$H_A: \beta_{0A} > \beta_{0B}$	$H_A: \beta_{0A} < \beta_{0B}$	$H_A: \beta_{0A} \neq \beta_{0B}$

where
A is the IPA product and
B is the IPA + CHG product

Step 2: Set α, choose n_A and n_B.

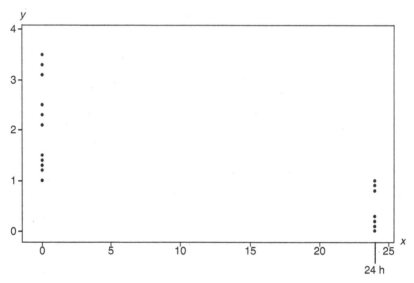

FIGURE 9.7 IPA product $\log_{10}$ reductions, all sites, Example 9.1.

Step 3: The test statistic is a t test of the form

$$t_c = \frac{\hat{b}_{0(A)} - \hat{b}_{0(B)}}{s_{\hat{b}_{0(A)} - \hat{b}_{0(B)}}}, \tag{9.7}$$

TABLE 9.10
Linear Regression Analysis for IPA at All Sites, Example 9.1

Predictor	Coef	St. Dev	t-Ratio	p	
b_0	2.0417	0.1948	10.48	0.000	
b_1	−0.07049	0.01148	−6.14	0.000	
$s = 0.6748$		R-sq $= 63.2\%$		R-sq(adj) $= 61.5\%$	

Analysis of Variance

Source	DF	SS	MS	F	P
Regression	1	17.170	17.170	37.70	0.000
Error	22	10.019	0.455		
Total	23	27.190			

The regression equation is $\hat{y} = 2.04 - 0.0705x$.

where

$$s^2_{\hat{b}_{0(A)} - \hat{b}_{0(B)}} = s^2_{\widehat{y,x}} \left[\frac{1}{n_A} + \frac{1}{n_B} + \frac{\bar{x}^2_A}{(n_A - 1)s^2_{x_{(A)}}} + \frac{\bar{x}^2_B}{(n_B - 1)s^2_{x_{(B)}}} \right],$$ (9.8)

where

$$s^2_{\widehat{y,x}} = \left[\frac{(n_A - 2)s^2_{y,x_A} + (n_B - 2)s^2_{y,x_B}}{n_A + n_B - 4} \right].$$ (9.9)

Note that

$$s^2_{\widehat{y,x}} = \frac{\sum (y_i - \hat{y})^2}{n - 2},$$ (9.10)

and

$$s^2_x = \frac{\sum (x_i - \bar{x})^2}{n - 1}.$$ (9.11)

Step 4: Decision rule.
Recall that there are three hypotheses available.

Upper Tail	Lower Tail	Two Tail
$H_0: \beta_{0(A)} \leq \beta_{0(B)}$	$H_0: \beta_{0(A)} \geq \beta_{0(B)}$	$H_0: \beta_{0(A)} = \beta_{0(B)}$
$H_A: \beta_{0(A)} > \beta_{0(B)}$	$H_A: \beta_{0(A)} < \beta_{0(B)}$	$H_A: \beta_{0(A)} \neq \beta_{0(B)}$
Test statistic: If	Test statistic: If	Test statistic: If
$t_c > t_{t(\alpha, n_A + n_B - 4)}$, then H_0 is rejected at α.	$t_c < -t_{t(\alpha, n_A + n_B - 4)}$, then H_0 is rejected at α.	$|t_c| > |t_{t(\alpha/2, n_A + n_B - 4)}|$, then H_0 is rejected at α.

Step 5: Perform the experiment.

Step 6: Make the decision based on the hypotheses (Step 4).
Let us perform a two-tail test to compare the IPA and the IPA + CHG products, where A is IPA and B is IPA + CHG.

Step 1: Formulate the test hypotheses.

$H_0: \beta_{0(A)} = \beta_{0(B)}$; the intercepts for IPA and IPA + CHG are the same,
$H_A: \beta_{0(A)} \neq \beta_{0(B)}$; the intercepts are not the same.

Step 2: Set α and n.
Let us set α at 0.10, so $\alpha/2 = 0.05$ because this is a two-tail test, and $n_A = n_B = 24$.

Step 3: Write the test statistic to be used.

$$t_c = \frac{\hat{b}_{0(A)} - \hat{b}_{0(B)}}{s_{\hat{b}_{0(A)} - \hat{b}_{0(B)}}}. \tag{9.7}$$

Step 4: Decision rule.

If $|t_c| > |t_t|$, reject H_0 at $\alpha = 0.10$.

$t_t = t_{t(\alpha/2;\, n_A + n_B - 4)} = t_{(0.10/2;\, 24 + 24 - 4)} = t_{(0.05, 44)} = 1.684$ (from Table B, the Student's t table). Because this is a two-tail test, 1.684 will be both negative and positive.

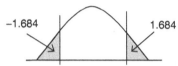

-1.684   1.684

If $|t_c| > |t_t = 1.684|$, reject H_0 at $\alpha = 0.10$, and conclude that the y-intercepts are not equivalent.

Step 5: Perform the experiment and the calculations.

$b_{0(A)}$, the intercept of IPA (Table 9.10) $= 2.0417$.

$b_{0(B)}$, the intercept of IPA + CHG (Table 9.8) $= 2.0667$.

$$s^2_{\hat{b}_{0(A)} - \hat{b}_{0(B)}} = s^2_{y,x}\left[\frac{1}{n_A} + \frac{1}{n_B} + \frac{\bar{x}_A^2}{(n_A - 1)s^2_{x(A)}} + \frac{\bar{x}_B^2}{(n_B - 1)s^2_{x(B)}}\right].$$

First, solving for $s^2_{y,x}$,

$$s^2_{y,x} = \frac{(n_A - 2)s^2_{y,x_A} + (n_B - 2)s^2_{y,x_B}}{n_A + n_B - 4} = \frac{(24 - 2)0.6802 + (24 - 2)0.455}{24 + 24 - 4}$$

$$= 0.5676.$$

Therefore,

$$s^2_{\hat{b}_{0(A)} - \hat{b}_{0(B)}} = 0.5676\left[\frac{1}{24} + \frac{1}{24} + \frac{12^2}{24 - 1(150.3076)} + \frac{12^2}{24 - 1(150.3076)}\right],$$

$$s^2_{\hat{b}_{0(A)} - \hat{b}_{0(B)}} = 0.0946,$$

and

$$s^2_{y,x_A} = \frac{\sum(y_i - \hat{y})^2}{n - 2} = MS_E = 0.6802 \text{ (Table 9.8), for IPA + CHG.}$$

$$s^2_{y,x_B} = MS_E = 0.455 \text{ (Table 9.10), for IPA only.}$$

Summary data for the x values (0 or 24) are for IPA and for IPA + CHG. Because the x_i values are identical, we only need one table (Table 9.11) to compute $s^2_{x_A}$ and $s^2_{x_B}$.

TABLE 9.11
x Values for the IPA and the IPA + CHG

Variable	n	Mean	Median	Tr Mean	St. Dev	SE Mean
$x =$ Time	24	12.00	12.00	12.00	12.26	2.50

Variable	Min	Max	Q1	Q3
$x =$ Time	0.00	24.00	0.00	24.00

$$s^2_{x_A} = \frac{\sum (x_i - \bar{x})^2}{n - 1} = (12.26)^2 = 150.3076,$$

$$s^2_{x_B} = \frac{\sum (x_i - \bar{x})^2}{n - 1} = (12.26)^2 = 150.3076.$$

Note that this variance for both IPA and IPA + CHG, $s^2_{x_j}$, is large, because the x_i range for both is 0 to 24. If the range had been much greater, some would normalize the x_i values, but these values are not so excessive as to cause problems. Finally,

$$t_c = \frac{\hat{b}_{0(A)} - \hat{b}_{0(B)}}{s^2_{\hat{b}_{0(A)} - \hat{b}_{0(B)}}} = \frac{2.0667 - 2.0417}{\sqrt{0.0946}} = 0.0813.$$

Step 6: Decision.
Because $|t_c| = 0.0813 \not> 1.684$, one cannot reject H_0 at $\alpha = 0.10$. Hence, we conclude that the b_0-intercepts for the 2% CHG + IPA and the IPA product, alone, are the same. In the context of our current problem, we note that both the products are equal in antimicrobial kill ($\log_{10}$ reductions) at the immediate time point. However, what about after time 0?

TEST OF B_1S OR SLOPES: PARALLELISM

In this test, we are interested in seeing if the slopes for microbial reductions are the same for the two compared groups, the IPA + CHG and the IPA, alone. If the slopes are the same, this would not mean the intercepts necessarily are.

The six-step procedure is as follows.

Step 1: State the hypotheses (three can be made).

Upper Tail	Lower Tail	Two Tail
$H_0: \beta_{1(A)} \leq \beta_{1(B)}$	$H_0: \beta_{1(A)} \geq \beta_{1(B)}$	$H_0: \beta_{1(A)} = \beta_{1(B)}$
$H_A: \beta_{1(A)} > \beta_{1(B)}$	$H_A: \beta_{1(A)} < \beta_{1(B)}$	$H_A: \beta_{1(A)} \neq \beta_{1(B)}$

Step 2: Set sample sizes and the α level.

Step 3: Write out the test statistic to be used

$$t_c = \frac{b_{1(A)} - b_{1(B)}}{s_{b_{1(A)} - b_{1(B)}}},$$

where

$$s^2_{b_{1(A)} - b_{1(B)}} = s^2_{\widehat{y,x}} \left[\frac{1}{(n_A - 1)s_{x(A)}} + \frac{1}{(n_B - 1)s_{x(B)}} \right],$$

$$s^2_{\widehat{y,x}} = \frac{(n_A - 2)s^2_{y,x_A} + (n_B - 2)s^2_{y,x_B}}{n_A + n_B - 4},$$

$$s^2_{y,x} = \frac{\sum(y_i - \hat{y}_i)^2}{n - 2},$$

$$s^2_{(x)} = \frac{\sum(x_i - \bar{x})^2}{n - 1}.$$

Step 4: Decision rule.
Upper tail:
If $t_c > t_{t(\alpha; n_A + n_B - 4)}$, reject H_0 at α.
Lower tail:
If $t_c < -t_{t(\alpha; n_A + n_B - 4)}$, reject H_0 at α.
Two tail:
If $|t_c| > |t_{t(\alpha/2; n_A + n_B - 4)}|$, reject H_0 at α.

Step 5: Perform experiment.

Step 6: Make the decision, based on Step 4.
Let us perform a two-tail test at $\alpha = 0.05$, using the data in Table 9.7 and Table 9.9.

Step 1: Set the hypotheses. We will perform a two-tail test for parallel slopes, where A represents IPA + CHG and B IPA.

$$H_0: \beta_{1(A)} = \beta_{1(B)},$$
$$H_A: \beta_{1(A)} \neq \beta_{1(B)}.$$

Step 2: $n_A = n_B = 24$ and $\alpha = 0.05$.

Step 3: Choose the test statistic to be used

$$t_c = \frac{b_{1(A)} - b_{1(B)}}{s_{b_{1(A)} - b_{1(B)}}}.$$

Step 4: Decision rule.

$t_t = t_{t(0.05/2;24+24-4)} = t_{t(0.025,44)} = 2.021$, from Table B, the student's t table.
If $|t_c| > |t_t = 2.021|$, reject H_0 at $\alpha = 0.05$.

Step 5: Perform experiment.
A = IPA + CHG and
B = IPA

$$s^2_{x_A} = \frac{\sum(x_i - \bar{x})^2}{n-1} = 12.26^2 = 150.3076, \text{ from Table 9.11, as given earlier,}$$

and

$$s^2_{x_B} = 12.26^2 = 150.3076, \text{ also as given earlier.}$$

$$s^2_{y,x_A} = \frac{\sum(y_i - \hat{y}_i)^2}{n-2} = MS_E = 0.6802, \text{ from Table 9.8.}$$

$$s^2_{y,x_B} = 0.455, \text{ from Table 9.10.}$$

$$s^2_{\widehat{y,x}} = \frac{(n_A - 2)s^2_{y,x_A} + (n_B - 2)s^2_{y,x_B}}{n_A + n_B - 4} = \frac{22(0.6802) + 22(0.455)}{24 + 24 - 4} = 0.5676.$$

$$s^2_{b_{1(A)} - b_{1(B)}} = s^2_{\widehat{y,x}}\left[\frac{1}{(n_A-1)s^2_{x(A)}} + \frac{1}{(n_B-1)s^2_{x(B)}}\right] = 0.5676\left[\frac{1}{23(150.31)} + \frac{1}{23(150.31)}\right] = 0.00033.$$

$$t_c = \frac{0.00208 - (-0.0711)}{\sqrt{0.00033}} = 4.03.$$

Step 6: Decision.
As $t_c = 4.03 > 2.021$, reject H_0 at $\alpha = 0.05$. The IPA + CHG product $\log_{10}$ microbial reduction rate (slope) is different from that produced by the IPA product, alone. The CHG provides a persistent antimicrobial effect that the IPA, by itself, does not have.

Let us compute the same problem using only one regression equation with an indicator variable. Let

$$x_2 = \begin{cases} 0, & \text{if IPA + CHG product} \\ 1, & \text{if IPA product} \end{cases}.$$

Table 9.12 presents the example in one equation.

We note that the r^2 is incredibly low, 34.2%. We also remember that the two equations for each product previously computed had different slopes. Therefore, the interaction between x_1 and x_2 is important. Table 9.13 presents the data without an interaction term and the large error, $e_i = y - \hat{y}$.

To correct this, we will use an interaction term, $x_3 = x_1 * x_2$, or x_1 times x_2, or $x_1 x_2$. Table 9.14 presents this.

The regression equation b_i is

$$\hat{y} = 2.07 + 0.0021x_1 - 0.025x_2 - 0.0726x_3.$$

TABLE 9.12
Regression Analysis (Reduced Model), Example 9.1

Predictor	Coef	St. Dev	t-Ratio	p
b_0	2.5021	0.2176	11.50	0.000
b_1	−0.03420	0.01047	−3.27	0.002
b_2	−0.8958	0.2512	−3.57	0.001
$s = 0.870284$		$R\text{-sq} = 34.2\%$		$R\text{-sq(adj)} = 31.3\%$

Analysis of Variance

Source	DF	SS	MS	F	p
Regression	2	17.7154	8.8577	11.69	0.000
Error	45	34.0827	0.7574		
Total	47	51.7981			

The regression equation is $\hat{y} = 2.50 - 0.0342x_1 - 0.896x_2$.

For the IPA + CHG formulation, where $x_2 = 0$, the equation is

$$\hat{y} = 2.07 + 0.0021x_1 - 0.0726x_3,$$
$$= 2.07 + 0.0021x_1.$$

For the IPA formulation, where $x_2 = 1$, the equation is

$$\hat{y} = 2.07 + 0.0021x_1 - 0.025(1) - 0.0726x_3,$$
$$= (2.07 - 0.025) + 0.0021x_1 - 0.0726x_3,$$
$$= 2.045 + 0.0021x_1 - 0.0726x_3.$$

PARALLEL SLOPE TEST USING INDICATOR VARIABLES

If the slopes are parallel, this is the same thing as saying $x_3 = x_1x_2 = 0$; that is, there is no significant interaction between x_1 and x_2. The model, $\hat{y} = b_0 + b_1x_1 + b_2x_2 + b_3x_3$, can be used to determine interaction between multiple products. Using the previous example and the six-step procedure,

Step 1: State the hypothesis.

$$H_0: \beta_3 = 0,$$
$$H_A: \beta_3 \neq 0.$$

Step 2: Set n_1 and n_2, as well as α.
$n_1 = n_2 = 24$; set $\alpha = 0.05$.

TABLE 9.13
$\hat{y}$ Predicting y, Example 9.1

Row	y	x_1	x_2	$\hat{y}$	$y - \hat{y}$
1	3.10	0	1	1.60625	1.49375
2	3.50	0	1	1.60625	1.89375
3	3.30	0	1	1.60625	1.69375
4	3.30	0	0	2.50208	0.79792
5	3.40	0	0	2.50208	0.89792
6	3.60	0	0	2.50208	1.09792
7	0.90	24	1	0.78542	0.11458
8	1.00	24	1	0.78542	0.21458
9	0.80	24	1	0.78542	0.01458
10	3.00	24	0	1.68125	1.31875
11	3.10	24	0	1.68125	1.41875
12	3.20	24	0	1.68125	1.51875
13	1.20	0	1	1.60625	−0.40625
14	1.00	0	1	1.60625	−0.60625
15	1.30	0	1	1.60625	−0.30625
16	1.30	0	0	2.50208	−1.20208
17	1.20	0	0	2.50208	−1.30208
18	1.10	0	0	2.50208	−1.40208
19	0.00	24	1	0.78542	−0.78542
20	0.10	24	1	0.78542	−0.68542
21	0.20	24	1	0.78542	−0.58542
22	1.40	24	0	1.68125	−0.28125
23	1.50	24	0	1.68125	−0.18125
24	1.20	24	0	1.68125	−0.48125
25	1.50	0	1	1.60625	−0.10625
26	1.30	0	1	1.60625	−0.30625
27	1.40	0	1	1.60625	−0.20625
28	1.60	0	0	2.50208	−0.90208
29	1.20	0	0	2.50208	−1.30208
30	1.40	0	0	2.50208	−1.10208
31	0.10	24	1	0.78542	−0.68542
32	0.20	24	1	0.78542	−0.58542
33	0.10	24	1	0.78542	−0.68542
34	1.70	24	0	1.68125	0.01875
35	1.80	24	0	1.68125	0.11875
36	1.50	24	0	1.68125	−0.18125
37	2.30	0	1	1.60625	0.69375
38	2.50	0	1	1.60625	0.89375
39	2.10	0	1	1.60625	0.49375
40	2.40	0	0	2.50208	−0.10208
41	2.10	0	0	2.50208	−0.40208

(continued)

TABLE 9.13 (continued)
$\hat{y}$ **Predicting y, Example 9.1**

Row	y	x_1	x_2	$\hat{y}$	$y - \hat{y}$
42	2.20	0	0	2.50208	-0.30208
43	0.30	24	1	0.78542	-0.48542
44	0.20	24	1	0.78542	-0.58542
45	0.30	24	1	0.78542	-0.48542
46	2.30	24	0	1.68125	0.61875
47	2.50	24	0	1.68125	0.81875
48	2.20	24	0	1.68125	0.51875

Step 3: Specify the test statistic.
We will use the partial F test.

$$F_{c(x_3|x_1,x_2)} = \frac{\dfrac{SS_{R(full)} - SS_{R(partial)}}{\nu}}{MS_{E(full)}} = \frac{\dfrac{SS_{R(x_1,x_2,x_3)} - SS_{R(x_1,x_2)}}{1}}{MS_{E(x_1,x_2,x_3)}}, \qquad (9.12)$$

TABLE 9.14
Regression Analysis with Interaction Term, Example 9.1

Predictor	Coef	St. Dev	t-Ratio	p
b_0	2.0667	0.2175	9.50	0.000
b_1	0.00208	0.01282	0.16	0.872
b_2	-0.0250	0.3076	-0.08	0.936
b_3	-0.07257	0.01813	-4.00	0.000

| $s = 0.753514$ | | R-sq $= 51.8\%$ | | R-sq(adj) $= 48.5\%$ |

Analysis of Variance

Source	DF	SS	MS	F	p
Regression	3	26.8156	8.9385	15.74	0.000
Error	44	24.9825	0.5678		
Total	47	51.7981			

where
$x_1 =$ sample time,

$x_2 = $ product $\begin{cases} 0, & \text{if IPA + CHG,} \\ 1, & \text{if IPA.} \end{cases}$

$x_3 = x_1 * x_2$, interaction of x_1 and x_2, or x_1x_2.
The regression equation is $\hat{y} = 2.07 + 0.0021x_1 - 0.025x_2 - 0.0726x_3$.

where

$$SS_{R(full)} = x_1, x_2, x_3,$$
$$SS_{R(partial)} = x_1, x_2,$$

where x_3, the interaction term, is removed,

$$n = n_A + n_B,$$

k is the number of b_is, not including b_0, and

$$y = df_{(full)} - df_{(partial)}.$$

Step 4: State the decision rule.
If $F_c > F_{T(\alpha, 1; n-k-1)}$, reject H_0 at α.
$F_T = df_{(full)} - df_{(partial)}$ for regression = numerator degrees of freedom
$df_{(full)}$ model error = denominator degrees of freedom
$F_T = 3 - 2 = 1 =$ numerator
$= 44 =$ denominator
$F_{T(0.05; 1, 44)} = 4.06$ (from Table C, the F distribution table)
So, if $F_c > 4.06$, reject H_0 at $\alpha = 0.05$.

Step 5: Compute the statistic.
From Table 9.14, the full model, including interaction, $SS_R = 26.8156$ and $MS_E = 0.5678$.
    From Table 9.12, the reduced model, $SS_R = 17.7154$.

$$F_c = \frac{\left(\dfrac{SS_{R(x_1, x_2, x_3)} - SS_{R(x_1, x_2)}}{1}\right)}{MS_{E(x_1, x_2, x_3)}} = \frac{\left(\dfrac{26.8156 - 17.7154}{1}\right)}{0.5678} = 16.03.$$

Step 6: Make the decision.
Because $F_c(16.03) > F_T(4.06)$, reject H_0 at $\alpha = 0.05$. Conclude that the interaction term is significant, and that the slopes of the two models differ at $\alpha = 0.05$.

INTERCEPT TEST USING AN INDICATOR VARIABLE MODEL

We will use the previous full model again,

$$\hat{y} = b_0 + b_1 x_1 + b_2 x_2 + b_3 x_3,$$

where

$x_1 = $ sample time,

$$x_2 = \text{product} = \begin{cases} 0, & \text{if IPA} + \text{CHG}, \\ 1, & \text{if IPA, and} \end{cases}$$

$x_3 = x_1 x_2$ interaction.

We can employ the six-step procedure to measure whether the intercepts are equivalent for multiple products.

Step 1: State the hypothesis.

Remember, where $\text{IPA} = x_2 = 1$, the full model is

$$\hat{y} = b_0 + b_1 x_1 + b_2(1) + b_3 x_3 = (b_0 + b_2) + b_1 x_1 + b_3 x_3,$$

and where $\text{IPA} + \text{CHG} = x_2 = 0$, the reduced model is

$$\hat{y} = b_0 + b_1 x_1 + b_3 x_3.$$

So, in order to have the same intercept, b_2 must equal zero.

H_0: Intercepts are the same for the microbial data for both products if $b_2 = 0$.
H_A: Intercepts are not the same if $b_2 \neq 0$.

Step 2: Set α and n.

Step 3: Write out the test statistic. In Case 1, for unequal slopes (interaction is significant), the formula is

$$F_c = \frac{\text{SS}_{R(x_1, x_2, x_3)} - \text{SS}_{R(x_1, x_3)}}{\text{MS}_{E(x_1, x_2, x_3)}}. \tag{9.13}$$

Note: If the test for parallelism is not rejected, and the slopes are equivalent, the F_c value for the intercept test is computed as

$$F_c = \frac{\text{SS}_{R(x_1, x_2)} - \text{SS}_{R(x_1)}}{\text{MS}_{E(x_1, x_2)}}. \tag{9.14}$$

Step 4: Make the decision rule.

If $F_c > F_{T(\alpha, v; n-k-1)}$, reject H_0 at α,

where

$v = \text{df}_{(\text{full})} - \text{df}_{(\text{partial})}$,
$n = n_A + n_B$,
$k = $ number of b_is, not including b_0.

Step 5: Perform the experiment.

Step 6: Make decision.
Using the same data schema for y, x_1, x_2, and x_3 (Table 9.14) and a two-tail test strategy, let us test the intercepts for equivalency.
   The model is

$$\hat{y} = b_0 + b_1 x_1 + b_2 x_2 + b_3 x_3,$$

where
   $x_1 =$ sample time (0 or 24 h),

$$x_2 = \text{product} = \begin{cases} 0, & \text{if IPA} + \text{CHG}, \\ 1, & \text{if IPA}, \end{cases}$$

   $x_3 = x_1 x_2$.
   Table 9.14 provides the regression equation, so the b_i values are

$$\hat{y} = 2.0667 + 0.0021 x_1 - 0.025 x_2 - 0.073 x_3.$$

For $x_2 = \text{IPA} = 1$, the model is

$$\hat{y} = 2.0667 + 0.0021 x_1 - 0.025(1) - 0.073 x_3,$$
$$\hat{y} = (2.0667 - 0.025) + 0.0021 x_1 - 0.073 x_3,$$
$$\hat{y} = 2.0417 + 0.0021 x_1 - 0.073 x_3,$$

for IPA only.
The intercept is 2.0417 for IPA.
For IPA + CHG, $x_2 = 0$

$$\hat{y} = 2.0667 + 0.0021 x_1 - 0.025(0) - 0.073 x_3,$$
$$\hat{y} = 2.0667 + 0.0021 x_1 - 0.073 x_3,$$

for IPA + CHG
The intercept is 2.0667.
Let us again use the six-step procedure. If the intercepts are the same, then $b_2 = 0$.

Step 1: State the test hypothesis, which we have made as a two-tail test.

   $H_0: b_2 = 0,$
   $H_A: b_2 \neq 0.$

Step 2: Set α and n.

$$n_1 = n_2 = 24.$$

Let us set $\alpha = 0.05$.

Step 3: State the test statistic.

$$F_c = \frac{SS_{R(full)} - SS_{R(partial)}}{MS_{E(full)}},$$

$$F_c = \frac{SS_{R(x_1,x_2,x_3)} - SS_{R(x_1,x_3)}}{MS_{E(x_1,x_2,x_3)}}.$$

Step 4: State decision rule.
If $F_c > F_{T(\alpha,v;\, n-k-1)}$,

$v = df_{(full)} - df_{(partial)}$ for regression = numerator, which is the number of x_is in the full model minus the number of x_is in the partial model,
$v = 3 - 1 = 2$ for the numerator,
$df = 48 - 3 - 1 = 44 =$ denominator,
$n - k - 1 =$ denominator for the full model,
where
$n = n_A + n_B$,
$k =$ number of b_i values, excluding b_0, and
$F_{T(0.05;1,44)} = 4.06$ (Table C, the F distribution table).
So, if $F_c > 4.06$, reject H_0 at $\alpha = 0.05$.

Step 5: Conduct the study and perform the computations.
$SS_{R(x_1,x_2,x_3)} = 26.8156$ and $MS_{E(x_1,x_2,x_3)} = 0.5678$ (Table 9.14).
$SS_{R(x_1,x_3)} = 26.801$ (Table 9.15).

$$F_c = \frac{SS_{R(x_1,x_2,x_3)} - SS_{R(x_1,x_3)}}{MS_{E(x_1,x_2,x_3)}} = \frac{26.8156 - 26.801}{0.5678} = 0.0257.$$

Step 6: Decision.
Because $F_c(0.0257) \not> F_T(4.06)$, one cannot reject H_0 at $\alpha = 0.05$. The intercept for both products are the same point.

PARALLEL SLOPE TEST USING A SINGLE REGRESSION MODEL

The test for parallel slopes also can be easily performed using indicator variables. Using the same model again,

$$\hat{y} = b_0 + b_1 x_1 + b_2 x_2 + b_3 x_3,$$

TABLE 9.15
Regression Analysis, Intercept Equivalency, Example 9.1

Predictor	Coef	SE Coef	T	p
b_0	2.0917	0.1521	13.75	0.000
b_1	−0.0500	0.2635	−0.19	0.850
b_3	−0.07049	0.01268	−5.56	0.000
$s = 0.745319$		R-sq $= 51.7\%$		R-sq(adj) $= 49.6\%$

Analysis of Variance

Source	DF	SS	MS	F	p
Regression	2	26.801	13.400	24.12	0.000
Error	45	24.998	0.556		
Total	47	51.798			

The regression equation is $\hat{y} = 2.09 - 0.050x_1 - 0.0705x_3$.

where

$x_1 = $ sample time,

$$x_2 = \text{product} = \begin{cases} 0, & \text{if CHG + IPA,} \\ 1, & \text{if IPA,} \end{cases}$$

$x_3 = x_1 x_2$, interaction.
If the slopes are parallel, then $x_3 = 0$.
Let us test the parallel hypothesis, using the six-step procedure.

Step 1: Set the test hypothesis.

H_0: Slopes are the same for microbial data for both products $= b_3 = 0$,
H_A: Slopes are not the same $= b_3 \neq 0$.

Step 2: Set α and n.

Step 3: Write out the test statistic. For unequal slopes, the formula is

$$F_c = \frac{SS_{R(full)} - SS_{R(partial)}}{MS_{E(full)}}. \tag{9.15}$$

The full model contains the interaction, x_3. The partial model does not.

$$F_c = \frac{SS_{R(x_1, x_2, x_3)} - SS_{R(x_1, x_2)}}{MS_{E(x_1, x_2, x_3)}}. \tag{9.16}$$

Step 4: Make the decision rule.

If $F_c > F_{T(\alpha,1;\,n-k-1)}$, reject H_0 at α, where

$n = n_A + n_B$,

$k =$ number of b_is, not including b_0.

Step 5: Perform the experiment.

Step 6: Make the decision.

Using the data for Example 9.1 and a two-tail test, let us test the slopes for equivalence, or that they are parallel. The full model is

$$\hat{y} = b_0 + b_1 x_1 + b_2 x_2 + b_3 x_3.$$

The partial model is the model without interaction

$$\hat{y} = b_0 + b_1 x_1 + b_2 x_2,$$

where

$x_1 =$ sample time (0 or 24 h),

$$x_2 = \text{product} = \begin{cases} 0, & \text{if CHG + IPA,} \\ 1, & \text{if IPA,} \end{cases}$$

$x_3 = x_1 x_2$ interaction.

Table 9.14 provides the actual b_i values for the full model

$$\hat{y} = 2.07 + 0.0021 x_1 - 0.025 x_2 - 0.073 x_3.$$

IPA PRODUCT

For $x_2 = \text{IPA} = 1$, the full model is

$$
\begin{aligned}
\hat{y} &= b_0 + b_1 x_1 + b_2 x_2 + b_3 x_3, \\
&= b_0 + b_1 x_1 + b_2(1) + b_3 x_3, \\
&= (b_0 + b_2) + b_1 x_1 + b_3 x_3, \\
&= (2.07 - 0.25) + 0.0021 x_1 - 0.073 x_3, \\
&= 1.82 + 0.0021 x_1 - 0.073 x_3.
\end{aligned}
$$

IPA + CHG PRODUCT

For $x_2 = \text{IPA} + \text{CHG} = 0$, the full model is

$$
\begin{aligned}
\hat{y} &= b_0 + b_1 x_1 + b_2 x_2 + b_3 x_3, \\
&= b_0 + b_1 x_1 + b_2(0) + b_3 x_3, \\
&= b_0 + b_1 x_1 + b_3 x_3, \\
&= 2.07 + 0.0021 x_1 - 0.025(0) - 0.073 x_3, \\
&= 2.07 + 0.0021 x_1 - 0.073 x_3.
\end{aligned}
$$

If the interaction is 0, or the slopes are parallel, then $b_3 = 0$.

Step 1: State the test hypothesis.

H_0: $\beta_3 = 0$,
H_A: $\beta_3 \neq 0$.

Step 2: Set α and n.
Let us set $\alpha = 0.05$ and $n_A = n_B = 24$.

Step 3: State the test statistic.

$$F_c = \frac{SS_{R(full)} - SS_{R(reduced)}}{MS_{E(full)}} = \frac{SS_{R(x_1,x_2,x_3)} - SS_{R(x_1,x_2)}}{MS_{E(x_1,x_2,x_3)}}.$$

Step 4: Make the decision rule.
If $F_c > F_{T(\alpha,1;\ n-k-1)} = F_{T(0.05,1;\ 48-3-1)} = F_{T(0.05;\ 1,44)} = 4.06$ (Table C, the F distribution table), reject H_0 at $\alpha = 0.05$.

Step 5: Perform the calculations.
From Table 9.15, the full model is

$$SS_{R(x_1,x_2,x_3)} = 26.801.$$

From Table 9.12, the partial model (without the x_1x_2 interaction term) is

$$SS_{R(x_1,x_2)} = 17.7154.$$

From Table 9.15, the full model is

$$MS_{E(x_1,x_2,x_3)} = 0.556.$$

$$F_c = \frac{26.801 - 17.7154}{0.556} = 16.3410.$$

Step 6: Make decision.
Because $F_c = 16.3410 > F_T = 4.06$, reject the null hypothesis at $\alpha = 0.05$. The slopes are not parallel.

TEST FOR COINCIDENCE USING A SINGLE REGRESSION MODEL

Remember that the test for coincidence tests both the intercepts and the slopes for equivalence. The full model is

$$\hat{y} = b_0 + b_1x_1 + b_2x_2 + b_3x_3.$$

For the IPA product, $x_2 = 1$,

$$\hat{y} = b_0 + b_1x_1 + b_2(1) + b_3x_3.$$

The full model, deconstructed for IPA, is

$$\hat{y} = \underbrace{(b_0 + b_2)}_{\text{intercept}} + \underbrace{(b_1 x_1 + b_3 x_3)}_{\text{slope}}.$$

For the IPA + CHG product, $x_2 = 0$. So the full model, deconstructed for IPA + CHG, is

$$\hat{y} = \underbrace{(b_0)}_{\text{intercept}} + \underbrace{(b_1 x_1 + b_3 x_3)}_{\text{slope}}.$$

If both of these models have the same intercepts and same slopes, then both b_2 and b_3 must be 0 ($b_2 = 0$) and ($b_3 = 0$).

Hence, the test hypothesis is whether $b_2 = b_3 = 0$. The partial or reduced model, then, is

$$\hat{y} = b_0 + b_1 x_1 + b_2(0) + b_3(0),$$
$$\hat{y} = b_0 + b_1 x_1.$$

Step 1: State the hypothesis.

H_0: $b_2 = b_3 = 0$. (The microbial reduction data for the two products have the same slope and intercepts.)

H_A: b_2 and/or $b_3 \neq 0$. (The two data sets differ in intercepts and/or slopes.)

Step 2: Set α and n.
We will set $\alpha = 0.05$.
$n_A = n_B = 24$.

Step 3: Write the test statistic.

$$F_c = \frac{\left(\dfrac{SS_{R(\text{full})} - SS_{R(\text{partial})}}{v}\right)}{MS_{E(\text{full})}},$$

where

$v = df$ numerator, or number of x_i variables in the full model minus the number of x_i variables in the partial model.

$v = 3 - 1 = 2$.

$$F_c = \frac{\left(\dfrac{SS_{R(x_1, x_2, x_3)} - SS_{R(x_1)}}{2}\right)}{MS_{E(x_1, x_2, x_3)}}.$$

One must divide by 2 in the numerator because $x_1, x_2, x_3 = 3$ values, and $x_1 = 1$ value, $3 - 1 = 2$.

Step 4: Make the decision rule.

If $F_c > F_{T(\alpha;\, v;\, n-k-1)} = F_{T(0.05;\, 2;\, 44)} = 3.22$ (Table C, the F distribution table), where $n = n_A + n_B$, reject H_0 at α. The regression differs in intercepts and/or slopes.

Step 5: Perform the calculations.

$$SS_{R(x_1, x_2, x_3)} = 26.8156 \quad \text{and} \quad MS_{E(x_1, x_2, x_3)} = 0.5678 \text{ (Table 9.14)}$$
$$SS_{R(x_1)} = 8.0852 \text{ (Table 9.16)}$$

So,

$$F_c = \frac{\dfrac{26.8156 - 8.0852}{2}}{0.5678} = 16.4938.$$

Step 6: Make decision.

Because $F_c = 16.4938 > F_T = 3.22$, one rejects H_0 at $\alpha = 0.05$. The slopes and/or intercepts differ.

LARGER VARIABLE MODELS

The same general strategy can be used to measure parallel slopes, intercepts, and coincidence for larger models.

$$F_c = \frac{\dfrac{SS_{R(\text{full})} - SS_{R(\text{partial})}}{v}}{MS_{R(\text{full})}},$$

where v is the number of x_i values in the full model minus the number of x_i values in the partial model.

TABLE 9.16
Regression Equation Test for Coincidence, Example 9.1

Predictor	Coef	St. Dev	t-Ratio	p
b_0	2.0542	0.1990	10.32	0.000
b_1	−0.03420	0.01173	−2.92	0.005
$s = 0.974823$		R-sq = 15.6%		R-sq(adj) = 13.8%

Analysis of Variance

Source	DF	SS	MS	F	p
Regression	1	8.0852	8.0852	8.51	0.005
Error	46	43.7129	0.9503		
Total	47	51.7981			

The regression equation is $\hat{y} = 2.05 - 0.0342x_1$.

MORE COMPLEX TESTING

Several points must be considered before going further in discussions of using a single regression model to evaluate more complex data.

1. If the slopes between the two or more regressions are not parallel (graph the averages of the (x, y) points of the regressions to see), include interaction terms.
2. Interaction occurs between the continuous predictor variables and between the continuous and the dummy predictor variables. Some authors use z_i values to indicate dummy variables, instead of x_i.
3. Testing for interaction between dummy variables generally is not useful and eats up degrees of freedom. For example, in Example 9.1, we would have 15 variables, if all possible interactions were considered.
4. The strategy to use in comparing regressions is to test for coincidence first. If the regressions are coincidental, then the testing is complete. If not, graph the average x, y values at the extreme high values, making sure to superimpose the different regression models onto the same graph. This will provide a general visual of what is going on. For example, if there are four test groups for which the extreme x, y average values are superimposed, connect the extreme x, y points, as in Figure 9.8.

Figure 9.8a shows equal intercepts, but unequal slopes; Figure 9.8b shows both unequal slopes and intercepts; and Figure 9.8c shows coincidence in two regressions, but inequality in the two intercepts.

Superimposing the values will help decide whether the intercepts, or parallels, or both are to be tested. If the model has more than one x_i value, sometimes checking for parallelism first is the easiest. If they are parallel (not significant), and you test for coincidence and it is significant (not the same regressions), then you know the intercepts are different.

Let us now perform a new twist to the experiment, Example 9.1. The IPA formulation and the IPA + CHG formulation have been used on four anatomical sites, and the $\log_{10}$ microbial reductions were evaluated at times

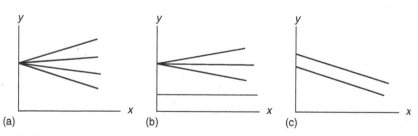

FIGURE 9.8 Superimposed x, y average values.

0 and 24 h after skin preparation. We will incorporate z_i for indicator variables at this time, because it is a common notation.

$y_i =$ microbial counts,

$x_1 =$ time $= 0$ or 24,

$$\text{product} = z_1 = \begin{cases} 1, & \text{if IPA}, \\ 0, & \text{if IPA} + \text{CHG}, \end{cases}$$

$$\text{inguinal} = z_2 = \begin{cases} 1, & \text{if yes}, \\ 0, & \text{if no}, \end{cases}$$

$$\text{forearm} = z_3 = \begin{cases} 1, & \text{if yes}, \\ 0, & \text{if no}, \end{cases}$$

$$\text{subclavian} = z_4 = \begin{cases} 1, & \text{if yes}, \\ 0, & \text{if no}. \end{cases}$$

By default, abdomen $= z_2 = z_3 = z_4 = 0$.

Let

$z_5 = x_1 z_1$, or time $\times$ product interaction.

The full model is

$$\hat{y} = b_0 + b_1 x_1 + b_2 z_1 + b_3 z_2 + b_4 z_3 + b_5 z_4 + b_6 z_5.$$

It is coded as

		x_1	z_1	z_2	z_3	z_4	z_5
IPA	Inguinal	0	1	1	0	0	0
	Inguinal	24	1	1	0	0	24
IPA + CHG	Inguinal	0	0	1	0	0	0
	Inguinal	24	0	1	0	0	0
IPA	Forearm	0	1	0	1	0	0
	Forearm	24	1	0	1	0	24
IPA + CHG	Forearm	0	0	0	1	0	0
	Forearm	24	0	0	1	0	0
IPA	Subclavian	0	1	0	0	1	0
	Subclavian	24	1	0	0	1	24
IPA + CHG	Subclavian	0	0	0	0	1	0
	Subclavian	24	0	0	0	1	0

Table 9.17 presents the actual data.

Table 9.18 provides the full regression analysis.

Much can be done with this model, as we will see.

TABLE 9.17
Example 9.1 Data, with Time × Product Interaction

n	y $\log_{10}$ Colony Counts	x_1 (time)	z_1 (product)	z_2 (inguinal)	z_3 (forearm)	z_4 subclavian	z_5 $x_1 z_1$
1	3.10	0	1	1	0	0	0
2	3.50	0	1	1	0	0	0
3	3.30	0	1	1	0	0	0
4	3.30	0	0	1	0	0	0
5	3.40	0	0	1	0	0	0
6	3.60	0	0	1	0	0	0
7	0.90	24	1	1	0	0	24
8	1.00	24	1	1	0	0	24
9	0.80	24	1	1	0	0	24
10	3.00	24	0	1	0	0	0
11	3.10	24	0	1	0	0	0
12	3.20	24	0	1	0	0	0
13	1.20	0	1	0	1	0	0
14	1.00	0	1	0	1	0	0
15	1.30	0	1	0	1	0	0
16	1.30	0	0	0	1	0	0
17	1.20	0	0	0	1	0	0
18	1.10	0	0	0	1	0	0
19	0.00	24	1	0	1	0	24
20	0.10	24	1	0	1	0	24
21	0.20	24	1	0	1	0	24
22	1.40	24	0	0	1	0	0
23	1.50	24	0	0	1	0	0
24	1.20	24	0	0	1	0	0
25	1.50	0	1	0	0	1	0
26	1.30	0	1	0	0	1	0
27	1.40	0	1	0	0	1	0
28	1.60	0	0	0	0	1	0
29	1.20	0	0	0	0	1	0
30	1.40	0	0	0	0	1	0
31	0.10	24	1	0	0	1	24
32	0.20	24	1	0	0	1	24
33	0.10	24	1	0	0	1	24
34	1.70	24	0	0	0	1	0
35	1.80	24	0	0	0	1	0
36	1.50	24	0	0	0	1	0
37	2.30	0	1	0	0	0	0
38	2.50	0	1	0	0	0	0
39	2.10	0	1	0	0	0	0
40	2.40	0	0	0	0	0	0
41	2.10	0	0	0	0	0	0

TABLE 9.17 (continued)
Example 9.1 Data, with Time × Product Interaction

n	y	x_1	z_1	z_2	z_3	z_4	z_5
42	2.20	0	0	0	0	0	0
43	0.30	24	1	0	0	0	24
44	0.20	24	1	0	0	0	24
45	0.30	24	1	0	0	0	24
46	2.30	24	0	0	0	0	0
47	2.50	24	0	0	0	0	0
48	2.20	24	0	0	0	0	0

GLOBAL TEST FOR COINCIDENCE

Sometimes, one will want to test components in one large model in one evaluation, as we have done. If the group is coincident, then one small model can be used to describe all. If not, one must test the inguinal, sub-clavian, forearm, or abdomen, with the IPA and IPA + CHG in individual components. First, extract the sub-models from the full model, $\hat{y} = b_0 + b_1 x_1 + b_2 z_1 + b_3 z_2 + b_4 z_3 + b_5 z_4 + b_6 z_5$.

TABLE 9.18
Regression Equation, with Time × Product Interaction, Example 9.1

Predictor	Coef	SE Coef	t-Ratio	p
b_0	2.2063	0.1070	20.63	0.000
b_1	0.002083	0.004765	0.44	0.664
b_2	−0.0250	0.1144	−0.22	0.828
b_3	0.9000	0.1144	7.87	0.000
b_4	−0.8250	0.1144	−7.21	0.000
b_5	−0.6333	0.1144	−5.54	0.000
b_6	−0.072569	0.006738	−10.77	0.000

$s = 0.280108$ R-Sq = 93.8%   R-Sq(adj) = 92.9%

Analysis of Variance

Source	DF	SS	MS	F	p
Regression	6	48.5813	8.0969	103.20	0.000
Error	41	3.2169	0.0785		
Total	47	51.7981			

The regression equation is $\hat{y} = 2.21 + 0.00208 x_1 - 0.025 z_1 + 0.900 z_2 - 0.825 z_3 - 0.633 z_4 - 0.0726 z_5$.

Inguinal site: $z_2 = 1$

IPA $= z_1 = 1$, $z_3 = 0$ (forearm), $z_4 = 0$ (subclavian), z_5 interaction, $x_1 z_1$.

$$\hat{y} = b_0 + b_1 x_1 + b_2(z_1) + b_3(z_2) + b_6(z_5),$$
$$\hat{y} = b_0 + b_1 x_1 + b_2(1) + b_3(1) + b_6 z_5,$$
$$\hat{y} = \underbrace{(b_0 + b_2 + b_3)}_{\text{intercept}} + \underbrace{(b_1 x_1 + b_6 z_5)}_{\text{slope}}.$$

IPA $+$ CHG $= z_1 = 0$, $z_3 = 0$ (forearm), $z_4 = 0$ (subclavian), z_5 interaction, $x_1 z_1$.

$$\hat{y} = b_0 + b_1 x_1 + b_3(z_2) + b_6(z_5),$$
$$\hat{y} = b_0 + b_1 x_1 + b_3(1) + b_6 z_5,$$
$$\hat{y} = \underbrace{(b_0 + b_3)}_{\text{intercept}} + \underbrace{(b_1 x_1 + b_6 z_5)}_{\text{slope}}.$$

Forearm site: $z_3 = 1$.

IPA $= z_1 = 1$, $z_2 = 0$ (inguinal), $z_4 = 0$ (subclavian), z_5 interaction, $x_1 z_1$.

$$\hat{y} = b_0 + b_1 x_1 + b_2(z_3) + b_4(z_3) + b_6(z_5),$$
$$\hat{y} = b_0 + b_1 x_1 + b_2(1) + b_4(1) + b_6 z_5,$$
$$\hat{y} = \underbrace{(b_0 + b_2 + b_4)}_{\text{intercept}} + \underbrace{(b_1 x_1 + b_6 z_5)}_{\text{slope}}.$$

IPA $+$ CHG $= z_1 = 0$, $z_2 = 0$, $z_4 = 0$, z_5 interaction, $x_1 z_1$.

$$\hat{y} = b_0 + b_1 x_1 + b_4(z_3) + b_6(z_5),$$
$$\hat{y} = b_0 + b_1 x_1 + b_4(1) + b_6 z_5,$$
$$\hat{y} = \underbrace{(b_0 + b_4)}_{\text{intercept}} + \underbrace{(b_1 x_1 + b_6 z_5)}_{\text{slope}}.$$

Subclavian site: $z_4 = 1$.

IPA $= z_1 = 1$ (product), $z_2 = 0$ (inguinal), $z_3 = 0$ (forearm), z_5 interaction, $x_1 z_1$.

$$\hat{y} = b_0 + b_1 x_1 + b_2(z_1) + b_5(z_4) + b_6(z_5),$$
$$\hat{y} = b_0 + b_1 x_1 + b_2(1) + b_5(1) + b_6 z_5,$$
$$\hat{y} = \underbrace{(b_0 + b_2 + b_5)}_{\text{intercept}} + \underbrace{(b_1 x_1 + b_6 z_5)}_{\text{slope}}.$$

IPA + CHG $= z_1 = 0$ (product), $z_2 = 0$ (inguinal), $z_3 = 0$ (forearm), z_5 interaction, $x_1 z_1$.

$$\hat{y} = b_0 + b_1 x_1 + b_5(z_4) + b_6(z_5),$$
$$\hat{y} = b_0 + b_1 x_1 + b_5(1) + b_6(z_5),$$
$$\hat{y} = \underbrace{(b_0 + b_5)}_{\text{intercept}} + \underbrace{(b_1 x_1 + b_6 z_5)}_{\text{slope}}.$$

Abdomen site

IPA $= z_1 = 1$ (product), $z_2 = 0$ (inguinal), $z_3 = 0$ (forearm), $z_4 = 0$ (subclavian), z_5 interaction, $x_1 z_1$.

$$\hat{y} = b_0 + b_1 x_1 + b_2(z_1) + b_6(z_5),$$
$$\hat{y} = b_0 + b_1 x_1 + b_2(1) + b_6 z_5,$$
$$\hat{y} = \underbrace{(b_0 + b_2)}_{\text{intercept}} + \underbrace{(b_1 x_1 + b_6 z_5)}_{\text{slope}}.$$

IPA + CHG $= z_1 = 0$ (product), $z_2 = 0$ (inguinal), $z_3 = 0$ (forearm), $z_4 = 0$ (subclavian), z_5 interaction, $x_1 z_1$.

$$\hat{y} = b_0 + b_1 x_1 + b_6 z_5,$$
$$\hat{y} = \underbrace{(b_0)}_{\text{intercept}} + \underbrace{(b_1 x_1 + b_6 z_5)}_{\text{slope}}.$$

The test for coincidence will be for all four test sites for both products. The only way the equation can be coincidental at all sites for both products is if the equation is to explain all that is the simplest; that is, $\hat{y} = b_0 + b_1 x_1$. So, if there is coincidence, then $b_2 = b_3 = b_4 = b_5 = b_6 = 0$. That is, all intercepts and slopes are identical.

So, let us perform the six-step procedure.

Step 1: State the hypothesis.

$H_0: b_2 = b_3 = b_4 = b_5 = b_6 = 0$.
$H_A:$ the above is not true; the multiple models are not coincidental.

Step 2: Set α and n.
Set $\alpha = 0.05$ and $n = 48$.

Step 3: Present the model.

$$F_c = \frac{\dfrac{SS_{R(\text{full})} - SS_{R(\text{partial})}}{\nu}}{MS_{E(\text{full})}},$$

where

v is the number of variables in the full model minus the number of variables in the partial model.

The full model is presented in Table 9.18.

$$\hat{y} = b_0 + b_1 x_1 + b_2 z_1 + b_3 z_2 + b_4 z_3 + b_5 z_4 + b_6 z_5.$$

The partial model is presented in Table 9.19.

$$\hat{y} = b_0 + b_1 x_1.$$

So,

$$F_c = \frac{\left(\dfrac{SS_{R(x_1, z_1, z_2, z_3, z_4, z_5)} - SS_{R(x_1)}}{v} \right)}{MS_{E(x_1, z_1, z_2, z_3, z_4, z_5)}}.$$

Step 4: Decision rule.

If $F_c > F_{T(\alpha, v; n-k-1)}$, reject H_0 at $\alpha = 0.05$.

For the denominator, we use $n - k - 1$ for the full model, where k is the number of b_is, excluding b_0.

For the numerator, v is the number of variables in full model minus the number of variables in the reduced model, $v = 6 - 1 = 5$.

So, $F_T = F_{T(0.05, 5; 48 - 6 - 1)} = F_{T(0.05, 5; 41)} = 2.34$ (Table C, the F distribution table).

TABLE 9.19
Partial Regression Equation, with Time × Product Interaction, Example 9.1

Predictor	Coef	SE Coef	t-Ratio	p
b_0	2.0542	0.1990	10.32	0.000
b_1	−0.03420	0.01173	−2.92	0.005
$s = 0.974823$		R-Sq = 15.6%		R-Sq(adj) = 13.8%

Analysis of Variance

Source	DF	SS	MS	F	p
Regression	1	8.0852	8.0852	8.51	0.005
Error	46	43.7129	0.9503		
Total	47	51.7981			

The regression equation is $\hat{y} = 2.05 - 0.0342 x_1$.

If $F_c > 2.34$, reject H_0 at $\alpha = 0.05$. All the regression equations are not coincidental.

Step 5: Perform the computation.
From Table 9.18,

$SS_{R(full)} = 48.5813$,
$MS_{E(full)} = 0.0785$.

From Table 9.19,

$SS_{R(partial)} = 8.0852$,
$v = 6 - 1 = 5$,

$$F_c = \frac{\left(\dfrac{48.5813 - 8.0852}{5}\right)}{0.0785} = 103.1748.$$

Step 6: Decision.
Because $F_c = 103.1748 > F_T = 2.34$, reject H_0. The equations are not coincidental at $\alpha = 0.05$. This certainly makes sense, because we know the slopes differ between IPA and IPA + CHG. The intercepts may also differ. Given that we want to find exactly where the differences are, it is easiest, then, to break the analyses into inguinal, subclavian, forearms, and abdomen, because they will have to be marked separately.

GLOBAL PARALLELISM

The next step is to evaluate parallelism from a very broad view: four anatomical sites, each treated with two different products. Recall that, if the slopes are parallel, no interaction terms are present. To evaluate whether the regression slopes are parallel on a grand scheme requires only that any interaction term be removed.

The full model, again, is

$$\hat{y} = b_0 + b_1 x_1 + b_2 z_1 + b_3 z_2 + b_4 z_3 + b_5 z_4 + b_6 z_5.$$

Looking at the model breakdown, the interaction term is $b_6 z_5$, where $z_5 = $ time $\times$ product. So, if the slopes are parallel, the interaction term must be equal to 0; that is, $b_6 = 0$.

Let us perform the six-step procedure.

Step 1: State the hypothesis.

H_0: $b_6 = 0$,
H_A: the above is not true; at least one slope is not parallel.

Step 2: Set α and n.
$\alpha = 0.05$ and $n = 48$

Step 3: Write out the model.

$$F_c = \frac{\left(\dfrac{SS_{R(full)} - SS_{R(partial)}}{v}\right)}{MS_{E(full)}},$$

$$SS_{R(full)} = SS_{R(x_1, z_1, z_2, z_3, z_4, z_5)},$$
$$SS_{R(partial)} = SS_{R(x_1, z_1, z_2, z_3, z_4)},$$
$$MS_{E(full)} = MS_{E(x_1, z_1, z_2, z_3, z_4, z_5)}.$$

Step 4: Write the decision rule.

If $F_c > F_T$, reject H_0 at $\alpha = 0.05$.

$F_T = F_{T(\alpha, v; n-k-1)}$

v is the number of indicator variables in full model minus number of indicator variables in partial model $= 6 - 5 = 1$.

$n - k - 1 = 48 - 6 - 1 = 41$.

$F_{T(0.05, 1; 41)} = 4.08$ (Table C, the F distribution table).

Step 5: Perform the computation. Table 9.20 presents the partial model.

$SS_{R(full)} = 48.5813$ (Table 9.18),
$MS_{E(full)} = 0.0785$ (Table 9.18),
$SS_{R(partial)} = 39.4810$ (Table 9.20),

$$F_c = \frac{\left(\dfrac{48.5813 - 39.4810}{1}\right)}{0.0785}$$

$$= 115.9274.$$

TABLE 9.20
Partial Model Parallel Test (x_1, z_1, z_2, z_3, z_4), Example 9.1

Predictor	Coef	SE Coef	t	p
b_0	2.6417	0.1915	13.80	0.000
b_1	−0.034201	0.006514	−5.25	0.000
b_2	−0.8958	0.1563	−5.73	0.000
b_3	0.9000	0.2211	4.07	0.000
b_4	−0.8250	0.2211	−3.73	0.001
b_5	−0.6333	0.2211	−2.86	0.006
$s = 0.541538$		R-sq $= 76.2\%$		R-sq(adj) $= 73.4\%$

Analysis of Variance

Source	DF	SS	MS	F	p
Regression	5	39.4810	7.8962	26.93	0.000
Error	42	12.3171	0.2933		
Total	47	51.7981			

The regression equation is $\hat{y} = 2.64 - 0.0342x_1 - 0.896z_1 + 0.900z_2 - 0.825z_3 - 0.633z_4$.

Step 6: Because $F_c = 115.9274 > F_T = 4.08$, reject H_0 at $\alpha = 0.05$. The slopes are not parallel at $\alpha = 0.05$. To determine which of the equations are not parallel, run the four anatomical sites as separate problems.

GLOBAL INTERCEPT TEST

The intercepts also can be checked from a global perspective. First, write out the full model

$$\hat{y} = b_0 + b_1 x_1 + b_2 z_1 + b_3 z_2 + b_4 z_3 + b_5 z_4 + b_6 z_5.$$

Looking at the model breakdown in the global coincidence test, we see that the variables that serve the intercept, other than b_0, are $b_2, b_3, b_4,$ and b_5. In order for the intercepts to meet at the same point, then $b_2, b_3, b_4,$ and b_5 all must be equal to 0.

Let us determine if the intercepts are all 0, using the six-step procedure.

Step 1: State the hypothesis.

$H_0: b_2 = b_3 = b_4 = b_5 = 0,$

$H_A:$ At least one of the above b_is is not 0.

Step 2: Set α and n.
$\alpha = 0.05$ and $n = 48$.

Step 3: Write out the test statistic.

$$F_c = \frac{\left(\dfrac{SS_{R(full)} - SS_{R(partial)}}{v} \right)}{MS_{E(full)}},$$

$$SS_{R(full)} = SS_{R(x_1, z_1, z_2, z_3, z_4, z_5)},$$
$$MS_{E(full)} = MS_{E(x_1, z_1, z_2, z_3, z_4, z_5)},$$
$$SS_{R(partial)} = SS_{R(x_1, z_5)},$$
$$v = 6 - 2 = 4.$$

Step 4: Determine the decision rule.
If $F_c > F_T$, reject H_0 at $\alpha = 0.05$.
$F_{T(\alpha, v; n-k-1)} = F_{T(0.05, 1; 41)} = 2.09$ (Table C, the F distribution table).

Step 5: Perform test computation.
$SS_{R(full)} = 48.5813$ (Table 9.18),
$MS_{E(full)} = 0.0785$ (Table 9.18),
$SS_{R(partial)} = 26.812$ (Table 9.21),

$$F_c = \frac{\left(\dfrac{48.5813 - 26.812}{4} \right)}{0.0785} = 69.329.$$

TABLE 9.21
Partial Model Intercept Test (x_1, z_5)

Predictor	Coef	SE Coef	T	p
b_0	2.0542	0.1521	13.51	0.000
b_1	0.00260	0.01098	0.24	0.814
b_6	−0.07361	0.01268	−5.81	0.000
s = 0.745151		R-sq = 51.8%		R-sq(adj) = 49.6%

Analysis of Variance

Source	DF	SS	MS	F	p
Regression	2	26.812	13.406	24.14	0.000
Error	45	24.986	0.555		
Total	47	51.798			

The regression equation is $\hat{y} = 2.05 + 0.0026 x_1 - 0.0736 z_5$.

Step 6: Make decision.

Because $F_c = 69.329 > F_T = 2.09$, reject H_0 at $\alpha = 0.05$. The equations (two products at z_2, z_3, z_4,—anatomical test sites—equals six equations) do not have the same intercept. Remember, the abdominal test site is evaluated when $z_2 = z_3 = z_4 = 0$, so it is still in the model. To find where the intercepts differ, break the problem into three: two regression equations at each of the three anatomical areas. Because the slopes were not parallel, nor the intercepts the same, the full model (Table 9.18) is the model of choice, at the moment.

CONFIDENCE INTERVALS FOR β_i VALUES

Determining the confidence intervals in indicator, or dummy variable analysis, is performed the same way as before.

$$\beta_i = \hat{b}_i \pm t_{\alpha/2, df} s_{b_i}, \tag{9.17}$$
$$df = n - k - 1,$$

where
   $\hat{b}_i$ is the ith regression coefficient,
   $t_{\alpha/2, df}$ is the tabled two-tail test,
   df is n minus number of b_is, including b_0,
   S_{b_i} is the standard error of values around b_i, and
   k is the number of b_i values, not including b_0.
For example, looking at Table 9.18, the full model is

$$\hat{y} = b_0 + b_1 x_1 + b_2 z_1 + b_3 z_2 + b_4 z_3 + b_5 z_4 + b_6 z_5.$$

For the value b_4,

$$\hat{b}_4 = -0.825, \quad s_{b_4} = 0.1144,$$
$$n = 48, \quad \alpha = 0.05,$$
$$\beta_4 = \hat{b}_4 \pm t_{\alpha/2, n-k-1} s_{b_4},$$
$$t_{0.05/2, 48-6-1} = t_{0.025, 41} = 2.021 \text{ (Student's } t \text{ Table)},$$
$$\beta_4 = -0.825 \pm 2.021(0.1144) = -0.825 \pm 0.2312,$$
$$-1.0562 \leq \beta_4 \leq -0.5938.$$

The 95% confidence intervals for the other b_is can be determined in the same way.

PIECEWISE LINEAR REGRESSION

A very useful application of dummy or indicator variable regression is in modeling regression functions that are nonlinear. For example, in steam sterilization death kinetic calculations, the thermal death curve for bacterial spores often looks sigmoidal (Figure 9.9).

One can fit this function using a polynomial regression or a linear piecewise model (Figure 9.10).

Hence, a piecewise linear model would require three different functions to explain this curve: functions A, B, and C.

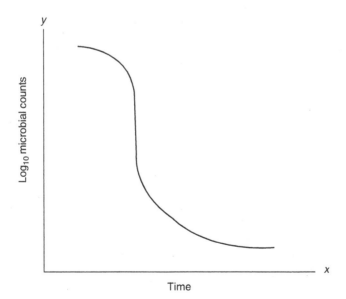

FIGURE 9.9 Thermal death curve.

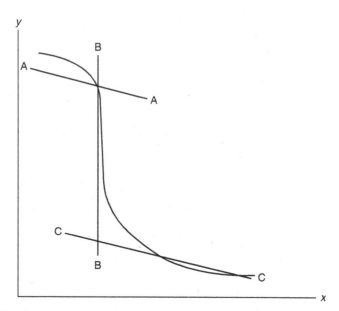

FIGURE 9.10 Linear piecewise model.

The goal in piecewise regression is to model a nonlinear model by linear pieces, for example, by conducting a microbial inactivation study that is nonlinear.

In Figure 9.11a, we see a representation of a thermal death curve for *Bacillus stearothermophilus* spores steam-sterilized at 121°C for x minutes. Figure 9.11b shows the piecewise delimiters. Generally, the shoulder values (near time 0) are not used. So, the actual regression intercept is near $8 \log_{10}$ scale. The slope changes at $x \approx 10$ min.

This function is easy to model using an indicator variable, because the function is merely two piecewise equations. Only one additional x_i is required.

$$\hat{y} = b_0 + b_1 x_1 + b_2(x_1 - 10)x_2,$$

where

x_1 is the time in minutes

$$x_2 = \begin{cases} 1, & \text{if } x_1 > 10 \text{ min,} \\ 0, & \text{if } x_1 \leq 10 \text{ min.} \end{cases}$$

When $x_2 = 0$, $x_1 \leq 10$, the model is $\hat{y} = b_0 + b_1 x_1$, which is the first component (Figure 9.11c).

When $x_2 > 10$, $x_1 = 1$, the second component is $\hat{y} = b_0 + b_1 x_1 + b_2(x - 10)$.

Let us work an example, Example 9.2.

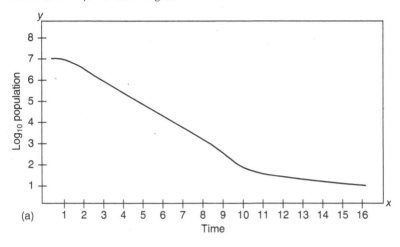

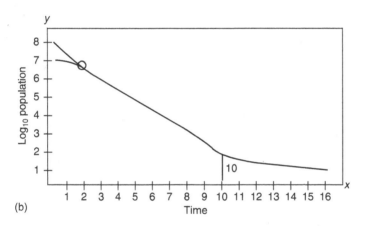

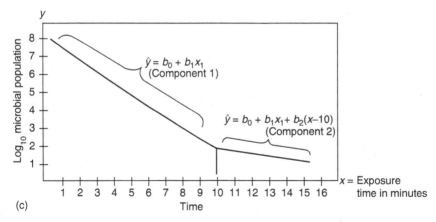

FIGURE 9.11 (a) Thermal death curve, *B. stearothermophilus* spores. (b) Piecewise model points, thermal death curve. (c) Piecewise fit, thermal death curve.

Example 9.2: In a steam sterilization experiment, three replicate biological indicators (*B. stearothermophilus* spore vials) are put in the sterilizer's "cold spot" over the course of 17 times of exposure. Each biological indicator has an inoculated population of 1×10^8 CFU spores per vial. The resulting data are displayed in Table 9.22.

The data plotted are presented in Figure 9.12.

These residual data $(y - \hat{y} = e)$ depict a definite trend (Figure 9.13) in residuals plotted over time. They are not randomly distributed.

From this plot, the value at $x = 7$ appears to be the residual pivot value, wherereas the slopes of e_is go from negative to positive. To get a better view, let us standardize the residuals by

$$S_t = \frac{e_i}{s},$$

where

$$s = \frac{\sum (y_i - \hat{y}_i)^2}{n - k - 1}.$$

This will give us a better picture, as presented in Figure 9.14.

Again, it seems that $x = 7$ is a good choice for the pivot point of a piecewise model.

Hence, the model will be

$$\hat{y} = b_0 + b_1 x_1 + b_2 (x_1 - 7) x_2,$$

where
$x_1 = \text{time},$

$$x_2 = \begin{cases} 1, & \text{if } x_i > 7, \\ 0, & \text{if } x_i \leq 7. \end{cases}$$

The model reduces to $\hat{y} = b_0 + b_1 x_1$, when $x_i \leq 7$.

Table 9.23 presents the data.

Table 9.24 presents the full regression analysis.

Figure 9.15 provides a residual plot (e vs. x_1) of the piecewise regression residuals, one that appears far better than the previous residual plot (Figure 9.13).

Figure 9.16 depicts schematically the piecewise regression functions.

Clearly, this model is better than without the piecewise component. Table 9.25 provides the data from regression without the piecewise procedure.

TABLE 9.22
Data, Example 9.2

n	$Y = \log_{10}$ Biological Indicator Population Recovered	$x =$ Exposure Time in min	n	$Y = \log_{10}$ Biological Indicator Population Recovered	$x =$ Exposure Time in min
1	8.3	0	28	4.2	9
2	8.2	0	29	4.0	9
3	8.3	0	30	3.8	9
4	7.7	1	31	3.5	10
5	7.5	1	32	3.2	10
6	7.6	1	33	3.4	10
7	6.9	2	34	3.2	11
8	7.1	2	35	3.3	11
9	7.0	2	36	3.4	11
10	6.3	3	37	3.3	12
11	6.5	3	38	3.2	12
12	6.4	3	39	2.9	12
13	5.9	4	40	2.8	13
14	5.9	4	41	2.7	13
15	5.7	4	42	2.7	13
16	5.3	5	43	2.6	14
17	5.4	5	44	2.5	14
18	5.2	5	45	2.6	14
19	5.0	6	46	2.4	15
20	4.8	6	47	2.3	15
21	5.0	6	48	2.5	15
22	4.6	7	49	2.2	16
23	4.3	7	50	2.3	16
24	4.4	7	51	2.2	16
25	4.5	8			
26	4.0	8			
27	4.1	8			

MORE COMPLEX PIECEWISE REGRESSION ANALYSIS

The extension of the piecewise regression to more complex designs is straight-forward. For example, in bioequivalence studies, absorption and elimination rates are often evaluated over time, and the collected data are not linear. Figure 9.17 shows one possibility.

The piecewise component model would look at three segments (Figure 9.18).

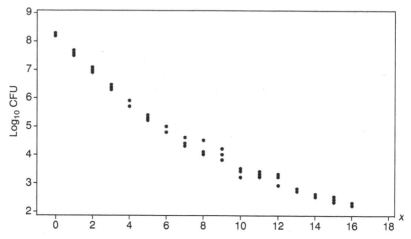

FIGURE 9.12 Data plot of $\log_{10}$ populations recovered, Example 9.2.

Example 9.3: In a study for absorption and elimination of oral drug 2121-B07, the following blood levels of the active Tinapticin-3 were determined by means of HPLC analysis (Table 9.26).

The plot of these data is presented in Figure 9.19.

It appears that the first pivot value is at $x = 5.0$ h and the second is at $x = 9.0$ h (see Figure 9.20).

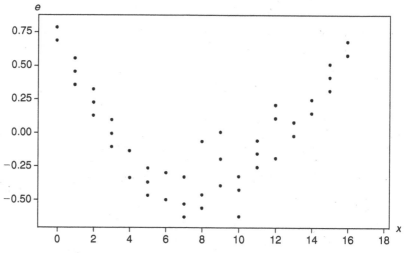

FIGURE 9.13 Residual plot, Example 9.2.

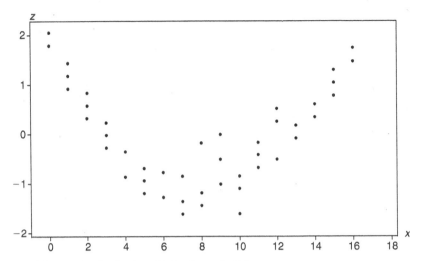

FIGURE 9.14 Studentized residuals, Example 9.2.

This approach to the pivotal points needs to be checked, ideally not just for this curve, but for application in other studies. That is, it is wise to keep the piece components as few as possible, because the idea is to create a model that can be used across studies, not just for one particular study. Technically, one could fit each value as a piecewise computation until one ran out of degrees of freedom, but this is not useful.

To build the model, we must create a b_i and an x_i for each pivot point, in addition to the first or original segment. The proposed model, then, is

$$\hat{y} = b_0 + b_1 x_1 + b_2 (x_1 - 5)x_2 + b_3 (x_1 - 9)x_3,$$

where

$x_1 =$ time in hours,

$$x_2 = \begin{cases} 1, & \text{if } x_1 > 5, \\ 0, & \text{if } x_1 \leq 5, \end{cases}$$

$$x_3 = \begin{cases} 1, & \text{if } x_1 > 9, \\ 0, & \text{if } x_1 \leq 9. \end{cases}$$

The results of regression using this model are presented in Table 9.27.

The model seems adequate, but the performance should be compared among other similar studies, if available. The actual input y, x, $x-5$, and $x-9$ data, as well as $\hat{y}$ and e are presented in Table 9.28.

TABLE 9.23
Data, Piecewise Model, Example 9.2

Row	y	x_1	$(x_1 - 7)x_2$	$\hat{y}$	e
1	8.3	0	0	8.12549	0.174510
2	8.2	0	0	8.12549	0.074510
3	8.3	0	0	8.12549	0.174510
4	7.7	1	0	7.58239	0.117612
5	7.5	1	0	7.58239	−0.082388
6	7.6	1	0	7.58239	0.017612
7	6.9	2	0	7.03929	−0.139286
8	7.1	2	0	7.03929	0.060714
9	7.0	2	0	7.03929	−0.039286
10	6.3	3	0	6.49618	−0.196183
11	6.5	3	0	6.49618	0.003817
12	6.4	3	0	6.49618	−0.096183
13	5.9	4	0	5.95308	−0.053081
14	5.9	4	0	5.95308	−0.053081
15	5.7	4	0	5.95308	−0.253081
16	5.3	5	0	5.40998	−0.109979
17	5.4	5	0	5.40998	−0.009979
18	5.2	5	0	5.40998	−0.209979
19	5.0	6	0	4.86688	0.133123
20	4.8	6	0	4.86688	−0.066876
21	5.0	6	0	4.86688	0.133123
22	4.6	7	0	4.32377	0.276226
23	4.3	7	0	4.32377	−0.023774
24	4.4	7	0	4.32377	0.076226
25	4.5	8	1	4.07908	0.420915
26	4.0	8	1	4.07908	−0.079085
27	4.1	8	1	4.07908	0.020915
28	4.2	9	2	3.83440	0.365604
29	4.0	9	2	3.83440	0.165605
30	3.8	9	2	3.83440	−0.034395
31	3.5	10	3	3.58971	−0.089706
32	3.2	10	3	3.58971	−0.389706
33	3.4	10	3	3.58971	−0.189706
34	3.2	11	4	3.34502	−0.145016
35	3.3	11	4	3.34502	−0.045016
36	3.4	11	4	3.34502	0.054984
37	3.3	12	5	3.10033	0.199673
38	3.2	12	5	3.10033	0.009673
39	2.9	12	5	3.10033	−0.200327
40	2.8	13	6	2.85564	−0.055637
41	2.7	13	6	2.85564	−0.155637

TABLE 9.23 (continued)
Data, Piecewise Model, Example 9.2

Row	y	x_1	$(x_1 - 7)x_2$	$\hat{y}$	e
42	2.7	13	6	2.85564	−0.155637
43	2.6	14	7	2.61095	−0.010948
44	2.5	14	7	2.61095	−0.110948
45	2.6	14	7	2.61095	−0.010948
46	2.4	15	8	2.36626	0.033742
47	2.3	15	8	2.36626	−0.066258
48	2.5	15	8	2.36626	0.133742
49	2.2	16	9	2.12157	0.078431
50	2.3	16	9	2.12157	0.178431
51	2.2	16	9	2.12157	0.078431

Figure 9.21 is a plot of the predicted ($\hat{y}$) values superimposed over the actual values. The fitted $\hat{y}_i$s are close to the actual $\hat{y}_i$ values.

However, what does this mean? What are the slopes and intercepts of each component?

Recall, the complete model is $\hat{y} = b_0 + b_1 x_1 + b_2(x_1 - 5)x_2 + b_3(x_1 - 9)x_3$. When $x_1 \leq 5$ (Component A), the regression model is $\hat{y} = b_0 + b_1 x_1$.

TABLE 9.24
Regression Analysis, Piecewise Model, Example 9.2

Predictor	Coef	St. Dev	t-Ratio	p
b_0	8.12549	0.05676	143.15	0.000
b_1	−0.54310	0.01170	−46.41	0.000
b_2	0.29841	0.01835	16.26	0.000
$s = 0.1580$		R-sq = 99.3%		R-sq(adj) = 99.3%

Analysis of Variance

Source	DF	SS	MS	F	p
Regression	2	171.968	85.984	3444.98	0.000
Error	48	1.198	0.025		
Total	50	173.166			

The regression equation is $\hat{y} = 8.13 - 0.543x_1 + 0.298\,(x_1 - 7)x_2$.

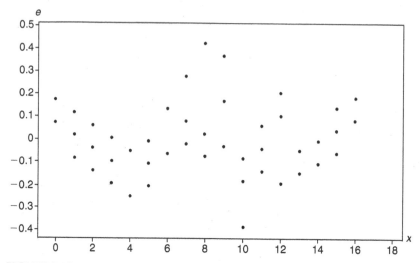

FIGURE 9.15 Residual plot, piecewise regression, Example 9.2.

Because $x_2 = x_3 = 0$ for this range, only a simple linear regression, $\hat{y} = 2.32 + 0.735x_1$, remains for Component A (Figure 9.18). Figure 9.22 shows the precise equation structure.

Component B (Figure 9.18)

When $x_1 > 5$, $x_2 = 1$, and $x_3 = 0$.

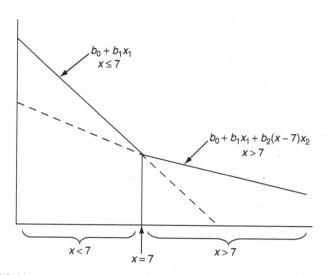

FIGURE 9.16 Piecewise regression breakdown into two regressions (one for data $\leq x = 7$ and one for data $> x = 7$), Example 9.2.

TABLE 9.25
Regression Without Piecewise Component, Example 9.2

Predictor	Coef	St. Dev	t-Ratio	p
b_0	7.5111	0.1070	70.22	0.000
b_1	−0.36757	0.01140	−32.23	0.000
$s = 0.3989$		R-sq = 95.5%		R-sq(adj) = 95.4%

Analysis of Variance

Source	DF	SS	MS	F	p
Regression	1	165.37	165.37	1039.08	0.000
Error	49	7.80	0.16		
Total	50	173.17	0.16		

The regression equation is $\hat{y} = 7.51 - 0.368x_1$.

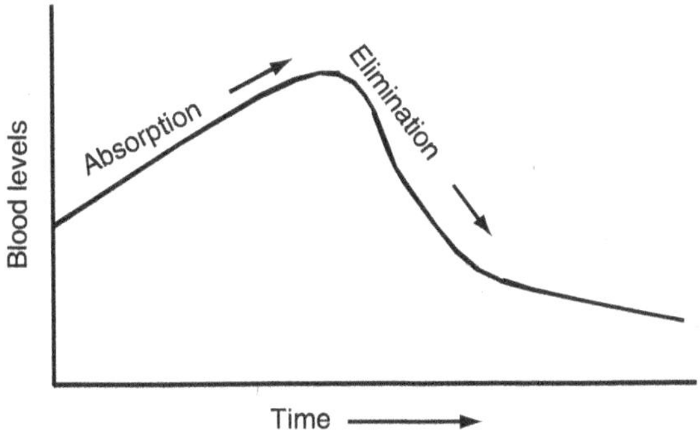

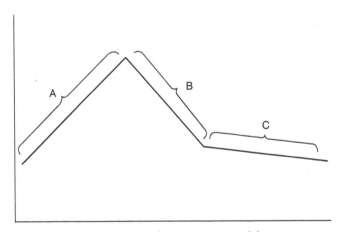

FIGURE 9.17 Absorption/elimination curve.

FIGURE 9.18 Segments of the piecewise component model.

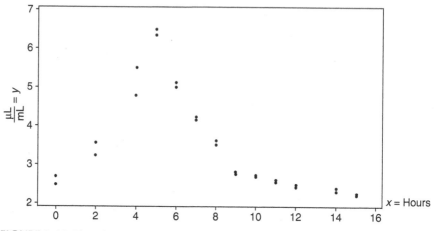

FIGURE 9.19 Plotted data, Example 9.3.

So the model is

$$\hat{y} = b_0 + b_1 x_1 + b_2(x_1 - 5)x_2,$$
$$= b_0 + b_1 x_1 + b_2(x_1 - 5),$$
$$= b_0 + b_1 x_1 + b_2 x_1 - 5b_2,$$
$$\hat{y} = \underbrace{(b_0 - 5b_2)}_{\text{intercept}} + \underbrace{(b_1 + b_2)x_1}_{\text{slope}},$$
$$b_0 - 5b_2 \approx 2.32 - 5(-1.55) \quad \text{(From Table 9.27)}.$$

Intercept ≈ 10.07.

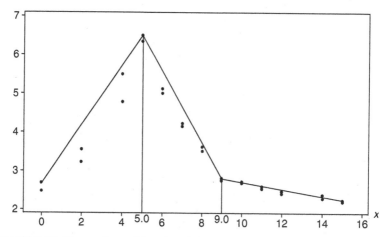

FIGURE 9.20 Pivot values of the plotted data, Example 9.3.

TABLE 9.26
HPLC Analysis of Blood Levels, Example 9.3

n	$\mu g/mL$	Time (h)
1	2.48	0
2	2.69	0
3	3.23	2
4	3.56	2
5	4.78	4
6	5.50	4
7	6.50	5
8	6.35	5
9	5.12	6
10	5.00	6
11	4.15	8
12	4.23	7
13	3.62	7
14	3.51	8
15	2.75	9
16	2.81	9
17	2.72	10
18	2.69	10
19	2.60	11
20	2.54	11
21	2.42	12
22	2.48	12
23	2.39	14
24	2.30	14
25	2.21	15
26	2.25	15

The y-intercept for Component B (Figure 9.18) is presented in Figure 9.22. The slope component of B is

$$b_1 + b_2 = 0.735 - 1.55 = -0.815.$$

Component C (Figure 9.18)

When $x_1 > 9$ and $x_2 = x_3 = 1$,

$$\hat{y} = b_0 + b_1 x_1 + b_2(x_1 - 5)x_2 + b_3(x_1 - 9)x_3,$$
$$= b_0 + b_1 x_1 + b_2(x_1 - 5) + b_3(x_1 - 9), \quad \text{because } x_2 = x_3 = 1.$$
$$= b_0 + b_1 x_1 + b_2 x_1 - 5b_2 + b_3 x_1 - 9b_3,$$
$$= \underbrace{(b_0 - 5b_2 - 9b_3)}_{\text{intercept}} + \underbrace{(b_1 + b_2 + b_3)x_1}_{\text{slope}}, \quad \text{where } x_1 > 9.$$

TABLE 9.27
Fitted Model, Example 9.3

Predictor	Coef	St. Dev	t-Ratio	p
b_0	2.3219	0.1503	15.45	0.000
b_1	0.73525	0.04103	17.92	0.000
b_2	−1.55386	0.07325	−21.21	0.000
b_3	0.73857	0.06467	11.42	0.000
$s = 0.245740$		$R\text{-sq} = 96.9\%$		$R\text{-sq(adj)} = 96.4\%$

Analysis of Variance

Source	DF	SS	MS	F	p
Regression	3	41.189	13.730	227.36	0.000
Error	22	1.329	0.060		
Total	25	42.518			

The regression equation is $\hat{y} = 2.32 + 0.735x_1 - 1.55(x_1 - 5)x_2 + 0.739(x_1 - 9)x_3$.

Plugging in the values from Table 9.27,
  Intercept $= 2.35 - 5(-1.55) - 9(0.739) = 3.449 \approx 3.45$.
  Slope $= 0.735 - 1.55 + 0.739 = -0.076$.
  So, the formula for Component C (Figure 9.18) is presented in Figure 9.22.
  $\hat{y} = 3.45 - 0.076x_1$, when $x_1 > 9$.
  The regressions are drawn in Figure 9.22.

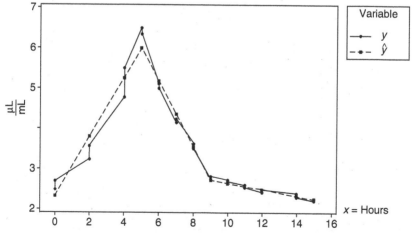

FIGURE 9.21 Fitted and actual values, piecewise regression, Example 9.3.

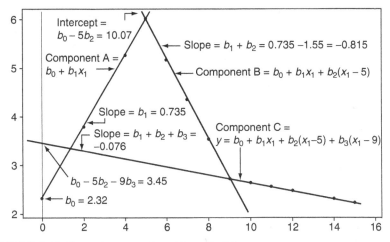

FIGURE 9.22 Piecewise regressions, Example 9.3.

The use of piecewise regression beyond two pivots is merely a continuation of the two-pivot model. The actual value $\hat{y}$ is, however, given at any one point on the entire equation range, without deconstructing it, as in Figure 9.22.

DISCONTINUOUS PIECEWISE REGRESSION

Sometimes, collected data are discontinuous, for example, the study of uptake levels of a drug when it is infused immediately into the blood stream via a central catheter by increasing the drip flow (Figure 9.23).

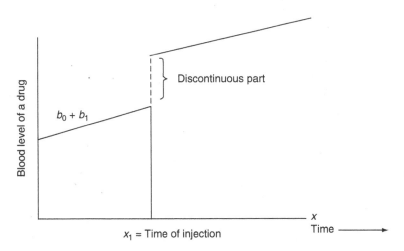

FIGURE 9.23 Uptake levels of a drug administered via central catheter.

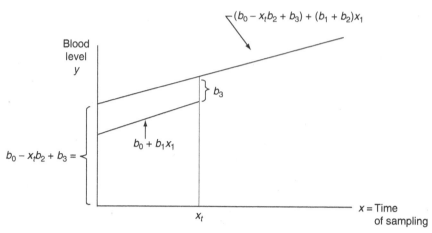

FIGURE 9.24 Piecewise regression analysis modeling.

This phenomenon can be modeled using piecewise regression analysis (Figure 9.24).

For example, let
y be the blood level of drug and
x_1 be the time in minutes of sample collection.

$$x_2 = \begin{cases} 1, & \text{if } x_1 > x_t, \\ 0, & \text{if } x_1 \leq x_t, \end{cases}$$

$$x_3 = \begin{cases} 1, & \text{if } x_1 > x_t, \\ 0, & \text{if } x_1 \leq x_t, \end{cases}$$

where
x_t is the discontinuous jump.
The full model is

$$\hat{y} = b_0 + b_1 x_1 + b_2(x_1 - x_t)x_2 + b_3 x_3.$$

Let us work an example.

Example 9.4: In a parenteral antibiotic study, blood levels are required to be greater than 20 μm/mL. A new device was developed to monitor blood levels and, in cases where levels were less than 15 μm/mL, for more than 4–5 min, the device spiked the dosage to bring it to 20–30 μm/mL, through a peripherally inserted central catheter. The validation on a nonhuman simulation study produced the resultant data (Table 9.29).

Figure 9.25 provides a graph of the data.

TABLE 9.28
Complete Data Set, Piecewise Regression, Example 9.3

n	y	x_1	$(x_1 - 5)x_2$	$(x_1 - 9)x_2$	$\hat{y}$	$y - \hat{y} = e$
1	2.48	0	0	0	2.32195	0.158052
2	2.69	0	0	0	2.32195	0.368052
3	3.23	2	0	0	3.79244	−0.562442
4	3.56	2	0	0	3.79244	−0.232442
5	4.78	4	0	0	5.26294	−0.482935
6	5.50	4	0	0	5.26294	0.237065
7	6.50	5	0	0	5.99818	0.501818
8	6.35	5	0	0	5.99818	0.351818
9	5.12	6	1	0	5.17957	−0.059570
10	5.00	6	1	0	5.17957	−0.179570
11	4.15	8	2	0	4.36096	−0.210958
12	4.23	7	2	0	4.36096	−0.130958
13	3.62	7	3	0	3.54235	0.077653
14	3.51	8	3	0	3.54235	−0.032347
15	2.75	9	4	0	2.72374	0.026265
16	2.81	9	4	0	2.72374	0.086265
17	2.72	10	5	1	2.64369	0.076311
18	2.69	10	5	1	2.64369	0.046311
19	2.60	11	6	2	2.56364	0.036358
20	2.54	11	6	2	2.56364	−0.023642
21	2.42	12	7	3	2.48360	−0.063595
22	2.48	12	7	3	2.48360	−0.003595
23	2.39	14	9	5	2.32350	0.066498
24	2.30	14	9	5	2.32350	−0.023502
25	2.21	15	10	6	2.24346	−0.033455
26	2.25	15	10	6	2.24346	0.006545

Because the auto-injector was activated between 4 and 5 min, we will estimate a spike at 4.5 min. Hence, let

x_1 be the sample time in minutes.

$$x_2 = \begin{cases} 1, & \text{if } x_1 > 4.5 \text{ min,} \\ 0, & \text{if } x_1 \leq 4.5 \text{ min,} \end{cases}$$

$$x_3 = \begin{cases} 1, & \text{if } x_1 > 4.5 \text{ min,} \\ 0, & \text{if } x_1 \leq 4.5 \text{ min.} \end{cases}$$

The entire model is

$$\hat{y} = b_0 + b_1 x_1 + b_2(x_1 - 4.5)x_2 + b_3 x_3.$$

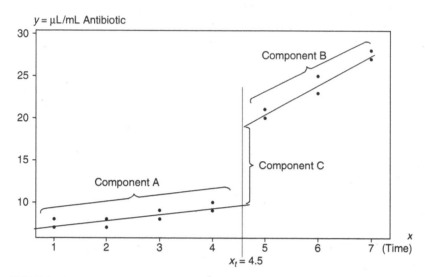

FIGURE 9.25 Data graph, Example 9.4.

TABLE 9.29
Analysis of Blood Levels of Antibiotic,
Example 9.4

$y = \mu g/mL$ of Drug	x = Time in min of Sample Collection
8	1
7	1
8	2
7	2
9	3
8	3
10	4
9	4
20	5
21	5
23	6
25	6
28	7
27	7

TABLE 9.30
Input Data, Piecewise Regression, Example 9.4

n	y	x_1	x_2	$(x_1 - 4.5) x_2$	x_3
1	8	1	0	0.0	0
2	7	1	0	0.0	0
3	8	2	0	0.0	0
4	7	2	0	0.0	0
5	9	3	0	0.0	0
6	8	3	0	0.0	0
7	10	4	0	0.0	0
8	9	4	0	0.0	0
9	20	5	1	0.5	1
10	21	5	1	0.5	1
11	23	6	1	1.5	1
12	25	6	1	1.5	1
13	28	7	1	2.5	1
14	27	7	1	2.5	1

The input data are presented in Table 9.30.
The regression analysis is presented in Table 9.31.
The complete data set is presented in Table 9.32.

TABLE 9.31
Piecewise Regression Analysis, Example 9.4

Predictor	Coef	St. Dev	t-Ratio	p
b_0	6.5000	0.6481	10.03	0.000
b_1	0.7000	0.2366	2.96	0.014
b_2	2.8000	0.4427	6.32	0.000
b_3	9.1000	0.8381	10.86	0.000
$s = 0.7483$		R-sq $= 99.4\%$		R-sq(adj) $= 99.2\%$

Analysis of Variance

Source	DF	SS	MS	F	p
Regression	3	904.40	301.47	538.33	0.000
Error	10	5.60	0.56		
Total	13	910.00			

The regression equation is $\hat{y} = 6.50 + 0.700x_1 + 2.80(x_1 - 4.5)x_2 + 9.10x_3$.

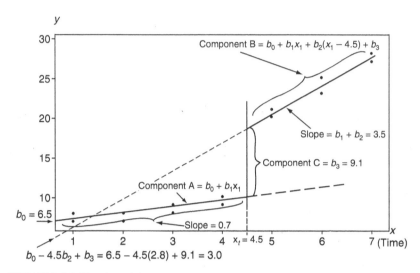

FIGURE 9.26 Fitted model.

The fitted model is presented in Figure 9.26.
The Component A ($x \leq 4.5$) model is

$$\hat{y} = b_0 + b_1 x_1 = 6.5 + 0.700 x_1.$$

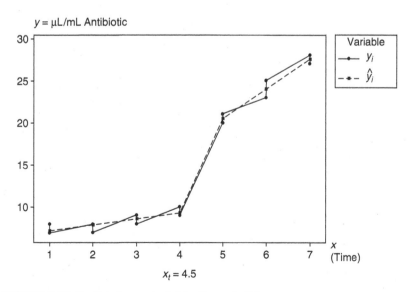

FIGURE 9.27 Predicted vs. actual data, Example 9.4.

TABLE 9.32
Complete Data Set, Piecewise Regression, Example 9.4

n	y	x_1	x_2	$(x_1 - 4.5)x_2$	x_3	$\hat{y}$	e
1	8	1	0	0.0	0	7.2	0.8
2	7	1	0	0.0	0	7.2	-0.2
3	8	2	0	0.0	0	7.9	0.1
4	7	2	0	0.0	0	7.9	-0.9
5	9	3	0	0.0	0	8.6	0.4
6	8	3	0	0.0	0	8.6	-0.6
7	10	4	0	0.0	0	9.3	0.7
8	9	4	0	0.0	0	9.3	-0.3
9	20	5	1	0.5	1	20.5	-0.5
10	21	5	1	0.5	1	20.5	0.5
11	23	6	1	1.5	1	24.0	-1.0
12	25	6	1	1.5	1	24.0	1.0
13	28	7	1	2.5	1	27.5	0.5
14	27	7	1	2.5	1	27.5	-0.5

The Component B $(x > 4.5)$ model is

$$\hat{y} = b_0 + b_1 x_1 + b_2(x_1 - 4.5)x_2 + b_3 x_3,$$
$$\hat{y} = b_0 + b_1 x_1 + b_2 x_1(1) - 4.5b_2(1) + b_3(1) = b_0 + b_1 x_1 + b_2 x_1 - 4.5b_2 + b_3,$$
$$\hat{y} = b_0 - 4.5b_2 + b_3 + b_1 x_1 + b_2 x_1,$$
$$= \underbrace{b_0 - 4.5b_2 + b_3}_{\text{intercept}} + \underbrace{(b_1 + b_2)}_{\text{slope}} x_1,$$
$$= \underbrace{6.5 - 4.5(2.8) + 9.1}_{3.0} + \underbrace{0.70 + 2.8 x_1}_{3.5}.$$

Figure 9.27 presents the final model of the predicted $\hat{y}$ values superimposed over the actual y_i values.

From this chapter, we have learned how extraordinarily flexible and useful the application of qualitative indicator variables can be.

10 Model Building and Model Selection

Regression model building, as we have seen, can not only be straightforward, but also tricky. Many times, if the researcher knows what variables are important and of interest, little effort is needed. However, when a researcher is exploring new areas or consulting for others, this is often not the case. In these situations, it can be valuable to collect wide data concerning variables thought to influence the outcome of the dependent variable, y. The entire process may be viewed as

1. Identifying independent predictor x_i variables of interest
2. Collecting measurements on those x_i variables related to the observed measurements of the y_i values
3. Selecting significant x_i variables by statistical procedures, in terms of increasing SS_R and decreasing SS_E
4. With the selected variables, validating the conditions under which the model is adequate

PREDICTOR VARIABLES

It is not uncommon for researchers to collect data on more variables than are practical for use in regression analysis. For example, in a laundry detergent validation study for which the author recently consulted, two methods were used—one for top-loading machines and another for front-loading machines. The main difference between the machines was water volume. Several micro-organism species were used in the study, against three concentrations of an antimicrobial laundry soap. Testing was conducted by two teams of techni-cians at each of six different laboratories over a five-day period. The number of variables to answer the research question, "Do significant differences in the data exist among the test laboratories," was extreme.

Yet, for "tightening" the variability within each laboratory, it proved valuable to have replicate data, day data, and machine data within each laboratory. Inter-laboratory variability was a moot point at this test level. In my opinion, it is generally a good idea to "overcollect" variables, particularly when one is not sure what will "pop up," as analysis unfolds. However, using methods that we have already learned, those variables need to be reduced to the ones that most relate to the research question.

For regression analysis, it is very important that potential for interaction between variables be considered during the process of model building. The interaction between variables can be accounted for simply as their product. Correcting for interactions among more than three variables generally is not that useful.

MEASUREMENT COLLECTION

A common experimental design used by applied researchers working in microbiology, medicine, and development of healthcare products is the controlled experiment, in which the x_i predictor variables are set at specified limits, and the response variable, y_i, is allowed to vary. Almost all the work we have covered in this book has been with fixed x_i values. However, in certain studies, the x_i values are not all preset, but are uncontrolled random variables themselves. For example, data on the age, blood pressure, disease state, and other conditions of a patient often are not set, but are collected as random x_i variables. In discussing the results of a study, conclusions must be limited to those values of the predictor variable in a preset, fixed-effects study. On the other hand, if predictor variables are randomly collected, then the study results can be generalized beyond those values to the range limits of the predictor values.

There are also studies that produce observations that are not found in a controlled experimental design. These studies can use x_i data that are collected based on intuition or hunches. For example, if a person wants to know if a water wash before the use of 70% alcohol as a hand rinse reduces the alcohol's antimicrobial effects, as compared with using 70% alcohol alone, an indicator (dummy) variable study may be required. That particular x_i variable may be coded as

$$x_i = \begin{cases} 0, & \text{if water rinse is used prior to alcohol rinse,} \\ 1, & \text{if no water rinse is used prior to alcohol rinse.} \end{cases}$$

Finally, there are times when an exploratory, observational study is necessary. For example, in evaluating the antimicrobial properties of different kinds of skin preparation for long-term venous catheterization, observational studies will be required, in which outcomes for patients are observed *in situ*, instead of in a controlled study.

SELECTION OF THE x_i PREDICTOR VARIABLES

In regression analysis, the selection of the most appropriate x_i variables will often be necessary. As was discussed, there are several approaches to determining the optimal number: backward elimination, forward selection, and stepwise regression. These use, as their basis, methods that were already discussed in this book. In review, including all x_i predictor variables in the model and eliminating sequentially the unnecessary variables are termed "backward elimination." The "forward selection" process begins with one x_i predictor variable and adds in others. And, "stepwise regression," a form of forward selection, is also a popular approach.

However, before selection procedures can be used effectively, the researcher should assure that the errors are normally distributed, and the model has no significant outliers, multicollinearity, or serial correlation. If any of these are problems, they must be addressed first.

ADEQUACY OF THE MODEL FIT

Checking the adequacy of the model fit before selecting x_i variables can save a great deal of time. If selection procedures are run, but the model is inappropriate, chances are that little will be gained. A simple way to check the model's adequacy is to perform a split-sample analysis. That is, one randomly partitions one half of the values into one group, and the remaining values into another group. It is easiest to do this by randomly assigning the n values to the groups. Suppose all the n values (there are only four here) are presented as

$$
\begin{array}{ccccccc}
n_1 & = & y_1 & x_1 & x_2 & x_3 & \cdots & x_k \\
n_2 & = & y_2 & x_1 & x_2 & x_3 & \cdots & x_k \\
n_3 & = & y_3 & x_1 & x_2 & x_3 & \cdots & x_k \\
n_4 & = & y_4 & x_1 & x_2 & x_3 & \cdots & x_k
\end{array}
$$

The randomization procedure here places n_1 and n_k in group 1, and n_2 and n_3 in group 2.

Group 1: n_1 and n_4	Group 2: n_2 and n_3
$n_1 = y_1\, x_1\, x_2\, x_3 \cdots x_k$	$n_2 = y_2\, x_1\, x_2\, x_3 \cdots x_k$
$n_4 = y_4\, x_1\, x_2\, x_3 \cdots x_k$	$n_3 = y_3\, x_1\, x_2\, x_3 \cdots x_k$

Regression models are then recalculated for each group. In the next step, an F test is conducted for: (1) y intercept equivalence, (2) parallel slopes, and (3) coincidence, as previously discussed. If the two regression functions are not different—that is, they are coincidental—the model is considered appropriate for evaluating the individual x_i variables. If they differ, one must determine where and in what way, and correct the data model, applying the methods discussed in previous chapters. If the split group regressions are equivalent, the evaluation of the actual x_i predictor variables can proceed. In previous chapters, we used a partial F test to do this. We use the same process but with different strategies: stepwise regression, forward selection, and backward elimination.

Let us now evaluate an applied problem.

Example 10.1: A researcher was interested in determining the $\log_{10}$ microbial counts obtained from a contaminated 2.3 cm^2 coupon at different temperatures and media concentrations. The researcher thought that temperature variation from 20°C to 45°C and media concentration would affect the microbial colony counts.

The initial regression model proposed was

$$\hat{y} = b_0 + b_1 x_1 + b_2 x_2, \tag{10.1}$$

where y is the $\log_{10}$ colony counts per 2.3 cm^2 coupon, x_1 is the temperature in °C, and x_2 is the media concentration.

After developing this model, the researcher discovered that the interaction term, $x_1 \cdot x_2 = x_3$, was omitted. Fifteen readings were collected, and the regression equation, $\hat{y} = b_0 + b_1 x_1 + b_2 x_2 + b_3 x_3$, was used. Table 10.1 provides the raw data (x_i, $\hat{y}$, and e_i). Table 10.2 provides the regression analysis.

Table 10.2 (regression equation Section A) provides the actual b_i values, the standard deviation of each b_i, the t-test value for each b_i, and the p-value for each b_i. In multiple regression, the t-ratio and p-value have limited use. The standard deviation of the regression equation, $s_{y|x_1, x_2, x_3} = 0.5949$, is just more than $\frac{1}{2}$ log value, and the coefficient of determination, $R^2_{(adj)y|x_1, x_2, x_3} = 86.1\%$, which means the regression equation explains about 86.1% of the variability in the model.

TABLE 10.1
Raw Data, Example 10.1

n	y	x_1	x_2	x_3	$\hat{y}$	e_i
1	2.1	20	1.0	20.0	2.15621	−0.056213
2	2.0	21	1.0	21.0	2.13800	−0.138000
3	2.4	27	1.0	27.0	2.02873	0.371271
4	2.0	26	1.8	46.8	2.78943	−0.789435
5	2.1	27	2.0	54.0	2.99373	−0.893733
6	2.8	29	2.1	60.9	3.13496	−0.334958
7	5.1	37	3.7	136.9	5.44805	−0.348047
8	2.0	37	1.0	37.0	1.84661	0.153391
9	1.0	45	0.5	22.5	0.88644	0.113565
10	3.7	20	2.0	40.0	2.86301	0.836987
11	4.1	20	3.0	60.0	3.56981	0.530187
12	3.0	25	2.8	70.0	3.66937	−0.669369
13	6.3	35	4.0	140.0	5.66331	0.636688
14	2.1	26	0.6	15.6	1.67569	0.424306
15	6.0	40	3.8	152.0	5.83664	0.163359

TABLE 10.2
Regression Analysis, Example 10.1

A
Predictor	Coef	St. Dev	t-Ratio	p
b_0	2.551	1.210	2.11	0.059
b_1	−0.05510	0.03694	−1.49	0.164
b_2	−0.0309	0.6179	−0.05	0.961
b_3	0.03689	0.01783	2.07	0.063

$s = 0.5949$ $R-\text{sq} = 89.1\%$ $R-\text{sq(adj)} = 86.1\%$

B
Analysis of Variance

Source	DF	SS	MS	F	p
Regression	3	31.744	10.581	29.89	0.000
Error	11	3.894	0.354		
Total	14	35.637			

C
Source	DF	Sequential SS	
x_1	1	$1.640 - SS_{R(x_1)}$	Because df $= 1$,
x_2	1	$28.589 - SS_{R(x_2\|x_1)}$	$SS_R = MS_R$
x_3	1	$1.515 - SS_{R(x_3\|x_1, x_2)}$	

The regression equation is $\hat{y} = 2.55 - 0.0551x_1 - 0.031x_2 + 0.0369x_3$.

Section B of Table 10.2 is the analysis of variance of the regression model

$$H_0 : b_1 = b_2 = b_3 = 0,$$
$$H_A : \text{at least one of the } b_i \text{ values is not 0.}$$

Section C provides a sequential analysis.

Source	Sequential SS		Sequential SS_R
x_1 = temperature	$SS_R(x_1)$	= amount of variability explained with x_1 in model	1.640
x_2 = media concentration	$SS_R(x_2\|x_1)$	= amount of variability explained by x_2 with x_1 in the model	28.589
$x_3 = x_1 \times x_2$	$SS_R(x_3\|x_1, x_2)$	= amount of variability explained by the addition of x_3 in the model	1.515
			31.744 (which is equal to the total SS_R in Part B)

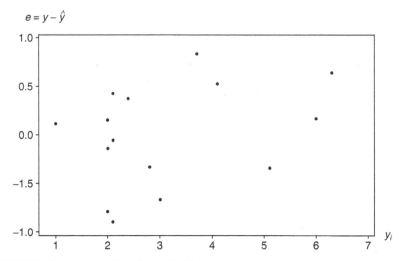

FIGURE 10.1 e_i vs. y_i plot, Example 10.1.

The researcher is mildly puzzled by these results, because the incubation temperature was expected to have more effect on the growth of the bacteria. In fact, it appears that media concentration has the main influence. Even so, this is not completely surprising, because the temperature range at which the organisms were cultured was optimal for growth and would not really be expected to produce varying and dramatic effects. The researcher, before continuing, decides to plot e_i vs. y_i, displayed in Figure 10.1.

Figure 10.1 does not look unusual, given the $n = 15$ sample size, which is small, so the researcher continues with the analysis.

STEPWISE REGRESSION

The first selection procedure we discuss is stepwise regression. We have done this earlier, but not with a software package. Instead, we did a number of partial regression contrasts. Briefly, the F-to-Enter value is set, which can be interpreted as an F_T value minimum for an x_i variable to be accepted into the final equation. That is, each x_i variable must contribute at least that level to be admitted into the equation. The variable is usually selected in terms of entering one variable at a time with $n - k - 1$ df. This would provide an F_T at $\alpha = 0.05$ of $F_{T(0.05, 1, 11)} = 4.84$. The F-to-Enter (sometimes referred to as "F in") is arbitrary. For more than one x_i variable, the test is the partial F test, exactly as we have done earlier. We already know that only x_2 would enter this model, because SS_R sequential for $x_2 = 28.580$ (Section C, Table 10.2).

$$F_c = \frac{MS_R}{MS_E} = \frac{28.589}{0.354} = 80.76 > F_T = 4.84.$$

TABLE 10.3
Stepwise Regression, Example 10.1

F-to-Enter:	4.00	F-to-Remove:	4.00
Response is	y	On three predictors,	with $n = 15$
Step	1		
Constant	0.6341		
x_2	1.23		
t-value	8.46		
s	0.649		
R^2	84.64		
$R^2_{(adj)}$	83.46		

Neither x_1 nor x_3 would enter the model, because their F_c values are less than $F_T = F_{(0.05, 1, 11)} = 4.84$, which is the cut-off value.

The F-to-Remove command is a set F_T value such that, if the F_c value is lesser than the F-to-Remove value, it is dropped from the model. The defaults for F-to-Enter and F-to-Remove are $F = 4.0$ in MiniTab, but can be easily changed. F-to-Remove, also known as F_{OUT}, is a value lesser than or equal to F-to-Enter; that is, F-to-Enter $\geq$ F-to-Remove.

Stepwise regression is a very popular regression procedure, because it evaluates both values going into and values removed from the regression model. The stepwise regression in Table 10.3, a standard MiniTab output, contains both F_{IN} and F_{OUT} set at 4.00. Note that only x_2 and b_0 (the constant) remain in the model after the stepwise procedure.

The constant $= 0.6341$ (Table 10.4) is the intercept value, b_0, with only x_2 in the model, and $x_2 = 1.23$ means that $b_2 = 1.23$. The t-ratio is the t-test value, T_c, $s =$ standard deviation of the regression equation, $s_{y|x_2} = 0.649$, and $R^2_{y|x_2} = 84.64\%$.

TABLE 10.4
Forward Selection Regression, Example 10.1

F-to-Enter:	4.00	F-to-Remove:	0.00
Response is	y	On three predictors,	with $n = 15$
Step	1		
Constant	0.6341		
x_2	1.23		
t-ratio	8.46		
s	0.649		
R^2	84.64		
$R^2_{(adj)}$	83.46		

TABLE 10.5
Regression Model, Single Independent Variable, Example 10.1

Predictor	Coef	St. Dev	t-Ratio	P
b_0	0.6341	0.3375	1.88	0.083
b_2	1.2273	0.1450	8.46	0.000

$s = 0.6489$ R-sq $= 84.6\%$ R-sq(adj) $= 83.5\%$

Analysis of Variance

Source	DF	SS	MS	F	P
Regression	1	30.163	30.163	71.63	0.000
Error	13	5.475	0.421		
Total	14	35.637			

The regression equation is $\hat{y} = 0.634 + 1.23x_2$.

The reader may wonder why a researcher would choose to use the stepwise regression model, which has both a smaller $s_{y|x}$ and a smaller R^2, when compared with the full model with the temperature and temperature–media concentration terms. The reason for this is that two degrees of freedom are gained in the error term with only media concentration in the model. We get one degree of freedom from the temperature x_i value and one degree of freedom from the interaction term. When SS_R is divided by a degree of freedom value of 1 instead of 3, the MS_R value is larger. When the larger MS_R value is divided by the MS_E value (which did not increase significantly), the F_c value increases. Note, in Table 10.2, Part B, that $F_c = 29.89$, and looking ahead to Table 10.5, $F_c = 71.63$. That is why the two independent variables were omitted. They "ate up" more degrees of freedom than the variables contributed to explaining that more of the variability is due to the regression.

FORWARD SELECTION

Forward selection operates using only the F-to-In value, bringing only those x_i variables into the equation that have F_c values exceeding the F-to-Enter value. It begins with b_0 in the model, then sequentially adds variables. In the example, we use F-to-Enter $= 4.0$, and set F-to-Remove $= 0$. That is, we are only bringing x_i variables into the model that contribute at least 4.0, using the F table. Table 10.4 presents that forward selection data.

Note that the results are exactly the same as those from the stepwise regression (Table 10.3). These values are again reflected in Table 10.5, the

TABLE 10.6
Original Data and Predicted and Error Values, Reduced Model,
Example 10.1

n	y	x_2	$\hat{y}$	e_i
1	2.1	1.0	1.86146	0.23854
2	2.0	1.0	1.86146	0.13854
3	2.4	1.0	1.86146	0.53854
4	2.0	1.8	2.84332	−0.84332
5	2.1	2.0	3.08879	−0.98879
6	2.8	2.1	3.21152	−0.41152
7	5.1	3.7	5.17524	−0.07524
8	2.0	1.0	1.86146	0.13854
9	1.0	0.5	1.24780	−0.24780
10	3.7	2.0	3.08879	0.61121
11	4.1	3.0	4.31611	−0.21611
12	3.0	2.8	4.07065	−1.07065
13	6.3	4.0	5.54344	0.75656
14	2.1	0.6	1.37053	0.72947
15	6.0	3.8	5.29798	0.70202

regression, $\hat{y} = b_0 + b_2 x_2$, where x_2 is the media concentration. Table 10.6 presents the y_i, x_i, $\hat{y}_i$, and e_i values.

BACKWARD ELIMINATION

In backward elimination, all x_i variables are initially entered into the model, but eliminated if their F_c value is not greater than the F-to-Remove value, or F_T. Table 10.7 presents the backward elimination process. Note that Step 1 included the entire model, and Step 2 provides the finished model, this time, with both temperature and interaction included in the model. The model is

$$\hat{y} = b_0 + b_1 x_1 + b_3 x_3,$$
$$\hat{y} = 2.499 - 0.54 x_1 + 0.036 x_3.$$

This procedure drops the most important x_i variable identified through forward selection, the media concentration, but then uses the interaction term, which is a meaningless variable without the media concentration value. Nevertheless, the regression equation is presented in Table 10.8. In practice, the researcher would undoubtedly drop the interaction term, because

TABLE 10.7
Backward Elimination Regression, Example 10.1

F-to-Enter:	4.00	F-to-Remove:	4.00
Response is	y	On three predictors,	with $n = 15$
Step	1	2	
Constant	2.551	2.499	
x_1	−0.055	−0.054	
t-value	−1.49	−2.49	
x_2	−0.03		
t-value	−0.05		
x_3	0.0369	0.0360	
t-value	2.07	9.63	
s	0.595	0.570	
R^2	89.07	89.07	
$R^2_{(adj)}$	86.09	87.25	

one of the two components of interaction, the media concentration, is not in the model. Table 10.9 provides the actual values of y, x_1, x_3, $\hat{y}$, and e in this model.

So what does one need to do? First, the three methods obviously may not provide the researcher with the same resultant model. To pick the best model requires experience in the field of study. In this case, using the backward elimination method, in which all x_i variables begin in the model and those less significant than F-to-Leave are removed, the media concentration was rejected. In some respects, the model was attractive in that $R^2_{(adj)}$ and s were more favorable. Yet, a smaller, more parsimonious model usually is more useful across studies than a larger, more complex one. The fact that the interaction term was left in the model when x_2 was rejected makes the interaction of $x_1 \times x_2$ a moot point. Hence, the model to select seems to be the one detected by both stepwise and forward selection, $\hat{y} = b_0 + b_2 x_2$, as presented in Table 10.5.

TABLE 10.8
Regression Equation, Double Independent Variable, Example 10.1

Predictor	Coef	St. Dev	t-Ratio	p
b_0	2.4989	0.5767	4.33	0.001
b_1	−0.05363	0.02157	−2.49	0.029
b_2	0.036016	0.003740	9.63	0.000
$s = 0.5697$		R-sq = 89.1%		R-sq(adj) = 87.3%

The regression equation is $\hat{y} = 2.50 - 0.0536 x_1 + 0.0360 x_3$.

TABLE 10.9
Original Data and Predicted and Error Values, Reduced Model, Example 10.1

n	y	x_1	x_3	$\hat{y}$	e_i
1	2.1	20	20.0	2.14652	−0.046521
2	2.0	21	21.0	2.12890	−0.128904
3	2.4	27	27.0	2.02320	0.376800
4	2.0	26	46.8	2.78994	−0.789942
5	2.1	27	54.0	2.99562	−0.895622
6	2.8	29	60.9	3.13686	−0.336864
7	5.1	37	136.9	5.44499	−0.344986
8	2.0	37	37.0	1.84703	0.152972
9	1.0	45	22.5	0.89574	0.104261
10	3.7	20	40.0	2.86683	0.833167
11	4.1	20	60.0	3.58714	0.512855
12	3.0	25	70.0	3.67914	−0.679137
13	6.3	35	140.0	5.66390	0.636100
14	2.1	26	15.6	1.66626	0.433744
15	6.0	40	152.0	5.82792	0.172077

It is generally recognized among statisticians that the forward selection procedure agrees with the stepwise when the subset number of independent variables is small, but when large subsets have been incorporated into a model, backward elimination and stepwise seem to agree more often. A problem with forward selection is that, once a variable is entered into the model, it is not released, which is not the case for backward or stepwise selection. This author recommends the use of all the three in one's research, selecting the one that seems to better portray what one is attempting to accomplish.

BEST SUBSET PROCEDURES

The first best subset we discuss is the evaluation of

$$R_k^2 = \frac{\mathrm{SS}_{R_k}}{\mathrm{SS}_T} = 1 - \frac{\mathrm{SS}_{E_k}}{\mathrm{SS}_T}. \tag{10.2}$$

As the number of k regression terms increases, so does R^2. However, as we saw earlier, this can be very inefficient, particularly when using the F test, because degrees of freedom are eaten up. The researcher can add x_i variables until the diminishing return is obvious (Figure 10.2). However, this process is inefficient. Aitkin (1974) proposed a solution using

$$R_A^2 = 1 - \left(1 - R_{k+1}^2\right)\left(1 + d_{\alpha;n,k}\right), \tag{10.3}$$

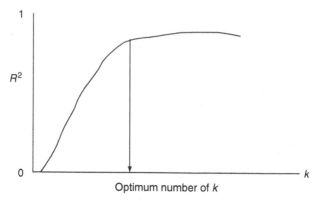

FIGURE 10.2 Obvious diminishing return.

where R_A^2 is the adequate R^2 subset of x_i values, R_{k+1}^2 is the full model, including b_0, and k is the number of b_is, excluding b_0.

R_k^2 and SS_{E_k}

R^2, the coefficient of determination, and SS_E, the sum of squares error term, can be used to help find the best subset (k) of x_i variables. R^2 and SS_E are denoted with a subscript k for the number of x_i variables in the model. When R_k^2 is large, SS_{E_k} tends to be small, because the regression variability is well explained by the regressors, so random error becomes smaller.

$$R_k^2 = 1 - \frac{SS_{E_k}}{SS_T}, \tag{10.4}$$

where SS_{E_k} is the SS_E with k predictors; SS_T is the total variability with all predictors in the model; and R_k^2 is the coefficient of determination with k predictors.

Adj R_k^2 and MS_{E_k}

Another way of determining the best k number of x_i variables is using Adj R_k^2 and MS_{E_k}. The model with the highest Adj R_k^2 also will be the model with the smallest MS_E. This method better takes into account the number of x_i variables in the model.

$$\text{Adj } R_k^2 = 1 - \frac{(n-1)SS_E}{(n-k)SS_T}, \tag{10.5}$$

where SS_E is the full model error sum of squares; SS_T is the full model total sum of squares; $n-1$ is the sample size less 1; and $n-k$ is the sample size minus the number of variables in the present model.

TABLE 10.10
Best Subsets Regression, Example 10.1

				Response Is Log_{10} Colony Count			
Vars	R-sq	R-sq(adj)	C_p	s	x_1	x_2	$x_2 \times x_1$
1	84.6	83.5	4.5	0.64894	—	X	—
1	83.4	82.2	5.7	0.67376	—	—	X
2	89.1	87.3	2.0	0.56968	X	—	X
2	86.9	84.7	4.2	0.62457	—	X	X
3	89.1	86.1	4.0	0.59495	X	X	X

MALLOW'S C_K CRITERIA

This value represents the total mean square error of the n fitted values for each k.

$$C_k = \frac{SS_{E_k}}{MS_E} - (n - 2k). \tag{10.6}$$

The goal is to determine the C_k value subset for which the C_k value is approximately equal ($\approx$) to k. If the model is adequate, the C_k value is equivalent to k, the number of x_i variables. A small C_k value indicates small variance, which will not decrease further with increased numbers of k.

Many software programs provide outputs for these subset predictors, as given in Table 10.10, for the data from Example 10.1.

Note that the R_k^2 terms for all the models are reasonably similar. The Adj R_k^2 values, too, are similar. The C_k ($= C_p$) value is the most useful here, but the model selected ($C_k = 2$) has two variables, temperature and interaction. This will not work, because there is no interaction unless temperature and media concentration both are in the model. Note that the value of s is $\sqrt{MS_{E_k}}$.

OTHER POINTS

All the tests and conditions we have discussed earlier should also be used, such as multicollinearity testing, serial correlation, and so on. The final model selected should be in terms of application to the "population," not just one sample. This caution, all too often, goes unheeded, so a new model must be developed for each new set of data. Therefore, when a final model is selected, it should be tested for its robustness.

11 Analysis of Covariance

Analysis of covariance (ANCOVA) employs both analysis of variance (ANOVA) and regression analyses in its procedures. In the present author's previous book (*Applied Statistical Designs for the Researcher*), ANCOVA was not reported mainly because it presented statistical analysis that did not require the use of a computer. For this book, a computer with statistical software is a requirement; hence, ANCOVA is discussed here, particularly because many statisticians refer to it as a special type of regression.

ANCOVA, in theory, is fairly straightforward. The statistical model includes qualitative independent factors as in ANOVA, say, three product formulations, A, B, and C, with corresponding quantitative response variables (Table 11.1). This is the ANOVA portion.

The regression portion employs quantitative values for the independent and the response variables (Table 11.2). The main value of ANCOVA is its ability to explain and adjust for variability attributed to variables that cannot be controlled easily and covary with one another, as in regression. For example, consider the case of catheter-related infection rates in three different hospitals. The skin of the groin region is baseline-sampled for normal microbial populations before prepping the proposed catheter site with a test product to evaluate its antimicrobial effectiveness in reducing the microbial counts. The baseline counts among subjects vary considerably (Figure 11.1).

The baseline counts tend to differ in various regions of the country—and hence, hospitals—an aspect that can potentially reduce the study's ability to compare the results and, therefore, different infection rates.

Using ANCOVA, the analysis would look like Figure 11.2. We can adjust or account for the unequal baselines and infection rates, and then compare the test products directly for antimicrobial effectiveness. Instead of using actual baseline values from the subjects at each hospital, the baseline populations minus the post-product-application populations—that is, the microbial reductions from baseline—are used.

Quantitative variables in the covariance model are termed concomitant variables or covariates. The covariate relationship is intended to provide reduction in error. If it does not, a covariance model should be replaced by an ANOVA, because one is losing degrees of freedom using covariates.

TABLE 11.1
Qualitative Variables

Qualitative Factors

A	B	C
x_{A_1}	x_{B_1}	x_{C_1}
x_{A_2}	x_{B_2}	x_{C_2}
⋮	⋮	⋮
x_{A_n}	x_{B_n}	x_{C_n}

Response variables within the factors

The best way to assure that the covariate is related to the dependent variable y is to have familiarity with the intended covariates before the study begins.

SINGLE-FACTOR COVARIANCE MODEL

Let us consider a single covariate and one qualitative factor in a fixed effects model. The basic model in regression is

$$\hat{Y} = \beta_0 + \beta_1 x_1 + \beta_2 z + e. \tag{11.1}$$

However, many statisticians favor writing the model equation in ANOVA form:

$$Y_{ij} = \mu + A_i + \beta(x_{ij} - \bar{x}..) + \varepsilon_{ij}, \tag{11.2}$$

where μ is the overall adjusted mean, A are the treatments or treatment effects, β is the covariance coefficient for y, x relationships, and ε_{ij} is the error term, which is independent and normally distributed, $N(0, \sigma^2)$.

The expected value of y, $E\lfloor y_{ij} \rfloor$, depends on the treatment effect and the covariate. A problem often encountered in ANCOVA is that the treatment effect slopes must be parallel; there can be no interaction (Figure 11.3).

TABLE 11.2
Quantitative Variables

Independent Variables Body Surface (cm²)	Response Variables Log₁₀ Microbial Counts
20	3.5
21	3.9
25	4.0
30	4.7
37	4.9
35	4.8
39	5.0

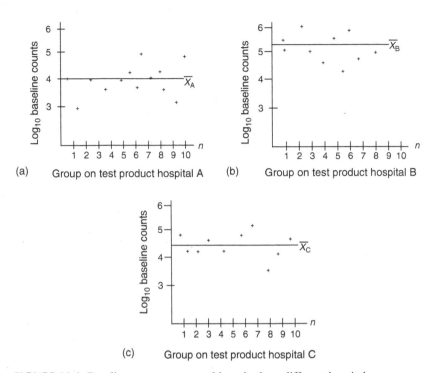

FIGURE 11.1 Baseline counts among subjects in three different hospitals.

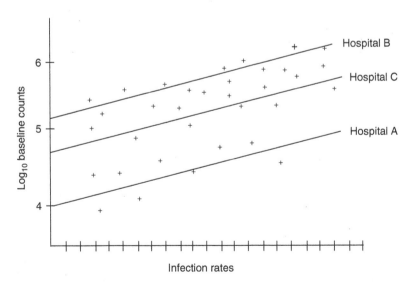

FIGURE 11.2 Covariance analysis.

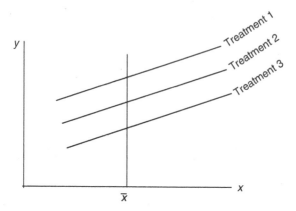

FIGURE 11.3 ANCOVA treatments.

This is a crucial requirement with ANCOVA, which sometimes cannot be met. If the treatment slopes are not parallel—that is, they interact—do not use ANCOVA. To test for parallelism, perform a parallelism test or plot out the covariates to determine this. If the slopes are not parallel, perform separate regression analyses on the single models.

SOME FURTHER CONSIDERATIONS

We have already applied the basic principles of ANCOVA in Chapter 9 on "dummy," or indicator variables. The common approach to the adjustment problem is using indicator variables as we have done. For example, the following equation

$$y = b_0 + b_1 x_1 + b_2 I + b_3 x_1 I \qquad (11.3)$$

presents an example with x_1 as the interaction term. Recall that if interaction is equal to 0, then the slopes are parallel and the model reduces to

$$y = b_0 + b_1 x_1 + b_2 I. \qquad (11.4)$$

Note that we are using I as the symbol in place of z. The ANCOVA model can be computed in ANOVA terms or as a regression. We look at both the approaches.

Let us consider a completely randomized design with one factor. A completely randomized design simply means that every possible observation is as likely to be run as any of the others. If there are k treatments in the factor, there will be $k - 1$ indicators (dummy variables).

The general schema is

$$I_1 = \begin{cases} 1, & \text{if treatment 1,} \\ -1, & \text{if treatment } k, \\ 0, & \text{if other,} \end{cases}$$

.
.
.

$$I_{k-1} = \begin{cases} 1, & \text{if treatment } k-1, \\ -1, & \text{if treatment } k, \\ 0, & \text{if other.} \end{cases}$$

For example, suppose we have four products (treatments) to test $k = 4$, and there will be $k - 1 = 3$ indicator variables:

$$I_1 = \begin{cases} 1, & \text{if treatment 1,} \\ -1, & \text{if treatment 4,} \\ 0, & \text{if otherwise,} \end{cases}$$

$$I_2 = \begin{cases} 1, & \text{if treatment 2,} \\ -1, & \text{if treatment 4,} \\ 0, & \text{if otherwise,} \end{cases}$$

$$I_3 = \begin{cases} 1, & \text{if treatment 3,} \\ -1, & \text{if treatment 4,} \\ 0, & \text{if otherwise.} \end{cases}$$

There will always be $k - 1$ dummy variables. This model would be written as

$$\hat{y}_{ij} = b_0 + b_1 x + b_2 I_1 + b_3 I_2 + b_3 I_3 + b_4(x_{ij} - \bar{x}),$$

where $\hat{y}_{ij}$ is the response variable, b_0 is the overall mean when $x_{ij} = X_{ij} - \bar{X}$, or centered values, which are the concomitant variables or covariates, and I is the indicator variable for the treatment of concern.

Note that the covariates are only adjustment variables to account for extraneous error, such as differing time 0 or baseline values. The main focus is among the treatments.

$$H_0: t_1 = t_2 = \cdots = t_k = 0,$$
$$H_A: \text{Not all treatments} = 0.$$

If H_0 is rejected, the researcher should perform contrasts—generally pairwise —to determine where the differences are.

REQUIREMENTS OF ANCOVA

1. Error terms, ε_{ij}, must be normally and independently distributed.
2. The variance components of the separate treatments must be equal.
3. The regression slopes among the treatments must be parallel.
4. Linearity between the covariates is necessary.

Let us work through the basic structure using the six-step procedure.

Step 1: Form the test hypothesis, which will be a two-tail test.

H_0: the treatments are of no effect $= 0$,

H_A: at least one treatment is not a zero effect.

Step 2: State the sample sizes and the α level.

Step 3: Choose the model configuration (covariates to control) and dummy variable configuration.

Step 4: Decision rule: The ANCOVA uses an F-test (Table C, the F distribution table).

The test statistic is

F_c is the calculated ANCOVA value for treatments. If done by regression, both full and reduced models are computed.

$$F_c = \frac{SS_{E(R)} - SS_{E(F)}}{df_{(R)} - df_{(F)}} \div \frac{SS_{E(E)}}{df_{(F)}}$$

F_T is the tabled value at the set α level with degrees of freedom in the numerator as df reduced model − df full model ÷ both error terms; the denominator portion of degrees of freedom is from the full model − error term.

Step 5: Perform ANCOVA.

Step 6: Decision rule is based on the values of F_c and F_T; reject H_0 at α, if $F_c > F_T$.

We perform a single-factor ANCOVA in two ways. This is because different computer software packages do it differently. Note, though, that one can also perform ANCOVA by using two regression analyses: one for the full model, and the other for a reduced model.

Let us begin with a very simple, yet often encountered evaluation comparing effects of three different topical antimicrobial products on two distinct groups—males and females—and how an ANCOVA model ultimately was used.

Example 11.1: In a small-scale surgical scrub product evaluation, three different products were evaluated—1%, 2%, and 4% chlorhexidine gluconate formulations. Only three (3) subjects were used in testing over the course of 5 consecutive days, one subject per product. Of interest were the cumulative antimicrobial effects over 5 days of product use. Obviously, the study was extremely underpowered in terms of sample size, but the sponsor would only pay for this sparse approach. Because ANCOVA might be used, the researcher decided to determine if the baseline and immediate microbial counts were associated. This was easily done via graphing. The researcher used the following codes:

$$Product = \begin{cases} 1, & \text{if } 1\% \text{ CHG}, \\ 2, & \text{if } 2\% \text{ CHG}, \\ 3, & \text{if } 4\% \text{ CHG}, \end{cases}$$

$$Day\ of\ test = \begin{cases} 1, & \text{if day 1}, \\ 2, & \text{if day 2}, \\ 3, & \text{if day 3}, \\ 4, & \text{if day 4}, \\ 5, & \text{if day 5}. \end{cases}$$

The three subjects were randomly assigned to use one of the three test products. The baseline counts were the number of microorganisms normally residing on one hand randomly selected. The immediate counts were the number of bacteria remaining on the other hand after the product application. All count data were presented in $\log_{10}$ scale (Table 11.3).

The researcher decided to determine whether interactions were significant via a regression model to view the repeated daily effect. It is important to plot the covariation to assure that the slopes are parallel. Figure 11.4 presents a multiple plot of the three-product baseline covariates.

It appears that a relationship between baseline and immediate reductions is present. If one was not present, the differences between baseline and immediate counts would not be useful. Table 11.4 presents the data, as modified to generate Figure 11.4.

Because ANCOVA requires that the covariant slopes be parallel, three regressions are performed, one on the data from the use of each of the three products (Table 11.5 through Table 11.7).

Note that the slopes—Product 1 = 1.0912, Product 2 = 0.9913, and Product 3 = 0.7337—seem to be parallel enough. But it is a good idea to check for parallelism in the slopes, using the methods described earlier. Recall that, when b_i slopes are not parallel, they have an interaction term within them. If that is the case, ANCOVA cannot be used. Once we determine that interaction is insignificant in the covariant among products, the ANCOVA can be performed. We do it using both the ANCOVA routine and regression analysis.

ANCOVA ROUTINE

Most statistical software packages offer an ANCOVA routine. We can use the six-step procedure to perform the test. In these cases, centering of the covariate may not be necessary.

TABLE 11.3
Microbial Count Data, Example 11.1

Daily Log$_{10}$ Microbial Baseline Counts	Daily Log$_{10}$ Microbial Immediate Counts	Test Product	Test Day
4.8	2.0	1	1
5.3	3.3	2	1
3.4	2.2	3	1
4.9	2.5	1	2
4.8	2.5	2	2
4.2	2.8	3	2
4.6	2.1	1	3
4.8	2.8	2	3
4.1	2.9	3	3
5.5	2.7	1	4
3.7	1.7	2	4
3.1	1.5	3	4
4.3	1.8	1	5
4.4	2.4	2	5
3.8	2.8	3	5

Step 1: State the hypothesis.

First, we want to make sure that the covariate is significant, that is, of value in the model. Then, we want to know if the treatments are significant.

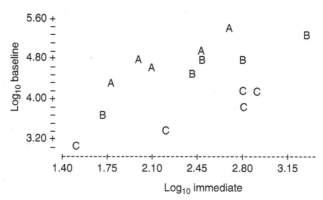

FIGURE 11.4 Multiple plot of baseline covariates, Example 11.1.
Product 1 = A = baseline A vs. immediate antimicrobial effects A,
Product 2 = B = baseline B vs. immediate antimicrobial effects B,
Product 3 = C = baseline C vs. immediate antimicrobial effects C.

TABLE 11.4
Baseline Covariates, Example 11.1

					Product 1 = A		Product 2 = B		Product 3 = C	
n	BL	IM	P	D	BL	IMM	BL	IMM	BL	IMM
1	4.8	2.0	1	1	4.8	2.0	5.3	3.3	3.4	2.2
2	5.3	3.3	2	1	4.9	2.5	4.8	2.5	4.2	2.8
3	3.4	2.2	3	1	4.6	2.1	4.8	2.8	4.1	2.9
1	4.9	2.5	1	2	5.5	2.7	3.7	1.7	3.1	1.5
2	4.8	2.5	2	2	4.3	1.8	4.4	2.4	3.8	2.8
3	4.2	2.8	3	2						
1	4.6	2.1	1	3						
2	4.8	2.8	2	3						
3	4.1	2.9	3	3						
1	5.5	2.7	1	4						
2	3.7	1.7	2	4						
3	3.1	1.5	3	4						
1	4.3	1.8	1	5						
2	4.4	2.4	2	5						
3	3.8	2.8	3	5						

Note: BL denotes baseline ($\log_{10}$ value), P denotes products 1, 2, or 3, IMM denotes immediate, and D represents days 1, 2, 3, 4, and 5.

The covariance model is

$$Y = \mu_. + A_i + \beta(x_i) + \varepsilon, \tag{11.5}$$

where A_i is the product effect and β is the covariate effect.
Hypothesis 1:

H_0: $\beta = 0$,
H_A: $\beta \neq 0$ (the covariate term explains sufficient variability).

TABLE 11.5
Product 1 Regression, Example 11.1

Predictor	Coef	St. Dev	t-Ratio	P
Constant (b_0)	2.3974	0.6442	3.72	0.034
b_1	1.0912	0.2870	3.80	0.032
$s = 0.2125$		R-sq $= 82.8\%$	R-sq(adj) $= 77.1\%$	

The regression equation is $\hat{y} = 2.40 + 1.09 b_1 x$.

TABLE 11.6
Product 2 Regression, Example 11.1

Predictor	Coef	St. Dev	t-Ratio	P
Constant (b_0)	2.0822	0.3428	6.07	0.009
b_1	0.9913	0.1322	7.50	0.005
$s = 0.1548$			R-sq = 94.9%	R-sq(adj) = 93.2%

The regression equation is $\hat{y} = 2.08 + 0.991b_1x$.

Hypothesis 2:

> $H_0: A = 0$,
>
> $H_A: A \neq 0$ (the data resulting from at least one of the products is significantly different from those of the other two).

Step 2: Set α, n.
Let us use $\alpha = 0.05$ for both contrasts, and $n = 15$.

Step 3: Select the statistical model (already done—Equation 11.5).

Step 4: Decision rule. There are two tests in this method.

Hypothesis 1:
If $F_c > F_T$, reject H_0; the covariate component is significant;
where

> $F_T = F_{T(\alpha;\ \text{number of covariates, df } MS_E)}$ and
>
> df $MS_E = n - a - b = 15 - 3 - 1 = 11$, where a is the number of treatments (3) and b is the number of covariates, 1
>
> $F_T = F_{T(0.05;\ 1,\ 11)} = 4.84$ (Table C, the F distribution table)

Hypothesis 2:
If $F_c > F_T$, reject H_0; at least one of the three treatments differs from the other two at $\alpha = 0.05$;

TABLE 11.7
Product 3 Regression, Example 11.1

Predictor	Coef	St. Dev	t-Ratio	P
Constant (b_0)	1.9297	0.3985	4.84	0.017
b_1	0.7337	0.1596	4.60	0.019
$s = 0.1896$		R-sq = 87.6%	R-sq(adj) = 83.4%	

The regression equation is $\hat{y} = 1.93 + 0.734b_1x$.

where

$$F_T = F_{T(\alpha; a-1, \text{df MS}_E)},$$
$$F_T = F_{T(0.05; 2, 11)} = 3.98 \text{ (Table C, the } F \text{ distribution table).}$$

Step 5: Perform computation (Table 11.8).

Step 6:

Hypothesis 1: (Covariance)
Because $F_c = 76.72$ (Table 11.8) > 4.84, one cannot reject H_0 at $\alpha = 0.05$. The covariate portion explains a significant amount of variability. This is good, because that means it explains a significant amount of variability that would have interfered with the analysis.

Recall that, in ANCOVA, the model has an ANOVA portion and a regression portion. The covariant is the regression portion. Hence, we have a b or slope for the covariate, which is $b = 0.9733$ (Table 11.8). This, in itself, can be used to determine if the covariate is significant in reducing overall error. If the b value is zero, then the use of a covariate is not of value in reducing error, and ANOVA would probably be a better application. A 95% confidence interval for the β value can be determined.

$$\beta = b \pm t_{(\alpha/2, n-a-b)} s_b. \tag{11.6}$$

In this case

$$\beta = b \pm t_{(\alpha/2, n-a-b)} s_b, \text{ where } b = 0.9733, t_{(\alpha/2; n-a-b)} = t_{(0.025; 15-3-1)}$$
$$= t_{(0.025, 11)} = 2.201, \text{ and}$$

TABLE 11.8
Analysis of Covariance, Example 11.1

Source	DF	ADJ SS	MS	F	P
Covariates (baseline)	1	2.9142	2.9142	76.72	0.000
A (treatment)	2	2.1202	1.0601	27.91	0.000
Error	11	0.4178	0.0380		
Total	14	3.6000			

Covariate	Coef	St dev	t-value	P	
B	0.9733	0.111	8.759	0.000	
Adjusted means					
C4	N	C3			
1	5	1.7917			
2	5	2.3259			
3	5	3.0824			

$s_b = 0.111$ (Table 11.8). $\beta = b \pm 2.201(0.111) = 0.9733 \pm 0.2443$.

$$0.7290 \le \beta \le 1.2176.$$

Because β does not include zero in the interval, the covariate is significant at $\alpha = 0.05$.

Hypothesis 2:

Because $F_c = 27.91 > 3.98$, the treatments are significantly different in at least one at $\alpha = 0.05$; where the difference will be determined by contrasts, as presented later in this chapter.

REGRESSION ROUTINE EXAMPLE

Let us now use the regression approach to covariance.

Referring to Table 11.3, there are $a = 3$ treatments, making $a - 1 = 2$ indicator variables, I.

$$I_1 = \begin{cases} 1, & \text{if treatment 1,} \\ -1, & \text{if treatment 3,} \\ 0, & \text{if otherwise,} \end{cases}$$

$$I_2 = \begin{cases} 1, & \text{if treatment 2,} \\ -1, & \text{if treatment 3,} \\ 0, & \text{if otherwise.} \end{cases}$$

As earlier, the regression when both I_1 and I_2 equal zero is for treatment 3. The new codes are presented in Table 11.9. The model is

$$y = b_0 + b_1 I_1 + b_2 I_2 + b_3(x - \bar{x}), \tag{11.7}$$

where $(x - \bar{x})$ is the centered covariate; the baseline $\bar{x} = 4.3800$. In the regression approach, two models are developed: the full model and the reduced model. The full model is as shown in Equation 11.7. The reduced model (H_0, no treatment effect) is

$$y = b_0 + b_1(x - \bar{x}). \tag{11.8}$$

Let us use the six-step procedure:

Step 1: State the hypothesis.
    H_0: Treatment effects are equal to 0,
    H_A: At least one treatment is not 0.

Step 2: Set α and n.
Let us use $\alpha = 0.05$, and $n = 15$.

TABLE 11.9
Data for Analysis of Covariance by Regression, Example 11.1

n	Y	x	I_1	I_2	$x - \bar{x}$
1	2.0	4.8	1	0	0.42
2	3.3	5.3	0	1	0.92
3	2.2	3.4	−1	−1	−0.98
4	2.5	4.9	1	0	0.52
5	2.5	4.8	0	1	0.42
6	2.8	4.2	−1	−1	−0.18
7	2.1	4.6	1	0	0.22
8	2.8	4.8	0	1	0.42
9	2.9	4.1	−1	−1	−0.28
10	2.7	5.5	1	0	1.12
11	1.7	3.7	0	1	−0.68
12	1.5	3.1	−1	−1	−1.28
13	1.8	4.3	1	0	−0.08
14	2.4	4.4	0	1	0.02
15	2.8	3.8	−1	−1	−0.58

Step 3: Select the test statistic.

$$F_c = \frac{SS_{E(R)} - SS_{E(F)}}{df_{(R)} - df_{(F)}} \div \frac{SS_{E(F)}}{df_{(F)}}, \tag{11.9}$$

where

$$df_{(R)} = n - 2,$$
$$df_{(F)} = n - (\text{number of treatments} + 1) = n - (a + 1).$$

Step 4: Decision rule.
If $F_c > F_T$, reject H_0 at α.

$$F_T = F_T \left(\underbrace{0.05; [df_{(R)} - df_{(F)}]}_{\text{numerator}}, \underbrace{[df_{(F)}]}_{\text{denominator}} \right)$$

$$df_{(R)} = n - 2 = 15 - 2 = 13,$$
$$df_{(F)} = n - (a + 1) = 15 - (3 + 1) = 11$$
$$= F_{T(0.05; \ 13-11, \ 11)}$$
$$= F_{T(0.05; \ 2, \ 11)} = 3.98 \text{ (Table C, the } F \text{ distribution table).}$$

TABLE 11.10
Full Model, Covariance by Regression, Example 11.1

Predictor	Coef	St. Dev	t-Ratio	P
b_0	2.40000	0.05032	47.69	0.000
b_1	−0.60827	0.08634	−7.04	0.000
b_2	−0.07414	0.07525	−0.99	0.346
b_3	0.9733	0.1111	8.76	0.000
s = 0.1949		R-sq = 88.4%		R-sq(adj) = 85.2%

Analysis of Variance

Source	DF	SS	MS	F	P
Regression	3	3.1822	1.0607	27.93	0.000
Error	11	0.4178	0.0380		
Total	14	3.6000			

The regression equation is $\hat{y} = 2.40 - 0.608I_1 - 0.0741I_2 + 0.973(x - \bar{x})$.

If $F_c > F_T$, reject H_0 at α.

Step 5: Perform computation.
Table 11.10 provides the full model. The reduced model is provided in Table 11.11.

$$F_c = \frac{SS_{E(R)} - SS_{E(F)}}{df_{(R)} - df_{(F)}} \div \frac{SS_{E(F)}}{df_{(F)}} = \frac{2.5381 - 0.4178}{13 - 11} \div \frac{0.4178}{11} = 27.91.$$

Step 6:
Because $F_c = 27.91 > F_T = 3.98$, reject H_0 at $\alpha = 0.05$. The treatments are significant.

TABLE 11.11
Reduced Model, Covariance by Regression, Example 11.1

Predictor	Coef	St. Dev	t-Ratio	P
Constant (b_0)	2.40000	0.1141	21.04	0.000
b_1	0.4053	0.1738	2.33	0.036
s = 0.4419		R-sq = 29.5%		R-sq(adj) = 24.1%

Analysis of Variance

Source	DF	SS	MS	F	P
Regression	1	1.0619	1.0619	5.44	0.036
Error	13	2.5381	0.1952		
Total	14	3.6000			

The regression equation is $\hat{y} = 2.40 + 0.405(x - \bar{x})$.

Note that F_c for treatment 27.91 is the same as determined from the covariance analysis.

TREATMENT EFFECTS

As in ANOVA, if a treatment effect has been determined significant, the task is to find which treatment(s) differ.

Recall that, in ANOVA, the treatment effects are determined as

$$\mu_i = \mu + T_i, \tag{11.10}$$

where μ is the common mean value, T_i is the treatment effect for the ith treatment, and μ_i is the population treatment i mean.

In ANCOVA, we must also account for the covariance effect.

$$\mu_i = \mu. + T_i + b(x - \bar{x}), \tag{11.11}$$

where $\mu.$ is the adjusted common average, T_i is the treatment effect for the ith treatment, b is the regression coefficient for covariance, and $(x - \bar{x})$ is the covariate centered about the mean.

We no longer discuss the mean effect from the ith treatment, because it varies with x_i. For example, suppose the graph in Figure 11.5 was derived.

The difference between T_1 and $T_3 = T_1 - T_3 = (\mu. + T_1) - (\mu. + T_3)$ anywhere on the graph for a given x or $(x - \bar{x})$, because the slopes are parallel. Hence, it is critical that the slopes are parallel.

Recall that the model we developed was

$$\hat{y} = b_0 + b_1 I_1 + b_2 I_2 + b_3(x - \bar{x}), \tag{11.7}$$

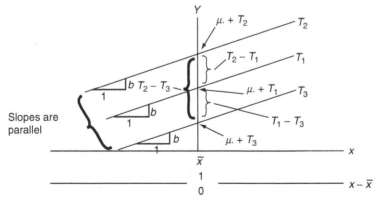

FIGURE 11.5 Possible treatment graph.

from Table 11.10, where

$$b_0 = \mu. = 2.40,$$
$$b_1 = -0.60827,$$
$$b_2 = -0.07414,$$
$$b_3 = 0.9733.$$

Therefore, $T_3 = -T_1 - T_2$ and $T_3 = 0$, if $T_1 = T_2 = 0$. Using the concept, $T_i - T_j$, we can determine the contrasts.

$T_1 - T_2, T_1 - T_3,$ and $T_2 - T_3,$ based on $T_3 = -T_1 - T_2.$

   Test   *Form*

$T_1 - T_2$ $T_1 - T_2 = -0.60872 - (-0.07414) = -0.5346,$

$T_1 - T_3$ using the form $\rightarrow T_3 = -T_1 - T_2,$

               $T_2 = -T_1 - T_3,$

               $2T_1 + T_2 = T_1 - T_3$ (add $2T_1$ to both sides of the equation).

So,

$T_1 - T_3$ $= 2T_1 + T_2 = 2(-0.60827) + (-0.07414) = -1.2907,$

$T_2 - T_3$ using the form $\rightarrow T_3 = -T_1 - T_2,$

               $T_1 = -T_3 - T_2,$

               $2T_2 + T_1 = -T_3 + T_2$ (add $2T_2$ to both sides of the equation),

               $2T_2 + T_1 = T_2 - T_3.$

So,

$T_2 - T_3$ $= 2T_2 + T_1 = 2(-0.07414) - 0.60827 = -0.7566.$

The variance estimator is

$$\sigma^2\{a_1Y_1 + a_2Y_2\} = a_1^2\sigma^2(y_1) + a_2^2\sigma^2(y_2) + 2a_1a_2\sigma(y_1, y_2), \qquad (11.12)$$

where a is a constant.

The variance of

$$T_1 - T_2 = (1)^2\sigma^2(T_1) + (1)^2\sigma^2(T_2) - 2(1)(1)\sigma(T_1T_2),$$
$$T_1 - T_3 = 2T_1 + T_2 = (1)^2 2\sigma^2(T_1) + (1)^2\sigma^2(T_2) - 2(2)(1)\sigma(T_1T_2),$$
$$T_2 - T_3 = T_1 + 2T_2 = (1)^2\sigma^2(T_1) + (1)^2 2\sigma^2(T_2) - 2(1)(2)\sigma(T_1T_2).$$

Before we can continue, we need a variance–covariance table for the betas or b_is

$$\sigma^2(\boldsymbol{b}) = \sigma^2(\boldsymbol{X}'\boldsymbol{X})^{-1}. \tag{11.13}$$

Table 11.12 presents the $\boldsymbol{X}$ matrix. Table 11.13 presents the $(\boldsymbol{X}'\boldsymbol{X})^{-1}$ matrix.

$$\sigma^2 = \mathrm{MS_E} = 0.0380 \quad \text{(from Table 11.10)}.$$

Table 11.14 presents the variance–covariance matrix for the betas. Hence, the variance–covariance of

$$T_1 - T_2 = 0.0074583 + 0.056646 - 2(-0.0013375),$$
$$T_1 - T_2 = 0.0668,$$
$$T_1 - T_3 = 2T_1 + T_2$$
$$\qquad = 2(0.007458) + (1)0.056646 - 2(2)(1)(-0.0013375)$$
$$\qquad = 0.0769,$$
$$T_2 - T_3 = T_1 + 2T_2$$
$$\qquad = 1(0.007458) + 2(0.056646) - 2(1)(2)(-0.0013375)$$
$$\qquad = 0.1261.$$

Table 11.15 presents the contrasts, the estimates, and the variances.

TABLE 11.12
X Matrix, Treatment Effects, Example 11.1

$$X_{(15 \times 4)}
\begin{bmatrix}
1.00000 & 1.00000 & 0.00000 & 0.42000 \\
1.00000 & 0.00000 & 1.00000 & 0.92000 \\
1.00000 & -1.00000 & -1.00000 & -0.98000 \\
1.00000 & 1.00000 & 0.00000 & 0.52000 \\
1.00000 & 0.00000 & 1.00000 & 0.42000 \\
1.00000 & -1.00000 & -1.00000 & -0.18000 \\
1.00000 & 1.00000 & 0.00000 & 0.22000 \\
1.00000 & 0.00000 & 1.00000 & 0.42000 \\
1.00000 & -1.00000 & -1.00000 & -0.28000 \\
1.00000 & 1.00000 & 0.00000 & 1.12000 \\
1.00000 & 0.00000 & 1.00000 & -0.68000 \\
1.00000 & -1.00000 & -1.00000 & -1.28000 \\
1.00000 & 1.00000 & 0.00000 & -0.08000 \\
1.00000 & 0.00000 & 1.00000 & 0.02000 \\
1.00000 & -1.00000 & -1.00000 & -0.58000
\end{bmatrix}$$

TABLE 11.13

$(X'X)^{-1}$ **Matrix, Treatment Effects, Example 11.1**

$$(X'X)^{-1} = \begin{bmatrix} 0.06667 & -0.00000 & -0.00000 & 0.00000 \\ -0.00000 & 0.196272 & -0.035197 & -0.143043 \\ -0.00000 & -0.035197 & 0.149068 & -0.071521 \\ 0.00000 & -0.143043 & -0.071521 & 0.325098 \end{bmatrix}$$

SINGLE INTERVAL ESTIMATE

$$T_i - T_i \pm t_{(\alpha/2;\, n-k-1)}\sqrt{s^2},$$

where k is the number of betas minus b_0, and s^2 is the appropriate variance (Table 11.15).

Rarely will a researcher want to use a t distribution for evaluating only one confidence interval. The researcher will want, more than likely, all contrasts.

SCHEFFE PROCEDURE—MULTIPLE CONTRASTS

$$C^2 = (a - 1)F_{T(\alpha,\, a-1;\, n-a-1)},$$

where a is the number of treatments and $\alpha = 0.05$.

$$C^2 = (3 - 1)F_{T(0.05,\, 3-1;\, 15-3-1)},$$
$$C^2 = 2F_{T(0.05;\, 2,\, 11)} = 2(3.98), \text{ from Table C, the } F$$
distribution table, so $C^2 = 7.96$
and $C = 2.8213.$

The interval form is

$$T_i - T_{i'} \pm c\sqrt{s^2},$$
$$T_1 - T_2 = -0.5346 \pm 2.8213\sqrt{0.0668}$$
$$= -0.5346 \pm 0.7292$$
$$-1.2638 \le T_1 - T_2 \le -0.1946.$$

TABLE 11.14

Variance–Covariance Matrix for the Betas, Example 11.1

		$b_0 = \mu.$	$b_1 = T_1 = I_1$	$b_2 = T_2 = I_2$	$b_3 = (x - \bar{x})$
$\sigma^2(X'X)^{-1} =$	$b_0 = \mu.$	0.0025333	-0.0000000	-0.0000000	0.0000000
	$b_1 = T_1$	-0.000000	0.0074583	-0.0013375	-0.0054356
	$b_2 = T_2$	-0.000000	-0.0013375	0.0056646	-0.0027178
	$b_3 = x$	0.000000	-0.0054356	-0.0027178	0.0123537

TABLE 11.15
Contrasts, Estimates, and Variances, Example 11.1

Contrast	Estimate	Variance
$T_1 - T_2$	$T_1 - T_2 = -0.5346$	0.0668
$T_1 - T_3$	$2T_1 + T_2 = -1.2907$	0.0769
$T_2 - T_3$	$T_1 + 2T_2 = -0.7566$	0.1261

Because 0 is included in the interval, T_1 and T_2 are not significantly different from one another at $\alpha = 0.05$.

$$T_1 - T_3 = -1.2907 \pm 2.8213\sqrt{0.0769}$$
$$= -1.2907 \pm 0.7824$$
$$-2.0731 \leq T_1 - T_3 \leq -0.5083.$$

Because 0 is not included in the interval, T_1 and T_2 are significantly different from one another at $\alpha = 0.05$.

$$T_2 - T_3 = -0.7566 \pm 2.8213\sqrt{0.1261}$$
$$= -0.7566 \pm 1.0019$$
$$-1.7585 \leq T_2 - T_3 \leq 0.2453.$$

Because 0 is included in the interval, T_2 and T_3 do not differ at $\alpha = 0.05$.
If the researcher wants to rank the treatments, $T_3 > T_2 > T_1$ (Figure 11.6).

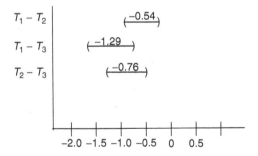

FIGURE 11.6 Treatment ranking.

BONFERRONI METHOD

The Bonferroni contrast procedure can also be used for g contrasts.

$$T_i - T_i = \hat{T}_i - \hat{T}_{i'} \pm \beta_T \sqrt{s^2},$$
$$\beta_T = t_{(\alpha/2g, n-a-1)}.$$

Suppose the researcher wants to evaluate $T_1 - T_2$ or $T_1 - T_3$ only, $g = 2$. Let us set $\alpha = 0.01$.

$$\beta_T = t_{(0.01/2(2), 15-3-1)} = t_{(0.0025, 11)} = 3.497 \text{ (Table B, the Student's } t \text{ table)}.$$

Contrast 1:

$$T_1 - T_2 = -0.5346 \pm 3.497\sqrt{0.0668}$$
$$= -0.5346 \pm 0.9038$$
$$-1.4384 \leq T_1 - T_2 \leq 0.3692.$$

Contrast 2:

$$T_1 - T_3 = -1.2907 \pm 3.497\sqrt{0.0769}$$
$$= -1.2907 \pm 0.970$$
$$-2.2607 \leq T_1 - T_3 \leq -0.3207.$$

The Scheffe method is recommended when the researcher desires to compare all possible contrasts, but the Bonferroni method is used when specific contrasts are desired.

ADJUSTED AVERAGE RESPONSE

There are times when a researcher desires to estimate an adjusted-by-covariance response. This is done by using the ith response, $x_i - \bar{x}$ as the estimate. It is an adjusted estimate because it takes into account the covariance effect (concomitant variable).

The full regression model used is

$$\hat{y} = b_0 + b_1 I_1 + b_2 I_2 + b_3(x - \bar{x}).$$

The mean responses in this example are:

$$\text{Treatment } 1 = \mu. + T_1 = b_0 + b_1,$$
$$\text{Treatment } 2 = \mu. + T_2 = b_0 + b_2,$$

Treatment $3 = \mu. + T_3 = b_0 - b_1 - b_2$ (recall that there are $a - 1$ indicator, or dummy, variables, in this case corresponding to $b_1 =$ treatment 1 and $b_2 =$ treatment 2. There is b_0, b_3 (or I_3) representing treatment 3. Hence, $T_3 = b_0 - b_1 - b_2$.

The variance estimates for the treatments are as follows, based on formula 11.12.

$$\text{var}(a_1 y_i a_2 x_2) = a_1^2 \sigma^2[y_1] + a_2^2 \sigma^2[y_2] + 2(a_1)(a_2)\sigma[y_1, y_2], \text{and}$$

$$\text{var}(\mu., T_1) = (1)^2 \sigma^2(\mu.) + (1)^2 \sigma^2(T_1) + 2(1)\sigma[\mu., T_1] \text{ using Table 11.16}$$

$$= (1)^2(0.0025333) + (1)^2(0.0074583) + 2(1)(1)(0),$$

$$\text{var}(\mu., T_1) = 0.0100,$$

$$\text{var}(\mu., T_2) = (1)^2 \sigma^2(\mu) + (1)^2 \sigma^2(T_2) + 2(1)(1)\sigma[\mu., T_2]$$

$$= (1)^2(0.0025333) + (1)^2(0.0056646) + 2[0],$$

$$\text{var}(\mu., T_2) = 0.0082,$$

$$\text{var}(\mu., T_3) = (1)^2 \sigma^2[\mu.] + (1)^2 \sigma^2[T_1] + (1)^2 \sigma^2[T_2] + (-1)2\sigma[\mu., T_1]$$
$$+ (-1)2\sigma[\mu., T_2] + (-1)(-1)2\sigma[T_1, T_2]$$

$$= (1)^2 \sigma^2[\mu.] + (-1)^2 \sigma^2[T_1] + (-1)^2 \sigma^2[T_2] - 2\sigma[\mu., T_1]$$
$$- 2\sigma[\mu., T_2] + 2\sigma^2[T_1, T_2]$$

$$= \sigma^2[\mu.] + \sigma^2[T_1] + \sigma^2[T_2] - 2\sigma[\mu., T_1] - 2\sigma[\mu., T_2]$$
$$+ 2\sigma^2[T_1, T_2]$$

$$= 0.0025333 + 0.0074583 + 0.0056646 - 2(0) - 2(0)$$
$$+ 2(-0.0013375),$$

$$\text{var}(\mu., T_3) = 0.0130.$$

Putting these together, the estimated adjusted mean responses are

	The Mean Response at $\bar{x}$	Var
Treatment 1	$b_0 + b_1 = 2.40 - 0.60827 = 1.7917$	0.0100
Treatment 2	$b_0 + b_2 = 2.40 - 0.07414 = 2.3259$	0.0082
Treatment 3	$b_0 - b_1 - b_2 = 2.40 + 0.6827 + 0.07414 = 3.15684$	0.0130

CONCLUSION

More complex models can be used, but present a problem to the researcher in that ever more restrictions make the design less applicable. This is particularly so when multiple covariates must be assured linear. If possible, the study should be designed as simply and directly as possible.

Appendix I

TABLE A
Cumulative Probabilities of the Standard Normal Distribution (z Table)

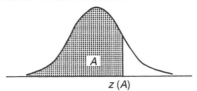

z (A)

z	0.00	0.01	0.02	0.03	0.04	0.05	0.06	0.07	0.08	0.09
0.0	0.5000	0.5040	0.5080	0.5120	0.5160	0.5199	0.5239	0.5279	0.5319	0.5359
0.1	0.5398	0.5438	0.5478	0.5517	0.5557	0.5596	0.5636	0.5675	0.5714	0.5753
0.2	0.5793	0.5832	0.5871	0.5910	0.5948	0.5987	0.6026	0.6064	0.6103	0.6141
0.3	0.6179	0.6217	0.6255	0.6293	0.6331	0.6368	0.6406	0.6443	0.6480	0.6517
0.4	0.6554	0.6591	0.6628	0.6664	0.6700	0.6736	0.6772	0.6808	0.6844	0.6879
0.5	0.6915	0.6950	0.6985	0.7019	0.7054	0.7088	0.7123	0.7157	0.7190	0.7224
0.6	0.7257	0.7291	0.7324	0.7357	0.7389	0.7422	0.7454	0.7486	0.7517	0.7549
0.7	0.7580	0.7611	0.7642	0.7673	0.7704	0.7734	0.7764	0.7794	0.7823	0.7852
0.8	0.7881	0.7910	0.7939	0.7967	0.7995	0.8023	0.8051	0.8078	0.8106	0.8133
0.9	0.8159	0.8186	0.8212	0.8238	0.8264	0.8289	0.8315	0.8340	0.8365	0.8389
1.0	0.8413	0.8438	0.8461	0.8485	0.8508	0.8531	0.8554	0.8577	0.8599	0.8621
1.1	0.8643	0.8665	0.8686	0.8708	0.8729	0.8749	0.8770	0.8790	0.8810	0.8830
1.2	0.8849	0.8869	0.8888	0.8907	0.8925	0.8944	0.8962	0.8980	0.8997	0.9015
1.3	0.9032	0.9049	0.9066	0.9082	0.9099	0.9115	0.9131	0.9147	0.9162	0.9177
1.4	0.9192	0.9207	0.9222	0.9236	0.9251	0.9265	0.9279	0.9292	0.9306	0.9319
1.5	0.9332	0.9345	0.9357	0.9370	0.9382	0.9394	0.9406	0.9418	0.9429	0.9441
1.6	0.9452	0.9463	0.9474	0.9484	0.9495	0.9505	0.9515	0.9525	0.9535	0.9545
1.7	0.9554	0.9564	0.9573	0.9582	0.9591	0.9599	0.9608	0.9616	0.9625	0.9633
1.8	0.9641	0.9649	0.9656	0.9664	0.9671	0.9678	0.9686	0.9693	0.9699	0.9706
1.9	0.9713	0.9719	0.9726	0.9732	0.9738	0.9744	0.9750	0.9756	0.9761	0.9767
2.0	0.9772	0.9778	0.9783	0.9788	0.9793	0.9798	0.9803	0.9808	0.9812	0.9817
2.1	0.9821	0.9826	0.9830	0.9834	0.9838	0.9842	0.9846	0.9850	0.9854	0.9857
2.2	0.9861	0.9864	0.9868	0.9871	0.9875	0.9878	0.9881	0.9884	0.9887	0.9890
2.3	0.9893	0.9896	0.9898	0.9901	0.9904	0.9906	0.9909	0.9911	0.9913	0.9916
2.4	0.9918	0.9920	0.9922	0.9925	0.9927	0.9929	0.9931	0.9932	0.9934	0.9936
2.5	0.9938	0.9940	0.9941	0.9943	0.9945	0.9946	0.9948	0.9949	0.9951	0.9952
2.6	0.9953	0.9955	0.9956	0.9957	0.9959	0.9960	0.9961	0.9962	0.9963	0.9964
2.7	0.9965	0.9966	0.9967	0.9968	0.9969	0.9970	0.9971	0.9972	0.9973	0.9974

(continued)

TABLE A (continued)
Cumulative Probabilities of the Standard Normal Distribution (z Table)

z	0.00	0.01	0.02	0.03	0.04	0.05	0.06	0.07	0.08	0.09
2.8	0.9974	0.9975	0.9976	0.9977	0.9977	0.9978	0.9979	0.9979	0.9980	0.9981
2.9	0.9981	0.9982	0.9982	0.9983	0.9984	0.9984	0.9985	0.9985	0.9986	0.9986
3.0	0.9987	0.9987	0.9987	0.9988	0.9988	0.9989	0.9989	0.9989	0.9990	0.9990
3.1	0.9990	0.9991	0.9991	0.9991	0.9992	0.9992	0.9992	0.9992	0.9993	0.9993
3.2	0.9993	0.9993	0.9994	0.9994	0.9994	0.9994	0.9994	0.9995	0.9995	0.9995
3.3	0.9995	0.9995	0.9995	0.9996	0.9996	0.9996	0.9996	0.9996	0.9996	0.9997
3.4	0.9997	0.9997	0.9997	0.9997	0.9997	0.9997	0.9997	0.9997	0.9997	0.9998

Cumulative probability A:	0.90	0.95	0.975	0.98	0.99	0.995	0.999
$z(A)$:	1.282	1.645	1.960	2.054	2.326	2.576	3.090

Note: Entry is area A under the standard normal curve from $-\infty$ to $z(A)$.

TABLE B
Percentiles of the t-Distribution

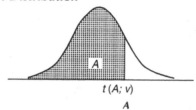

$t(A; v)$

A

v	0.60	0.70	0.80	0.85	0.90	0.95	0.975
1	0.325	0.727	1.376	1.963	3.078	6.314	12.706
2	0.289	0.617	1.061	1.386	1.886	2.920	4.303
3	0.277	0.584	0.978	1.250	1.638	2.353	3.182
4	0.271	0.569	0.941	1.190	1.533	2.132	2.776
5	0.267	0.559	0.920	1.156	1.476	2.015	2.571
6	0.265	0.553	0.906	1.134	1.440	1.943	2.447
7	0.263	0.549	0.896	1.119	1.415	1.895	2.365
8	0.262	0.546	0.889	1.108	1.397	1.860	2.306
9	0.261	0.543	0.883	1.100	1.383	1.833	2.262
10	0.260	0.542	0.879	1.093	1.372	1.812	2.228
11	0.260	0.540	0.876	1.088	1.363	1.796	2.201
12	0.259	0.539	0.873	1.083	1.356	1.782	2.179
13	0.259	0.537	0.870	1.079	1.350	1.771	2.160
14	0.258	0.537	0.868	1.076	1.345	1.761	2.145
15	0.258	0.536	0.866	1.074	1.341	1.753	2.131
16	0.258	0.535	0.865	1.071	1.337	1.746	2.120
17	0.257	0.534	0.863	1.069	1.333	1.740	2.110
18	0.257	0.534	0.862	1.067	1.330	1.734	2.101
19	0.257	0.533	0.861	1.066	1.328	1.729	2.093
20	0.257	0.533	0.860	1.064	1.325	1.725	2.086
21	0.257	0.532	0.859	1.063	1.323	1.721	2.080
22	0.256	0.532	0.858	1.061	1.321	1.717	2.074
23	0.256	0.532	0.858	1.060	1.319	1.714	2.069
24	0.256	0.531	0.857	1.059	1.318	1.711	2.064

(*continued*)

TABLE B (continued)
Percentiles of the t-Distribution

				A			
ν	0.60	0.70	0.80	0.85	0.90	0.95	0.975
25	0.256	0.531	0.856	1.058	1.316	1.708	2.060
26	0.256	0.531	0.856	1.058	1.315	1.706	2.056
27	0.256	0.531	0.855	1.057	1.314	1.703	2.052
28	0.256	0.530	0.855	1.056	1.313	1.701	2.048
29	0.256	0.530	0.854	1.055	1.311	1.699	2.045
30	0.256	0.530	0.854	1.055	1.310	1.697	2.042
40	0.255	0.529	0.851	1.050	1.303	1.684	2.021
60	0.254	0.527	0.848	1.045	1.296	1.671	2.000
120	0.254	0.526	0.845	1.041	1.289	1.658	1.980
∞	0.253	0.524	0.842	1.036	1.282	1.645	1.960

ν	0.98	0.985	0.99	0.9925	0.995	0.9975	0.9995
1	15.895	21.205	31.821	42.434	63.657	127.322	636.590
2	4.849	5.643	6.965	8.073	9.925	14.089	31.598
3	3.482	3.896	4.541	5.047	5.841	7.453	12.924
4	2.999	3.298	3.747	4.088	4.604	5.598	8.610
5	2.757	3.003	3.365	3.634	4.032	4.773	6.869
6	2.612	2.829	3.143	3.372	3.707	4.317	5.959
7	2.517	2.715	2.998	3.203	3.499	4.029	5.408
8	2.449	2.634	2.896	3.085	3.355	3.833	5.041
9	2.398	2.574	2.821	2.998	3.250	3.690	4.781
10	2.359	2.527	2.764	2.932	3.169	3.581	4.587
11	2.328	2.491	2.718	2.879	3.106	3.497	4.437
12	2.303	2.461	2.681	2.836	3.055	3.428	4.318
13	2.282	2.436	2.650	2.801	3.012	3.372	4.221
14	2.264	2.415	2.624	2.771	2.977	3.326	4.140
15	2.249	2.397	2.602	2.746	2.947	3.286	4.073
16	2.235	2.382	2.583	2.724	2.921	3.252	4.015
17	2.224	2.368	2.567	2.706	2.898	3.222	3.965
18	2.214	2.356	2.552	2.689	2.878	3.197	3.922
19	2.205	2.346	2.539	2.674	2.861	3.174	3.883
20	2.197	2.336	2.528	2.661	2.845	3.153	3.849
21	2.189	2.328	2.518	2.649	2.831	3.135	3.819
22	2.183	2.320	2.508	2.639	2.819	3.119	3.792
23	2.177	2.313	2.500	2.629	2.807	3.104	3.768
24	2.172	2.307	2.492	2.620	2.797	3.091	3.745
25	2.167	2.301	2.485	2.612	2.787	3.078	3.725
26	2.162	2.296	2.479	2.605	2.779	3.067	3.707
27	2.158	2.291	2.473	2.598	2.771	3.057	3.690
28	2.154	2.286	2.467	2.592	2.763	3.047	3.674
29	2.150	2.282	2.462	2.586	2.756	3.038	3.659
30	2.147	2.278	2.457	2.581	2.750	3.030	3.646
40	2.123	2.250	2.423	2.542	2.704	2.971	3.551
60	2.099	2.223	2.390	2.504	2.660	2.915	3.460
120	2.076	2.196	2.358	2.468	2.617	2.860	3.373
∞	2.054	2.170	2.326	2.432	2.576	2.807	3.291

Note: Entry is $t(A; ν)$, where $P\{t(ν) \leq t(A; ν)\} = A$.

TABLE C
F-Distribution Tables $F_{0.25}(v_1, v_2)$

v_2	v_1 1	2	3	4	5	6	7	8	9	10	12	15	20	24	30	40	60	120	∞
1	5.83	7.50	8.20	8.58	8.82	8.98	9.10	9.19	9.26	9.32	9.41	9.49	9.58	9.63	9.67	9.71	9.76	9.80	9.85
2	2.57	3.00	3.15	3.23	3.28	3.31	3.34	3.35	3.37	3.38	3.39	3.41	3.43	3.43	3.44	3.45	3.46	3.47	3.48
3	2.02	2.28	2.36	2.39	2.41	2.42	2.43	2.44	2.44	2.44	2.45	2.46	2.46	2.46	2.47	2.47	2.47	2.47	2.47
4	1.81	2.00	2.05	2.06	2.07	2.08	2.08	2.08	2.08	2.08	2.08	2.08	2.08	2.08	2.08	2.08	2.08	2.08	2.08
5	1.69	1.85	1.88	1.89	1.89	1.89	1.89	1.89	1.89	1.89	1.89	1.89	1.88	1.88	1.88	1.88	1.87	1.87	1.87
6	1.62	1.76	1.78	1.79	1.79	1.78	1.78	1.78	1.77	1.77	1.77	1.76	1.76	1.75	1.75	1.75	1.74	1.74	1.74
7	1.57	1.70	1.72	1.72	1.71	1.71	1.70	1.70	1.70	1.69	1.68	1.68	1.67	1.67	1.66	1.66	1.65	1.65	1.65
8	1.54	1.66	1.67	1.66	1.66	1.65	1.64	1.64	1.63	1.63	1.62	1.62	1.61	1.60	1.60	1.59	1.59	1.58	1.58
9	1.51	1.62	1.63	1.63	1.62	1.61	1.60	1.60	1.59	1.59	1.58	1.57	1.56	1.56	1.55	1.54	1.54	1.53	1.53
10	1.49	1.60	1.60	1.59	1.59	1.58	1.57	1.56	1.56	1.55	1.54	1.53	1.52	1.52	1.51	1.51	1.50	1.49	1.48
11	1.47	1.58	1.58	1.57	1.56	1.55	1.54	1.53	1.53	1.52	1.51	1.50	1.49	1.49	1.48	1.47	1.47	1.46	1.45
12	1.46	1.56	1.56	1.55	1.54	1.53	1.52	1.51	1.51	1.50	1.49	1.48	1.47	1.46	1.45	1.45	1.44	1.43	1.42
13	1.45	1.55	1.55	1.53	1.52	1.51	1.50	1.49	1.49	1.48	1.47	1.46	1.45	1.44	1.43	1.42	1.42	1.41	1.40
14	1.44	1.53	1.53	1.52	1.51	1.50	1.49	1.48	1.47	1.46	1.45	1.44	1.43	1.42	1.41	1.41	1.40	1.39	1.38
15	1.43	1.52	1.52	1.51	1.49	1.48	1.47	1.46	1.46	1.45	1.44	1.43	1.41	1.41	1.40	1.39	1.38	1.37	1.36

16	1.34	1.35	1.36	1.37	1.38	1.39	1.40	1.41	1.43	1.44	1.44	1.45	1.46	1.47	1.48	1.50	1.51	1.51	1.42
17	1.33	1.34	1.35	1.36	1.37	1.38	1.39	1.40	1.41	1.43	1.43	1.44	1.45	1.46	1.47	1.49	1.50	1.51	1.42
18	1.32	1.33	1.34	1.35	1.36	1.37	1.38	1.39	1.40	1.42	1.42	1.43	1.44	1.45	1.46	1.48	1.49	1.50	1.41
19	1.30	1.32	1.33	1.34	1.35	1.36	1.37	1.38	1.40	1.41	1.41	1.42	1.43	1.44	1.46	1.47	1.49	1.49	1.41
20	1.29	1.31	1.32	1.33	1.34	1.35	1.36	1.37	1.39	1.40	1.41	1.42	1.43	1.44	1.45	1.47	1.48	1.49	1.40
21	1.28	1.30	1.31	1.32	1.33	1.34	1.35	1.37	1.38	1.39	1.40	1.41	1.42	1.43	1.44	1.46	1.48	1.48	1.40
22	1.28	1.29	1.30	1.31	1.32	1.33	1.34	1.36	1.37	1.39	1.39	1.40	1.41	1.42	1.44	1.45	1.47	1.48	1.40
23	1.27	1.28	1.30	1.31	1.32	1.33	1.34	1.35	1.37	1.38	1.39	1.40	1.41	1.42	1.43	1.45	1.47	1.47	1.39
24	1.26	1.28	1.29	1.30	1.31	1.32	1.33	1.35	1.36	1.38	1.38	1.39	1.40	1.41	1.43	1.44	1.46	1.47	1.39
25	1.25	1.27	1.28	1.29	1.31	1.32	1.33	1.34	1.36	1.37	1.38	1.39	1.40	1.41	1.42	1.44	1.46	1.47	1.39
26	1.25	1.26	1.28	1.29	1.30	1.31	1.32	1.34	1.35	1.37	1.37	1.38	1.39	1.41	1.42	1.44	1.45	1.46	1.38
27	1.24	1.26	1.27	1.28	1.30	1.31	1.32	1.33	1.35	1.36	1.37	1.38	1.39	1.40	1.42	1.43	1.45	1.46	1.38
28	1.24	1.25	1.27	1.28	1.29	1.30	1.31	1.33	1.34	1.36	1.37	1.38	1.39	1.40	1.41	1.43	1.45	1.46	1.38
29	1.23	1.25	1.26	1.27	1.29	1.30	1.31	1.32	1.34	1.35	1.36	1.37	1.38	1.40	1.41	1.43	1.45	1.45	1.38
30	1.23	1.24	1.26	1.27	1.28	1.29	1.30	1.32	1.34	1.35	1.36	1.37	1.38	1.39	1.41	1.42	1.44	1.45	1.38
40	1.19	1.21	1.22	1.24	1.25	1.26	1.28	1.30	1.31	1.33	1.34	1.35	1.36	1.37	1.39	1.40	1.42	1.44	1.36
60	1.15	1.17	1.19	1.21	1.22	1.24	1.25	1.27	1.29	1.30	1.31	1.32	1.33	1.35	1.37	1.38	1.41	1.42	1.35
120	1.10	1.13	1.16	1.18	1.19	1.21	1.22	1.24	1.26	1.28	1.29	1.30	1.31	1.33	1.35	1.37	1.39	1.40	1.34
∞	1.00	1.08	1.12	1.14	1.16	1.18	1.19	1.22	1.24	1.25	1.27	1.28	1.29	1.31	1.33	1.35	1.37	1.39	1.32

Note: v_1 is the degrees of freedom for the numerator and v_2 is the degrees of freedom for the denominator.

(continued)

TABLE C (continued)
F-Distribution Tables $F_{0.10}(v_1, v_2)$

v_1

v_2	1	2	3	4	5	6	7	8	9	10	12	15	20	24	30	40	60	120	∞
1	39.86	49.50	53.59	55.83	57.24	58.20	58.91	59.44	59.86	60.19	60.71	61.22	61.74	62.00	62.26	62.53	62.79	63.06	63.33
2	8.53	9.00	9.16	9.24	9.29	9.33	9.35	9.37	9.38	9.39	9.41	9.42	9.44	9.45	9.46	9.47	9.47	9.48	9.49
3	5.54	5.46	5.39	5.34	5.31	5.28	5.27	5.25	5.24	5.23	5.22	5.20	5.18	5.18	5.17	5.16	5.15	5.14	5.13
4	4.54	4.32	4.19	4.11	4.05	4.01	3.98	3.95	3.94	3.92	3.90	3.87	3.84	3.83	3.82	3.80	3.79	3.78	3.76
5	4.06	3.78	3.62	3.52	3.45	3.40	3.37	3.34	3.32	3.30	3.27	3.24	3.21	3.19	3.17	3.16	3.14	3.12	3.10
6	3.78	3.46	3.29	3.18	3.11	3.05	3.01	2.98	2.96	2.94	2.90	2.87	2.84	2.82	2.80	2.78	2.76	2.74	2.72
7	3.59	3.26	3.07	2.96	2.88	2.83	2.78	2.75	2.72	2.70	2.67	2.63	2.59	2.58	2.56	2.54	2.51	2.49	2.47
8	3.46	3.11	2.92	2.81	2.73	2.67	2.62	2.59	2.56	2.54	2.50	2.46	2.42	2.40	2.38	2.36	2.34	2.32	2.29
9	3.36	3.01	2.81	2.69	2.61	2.55	2.51	2.47	2.44	2.42	2.38	2.34	2.30	2.28	2.25	2.23	2.21	2.18	2.16
10	3.29	2.92	2.73	2.61	2.52	2.46	2.41	2.38	2.35	2.32	2.28	2.24	2.20	2.18	2.16	2.13	2.11	2.08	2.06
11	3.23	2.86	2.66	2.54	2.45	2.39	2.34	2.30	2.27	2.25	2.21	2.17	2.12	2.10	2.08	2.05	2.03	2.00	1.97
12	3.18	2.81	2.61	2.48	2.39	2.33	2.28	2.24	2.21	2.19	2.15	2.10	2.06	2.04	2.01	1.99	1.96	1.93	1.90
13	3.14	2.76	2.56	2.43	2.35	2.28	2.23	2.20	2.16	2.14	2.10	2.05	2.01	1.98	1.96	1.93	1.90	1.88	1.85
14	3.10	2.73	2.52	2.39	2.31	2.24	2.19	2.15	2.12	2.10	2.05	2.01	1.96	1.94	1.91	1.89	1.86	1.83	1.80
15	3.07	2.70	2.49	2.36	2.27	2.21	2.16	2.12	2.09	2.06	2.02	1.97	1.92	1.90	1.87	1.85	1.82	1.79	1.76
16	3.05	2.67	2.46	2.33	2.24	2.18	2.13	2.09	2.06	2.03	1.99	1.94	1.89	1.87	1.84	1.81	1.78	1.75	1.72

v_2																		
17	3.03	2.64	2.44	2.31	2.22	2.15	2.10	2.06	2.03	2.00	1.96	1.91	1.86	1.84	1.81	1.78	1.75	1.72	1.69
18	3.01	2.62	2.42	2.29	2.20	2.13	2.08	2.04	2.00	1.98	1.93	1.89	1.84	1.81	1.78	1.75	1.72	1.69	1.66
19	2.99	2.61	2.40	2.27	2.18	2.11	2.06	2.02	1.98	1.96	1.91	1.86	1.81	1.79	1.76	1.73	1.70	1.67	1.63
20	2.97	2.59	2.38	2.25	2.16	2.09	2.04	2.00	1.96	1.94	1.89	1.84	1.79	1.77	1.74	1.71	1.68	1.64	1.61
21	2.96	2.57	2.36	2.23	2.14	2.08	2.02	1.98	1.95	1.92	1.87	1.83	1.78	1.75	1.72	1.69	1.66	1.62	1.59
22	2.95	2.56	2.35	2.22	2.13	2.06	2.01	1.97	1.93	1.90	1.86	1.81	1.76	1.73	1.70	1.67	1.64	1.60	1.57
23	2.94	2.55	2.34	2.21	2.11	2.05	1.99	1.96	1.92	1.89	1.84	1.80	1.74	1.72	1.69	1.66	1.62	1.59	1.55
24	2.93	2.54	2.33	2.19	2.10	2.04	1.98	1.94	1.91	1.88	1.83	1.78	1.73	1.70	1.67	1.64	1.61	1.57	1.53
25	2.92	2.53	2.32	2.18	2.09	2.02	1.97	1.93	1.89	1.87	1.82	1.77	1.72	1.69	1.66	1.63	1.59	1.56	1.52
26	2.91	2.52	2.31	2.17	2.08	2.01	1.96	1.92	1.88	1.86	1.81	1.76	1.71	1.68	1.65	1.61	1.58	1.54	1.50
27	2.90	2.51	2.30	2.17	2.07	2.00	1.95	1.91	1.87	1.85	1.80	1.75	1.70	1.67	1.64	1.60	1.57	1.53	1.49
28	2.89	2.50	2.29	2.16	2.06	2.00	1.94	1.90	1.87	1.84	1.79	1.74	1.69	1.66	1.63	1.59	1.56	1.52	1.48
29	2.89	2.50	2.28	2.15	2.06	1.99	1.93	1.89	1.86	1.83	1.78	1.73	1.68	1.65	1.62	1.58	1.55	1.51	1.47
30	2.88	2.49	2.28	2.14	2.03	1.98	1.93	1.88	1.85	1.82	1.77	1.72	1.67	1.64	1.61	1.57	1.54	1.50	1.46
40	2.84	2.44	2.23	2.09	2.00	1.93	1.87	1.83	1.79	1.76	1.71	1.66	1.61	1.57	1.54	1.51	1.47	1.42	1.38
60	2.79	2.39	2.18	2.04	1.95	1.87	1.82	1.77	1.74	1.71	1.66	1.60	1.54	1.51	1.48	1.44	1.40	1.35	1.29
120	2.75	2.35	2.13	1.99	1.90	1.82	1.77	1.72	1.68	1.65	1.60	1.55	1.48	1.45	1.41	1.37	1.32	1.26	1.19
∞	2.71	2.30	2.08	1.94	1.85	1.77	1.72	1.67	1.63	1.60	1.55	1.49	1.42	1.38	1.34	1.30	1.24	1.17	1.00

Note: v_1 is the degrees of freedom for the numerator and v_2 is the degrees of freedom for the denominator.

(continued)

TABLE C (continued)
F-Distribution Tables $F_{0.05}(v_1, v_2)$

v_1

v_2	1	2	3	4	5	6	7	8	9	10	12	15	20	24	30	40	60	120	∞
1	161.4	199.5	215.7	224.6	230.2	234.0	236.8	238.9	240.5	241.9	243.9	245.9	248.0	249.1	250.1	251.1	252.2	253.3	254.3
2	18.51	19.00	19.16	19.25	19.30	19.33	19.35	19.37	19.38	19.40	19.41	19.43	19.45	19.45	19.46	19.47	19.48	19.49	19.50
3	10.13	9.55	9.28	9.12	9.01	8.94	8.89	8.85	8.81	8.79	8.74	8.70	8.66	8.64	8.62	8.59	8.57	8.55	8.53
4	7.71	6.94	6.59	6.39	6.26	6.16	6.09	6.04	6.00	5.96	5.91	5.86	5.80	5.77	5.75	5.72	5.69	5.66	5.63
5	6.61	5.79	5.41	5.19	5.05	4.95	4.88	4.82	4.77	4.74	4.68	4.62	4.56	4.53	4.50	4.46	4.43	4.40	4.36
6	5.99	5.14	4.76	4.53	4.39	4.28	4.21	4.15	4.10	4.06	4.00	3.94	3.87	3.84	3.81	3.77	3.74	3.70	3.67
7	5.59	4.74	4.35	4.12	3.97	3.87	3.79	3.73	3.68	3.64	3.57	3.51	3.44	3.41	3.38	3.34	3.30	3.27	3.23
8	5.32	4.46	4.07	3.84	3.69	3.58	3.50	3.44	3.39	3.35	3.28	3.22	3.15	3.12	3.08	3.04	3.01	2.97	2.93
9	5.12	4.26	3.86	3.63	3.48	3.37	3.29	3.23	3.18	3.14	3.07	3.01	2.94	2.90	2.86	2.83	2.79	2.75	2.71
10	4.96	4.10	3.71	3.48	3.33	3.22	3.14	3.07	3.02	2.98	2.91	2.85	2.77	2.74	2.70	2.66	2.62	2.58	2.54
11	4.84	3.98	3.59	3.36	3.20	3.09	3.01	2.95	2.90	2.85	2.79	2.72	2.65	2.61	2.57	2.53	2.49	2.45	2.40
12	4.75	3.89	3.49	3.26	3.11	3.00	2.91	2.85	2.80	2.75	2.69	2.62	2.54	2.51	2.47	2.43	2.38	2.34	2.30
13	4.67	3.81	3.41	3.18	3.03	2.92	2.83	2.77	2.71	2.67	2.60	2.53	2.46	2.42	2.38	2.34	2.30	2.25	2.21
14	4.60	3.74	3.34	3.11	2.96	2.85	2.76	2.70	2.65	2.60	2.53	2.46	2.39	2.35	2.31	2.27	2.22	2.18	2.13
15	4.54	3.68	3.29	3.06	2.90	2.79	2.71	2.64	2.59	2.54	2.48	2.40	2.33	2.29	2.25	2.20	2.16	2.11	2.07

v_2																			
16	4.49	3.63	3.24	3.01	2.85	2.74	2.66	2.59	2.54	2.49	2.42	2.35	2.28	2.24	2.19	2.15	2.11	2.06	2.01
17	4.45	3.59	3.20	2.96	2.81	2.70	2.61	2.55	2.49	2.45	2.38	2.31	2.23	2.19	2.15	2.10	2.06	2.01	1.96
18	4.41	3.55	3.16	2.93	2.77	2.66	2.58	2.51	2.46	2.41	2.34	2.27	2.19	2.15	2.11	2.06	2.02	1.97	1.92
19	4.38	3.52	3.13	2.90	2.74	2.63	2.54	2.48	2.42	2.38	2.31	2.23	2.16	2.11	2.07	2.03	1.98	1.93	1.88
20	4.35	3.49	3.10	2.87	2.71	2.60	2.51	2.45	2.39	2.35	2.28	2.20	2.12	2.08	2.04	1.99	1.95	1.90	1.84
21	4.32	3.47	3.07	2.84	2.68	2.57	2.49	2.42	2.37	2.32	2.25	2.18	2.10	2.05	2.01	1.96	1.92	1.87	1.81
22	4.30	3.44	3.05	2.82	2.66	2.55	2.46	2.40	2.34	2.30	2.23	2.15	2.07	2.03	1.98	1.94	1.89	1.84	1.78
23	4.28	3.42	3.03	2.80	2.64	2.53	2.44	2.37	2.32	2.27	2.20	2.13	2.05	2.01	1.96	1.91	1.86	1.81	1.76
24	4.26	3.40	3.01	2.78	2.62	2.51	2.42	2.36	2.30	2.25	2.18	2.11	2.03	1.98	1.94	1.89	1.84	1.79	1.73
25	4.24	3.39	2.99	2.76	2.60	2.49	2.40	2.34	2.28	2.24	2.16	2.09	2.01	1.96	1.92	1.87	1.82	1.77	1.71
26	4.23	3.37	2.98	2.74	2.59	2.47	2.39	2.32	2.27	2.22	2.15	2.07	1.99	1.95	1.90	1.85	1.80	1.75	1.69
27	4.21	3.35	2.96	2.73	2.57	2.46	2.37	2.31	2.25	2.20	2.13	2.06	1.97	1.93	1.88	1.84	1.79	1.73	1.67
28	4.20	3.34	2.95	2.71	2.56	2.45	2.36	2.29	2.24	2.19	2.12	2.04	1.96	1.91	1.87	1.82	1.77	1.71	1.65
29	4.18	3.33	2.93	2.70	2.55	2.43	2.35	2.28	2.22	2.18	2.10	2.03	1.94	1.90	1.85	1.81	1.75	1.70	1.64
30	4.17	3.32	2.92	2.69	2.53	2.42	2.33	2.27	2.21	2.16	2.09	2.01	1.93	1.89	1.84	1.79	1.74	1.68	1.62
40	4.08	3.23	2.84	2.61	2.45	2.34	2.25	2.18	2.12	2.08	2.00	1.92	1.84	1.79	1.74	1.69	1.64	1.58	1.51
60	4.00	3.15	2.76	2.53	2.37	2.25	2.17	2.10	2.04	1.99	1.92	1.84	1.75	1.70	1.65	1.59	1.53	1.47	1.39
120	3.92	3.07	2.68	2.45	2.29	2.17	2.09	2.02	1.96	1.91	1.83	1.75	1.66	1.61	1.55	1.55	1.43	1.35	1.25
∞	3.84	3.00	2.60	2.37	2.21	2.10	2.01	1.94	1.88	1.83	1.75	1.67	1.57	1.52	1.46	1.39	1.32	1.22	1.00

Note: v_1 is the degrees of freedom for the numerator and v_2 is the degrees of freedom for the denominator.

(continued)

TABLE C (continued)
F-Distribution Tables $F_{0.025}(v_1, v_2)$

v_2	v_1																		
	1	2	3	4	5	6	7	8	9	10	12	15	20	24	30	40	60	120	∞
1	647.8	799.5	864.2	899.6	921.8	937.1	948.2	956.7	963.3	968.6	976.7	984.9	993.1	997.2	1001	1006	1010	1014	1018
2	38.51	39.00	39.17	39.25	39.30	39.33	39.36	39.37	39.39	39.40	39.41	39.43	39.45	39.46	39.46	39.47	39.48	39.49	39.50
3	17.44	16.04	15.44	15.10	14.88	14.73	14.62	14.54	14.47	14.42	14.34	14.25	14.17	14.12	14.08	14.04	13.99	13.95	13.90
4	12.22	10.65	9.98	9.60	9.36	9.20	9.07	8.98	8.90	8.84	8.75	8.66	8.56	8.51	8.46	8.41	8.36	8.31	8.26
5	10.01	8.43	7.76	7.39	7.15	6.98	6.85	6.76	6.68	6.62	6.52	6.43	6.33	6.28	6.23	6.18	6.12	6.07	6.02
6	8.81	7.26	6.60	6.23	5.99	5.82	5.70	5.60	5.52	5.46	5.37	5.27	5.17	5.12	5.07	5.01	4.96	4.90	4.85
7	8.07	6.54	5.89	5.52	5.29	5.12	4.99	4.90	4.82	4.76	4.67	4.57	4.47	4.42	4.36	4.31	4.25	4.20	4.14
8	7.57	6.06	5.42	5.05	4.82	4.65	4.53	4.43	4.36	4.30	4.20	4.10	4.00	3.95	3.89	3.84	3.78	3.73	3.67
9	7.21	5.71	5.08	4.72	4.48	4.32	4.20	4.10	4.03	3.96	3.87	3.77	3.67	3.61	3.56	3.51	3.45	3.39	3.33
10	6.94	5.46	4.83	4.47	4.24	4.07	3.95	3.85	3.78	3.72	3.62	3.52	3.42	3.37	3.31	3.26	3.20	3.14	3.08
11	6.72	5.26	4.63	4.28	4.04	3.88	3.76	3.66	3.59	3.53	3.43	3.33	3.23	3.17	3.12	3.06	3.00	2.94	2.88
12	6.55	5.10	4.47	4.12	3.89	3.73	3.61	3.51	3.44	3.37	3.28	3.18	3.07	3.02	2.96	2.91	2.85	2.79	2.72
13	6.41	4.97	4.35	4.00	3.77	3.60	3.48	3.39	3.31	3.25	3.15	3.05	2.95	2.89	2.84	2.78	2.72	2.66	2.60
14	6.30	4.86	4.24	3.89	3.66	3.50	3.38	3.29	3.21	3.15	3.05	2.95	2.84	2.79	2.73	2.67	2.61	2.55	2.49

v_2																			
15	6.20	4.77	4.15	3.80	3.58	3.41	3.29	3.20	3.12	3.06	2.96	2.86	2.76	2.70	2.64	2.59	2.52	2.46	2.40
16	6.12	4.69	4.08	3.73	3.50	3.34	3.22	3.12	3.05	2.99	2.89	2.79	2.68	2.63	2.57	2.51	2.45	2.38	2.32
17	6.04	4.62	4.01	3.66	3.44	3.28	3.16	3.06	2.98	2.92	2.82	2.72	2.62	2.56	2.50	2.44	2.38	2.32	2.25
18	5.98	4.56	3.95	3.61	3.38	3.22	3.10	3.01	2.93	2.87	2.77	2.67	2.56	2.50	2.44	2.38	2.32	2.26	2.19
19	5.92	4.51	3.90	3.56	3.33	3.17	3.05	2.96	2.88	2.82	2.72	2.62	2.51	2.45	2.39	2.33	2.27	2.20	2.13
20	5.87	4.46	3.86	3.51	3.29	3.13	3.01	2.91	2.84	2.77	2.68	2.57	2.46	2.41	2.35	2.29	2.22	2.16	2.09
21	5.83	4.42	3.82	3.48	3.25	3.09	2.97	2.87	2.80	2.73	2.64	2.53	2.42	2.37	2.31	2.25	2.18	2.11	2.04
22	5.79	4.38	3.78	3.44	3.22	3.05	2.93	2.84	2.76	2.70	2.60	2.50	2.39	2.33	2.27	2.21	2.14	2.08	2.00
23	5.75	4.35	3.75	3.41	3.18	3.02	2.90	2.81	2.73	2.67	2.57	2.47	2.36	2.30	2.24	2.18	2.11	2.04	1.97
24	5.72	4.32	3.72	3.38	3.15	2.99	2.87	2.78	2.70	2.64	2.54	2.44	2.33	2.27	2.21	2.15	2.08	2.01	1.94
25	5.69	4.29	3.69	3.35	3.13	2.97	2.85	2.75	2.68	2.61	2.51	2.41	2.30	2.24	2.18	2.12	2.05	1.98	1.91
26	5.66	4.27	3.67	3.33	3.10	2.94	2.82	2.73	2.65	2.59	2.49	2.39	2.28	2.22	2.16	2.09	2.03	1.95	1.88
27	5.63	4.24	3.65	3.31	3.08	2.92	2.80	2.71	2.63	2.57	2.47	2.36	2.25	2.19	2.13	2.07	2.00	1.93	1.85
28	5.61	4.22	3.63	3.29	3.06	2.90	2.78	2.69	2.61	2.55	2.45	2.34	2.23	2.17	2.11	2.05	1.98	1.91	1.83
29	5.59	4.20	1.61	3.27	3.04	2.88	2.76	2.67	2.59	2.53	2.43	2.32	2.21	2.15	2.09	2.03	1.96	1.89	1.81
30	5.57	4.18	3.59	3.25	3.03	2.87	2.75	2.65	2.57	2.51	2.41	2.31	2.20	2.14	2.07	2.01	1.94	1.87	1.79
40	5.42	4.05	3.46	3.13	2.90	2.74	2.62	2.53	2.45	2.39	2.29	2.18	2.07	2.01	1.94	1.88	1.80	1.72	1.64
60	5.29	3.93	3.34	3.01	2.79	2.63	2.51	2.41	2.33	2.27	2.17	2.06	1.94	1.88	1.82	1.74	1.67	1.58	1.48
120	5.15	3.80	3.23	2.89	2.67	2.52	2.39	2.30	2.22	2.16	2.05	1.94	1.82	1.76	1.69	1.61	1.53	1.43	1.31
∞	5.02	3.69	3.12	2.79	2.57	2.41	2.29	2.19	2.11	2.05	1.94	1.83	1.71	1.64	1.57	1.48	1.39	1.27	1.00

Note: v_1 is the degrees of freedom for the numerator and v_2 is the degrees of freedom for the denominator.

(continued)

TABLE C (continued)
F-Distribution Tables $F_{0.01(v_1, v_2)}$

v_1

v_2	1	2	3	4	5	6	7	8	9	10	12	15	20	24	30	40	60	120	∞
1	4052	4999.5	5403	5625	5764	5859	5928	5982	6022	6056	6106	6157	6209	6235	6261	6287	6313	6339	6366
2	98.50	99.00	99.17	99.25	99.30	99.33	99.36	99.37	99.39	99.40	99.42	99.43	99.45	99.46	99.47	99.47	99.48	99.49	99.50
3	34.12	30.82	29.46	28.71	28.24	27.91	27.67	27.49	27.35	27.23	27.05	26.87	26.69	26.00	26.50	26.41	26.32	26.22	26.13
4	21.20	18.00	16.69	15.98	15.52	15.21	14.98	14.80	14.66	14.55	14.37	14.20	14.02	13.93	13.84	13.75	13.65	13.56	13.46
5	16.26	13.27	12.06	11.39	10.97	10.67	10.46	10.29	10.16	10.05	9.89	9.72	9.55	9.47	9.38	9.29	9.20	9.11	9.02
6	13.75	10.92	9.78	9.15	8.75	8.47	8.26	8.10	7.98	7.87	7.72	7.56	7.40	7.31	7.23	7.14	7.06	6.97	6.88
7	12.25	9.55	8.45	7.85	7.46	7.19	6.99	6.84	6.72	6.62	6.47	6.31	6.16	6.07	5.99	5.91	5.82	5.74	5.65
8	11.26	8.65	7.59	7.01	6.63	6.37	6.18	6.03	5.91	5.81	5.67	5.52	5.36	5.28	5.20	5.12	5.03	4.95	4.86
9	10.56	8.02	6.99	6.42	6.06	5.80	5.61	5.47	5.35	5.26	5.11	4.96	4.81	4.73	4.65	4.57	4.48	4.40	4.31
10	10.04	7.56	6.55	5.99	5.64	5.39	5.20	5.06	4.94	4.85	4.71	4.56	4.41	4.33	4.25	4.17	4.08	4.00	3.91
11	9.65	7.21	6.22	5.67	5.32	5.07	4.89	4.74	4.63	4.54	4.40	4.25	4.10	4.02	3.94	3.86	3.78	3.69	3.60
12	9.33	6.93	5.95	5.41	5.06	4.82	4.64	4.50	4.39	4.30	4.16	4.01	3.86	3.78	3.70	3.62	3.54	3.45	3.36
13	9.07	6.70	5.74	5.21	4.86	4.62	4.44	4.30	4.19	4.10	3.96	3.82	3.66	3.59	3.51	3.43	3.34	3.25	3.17
14	8.86	6.51	5.56	5.04	4.69	4.46	4.28	4.14	4.03	3.94	3.80	3.66	3.51	3.43	3.35	3.27	3.18	3.09	3.00
15	8.68	6.36	5.42	4.89	4.36	4.32	4.14	4.00	3.89	3.80	3.67	3.52	3.37	3.29	3.21	3.13	3.05	2.96	2.87

16	8.53	6.23	5.29	4.77	4.44	4.20	4.03	3.89	3.78	3.69	3.55	3.41	3.26	3.18	3.10	3.02	2.93	2.84	2.75
17	8.40	6.11	5.18	4.67	4.34	4.10	3.93	3.79	3.68	3.59	3.46	3.31	3.16	3.08	3.00	2.92	2.83	2.75	2.65
18	8.29	6.01	5.09	4.58	4.25	4.01	3.84	3.71	3.60	3.51	3.37	3.23	3.08	3.00	2.92	2.84	2.75	2.66	2.57
19	8.18	5.93	5.01	4.50	4.17	3.94	3.77	3.63	3.52	3.43	3.30	3.15	3.00	2.92	2.84	2.76	2.67	2.58	2.49
20	8.10	5.85	4.94	4.43	4.10	3.87	3.70	3.56	3.46	3.37	3.23	3.09	2.94	2.86	2.78	2.69	2.61	2.52	2.42
21	8.02	5.78	4.87	4.37	4.04	3.81	3.64	3.51	3.40	3.31	3.17	3.03	2.88	2.80	2.72	2.64	2.55	2.46	2.36
22	7.95	5.72	4.82	4.31	3.99	3.76	3.59	3.45	3.35	3.26	3.12	2.98	2.83	2.75	2.67	2.58	2.50	2.40	2.31
23	7.88	5.66	4.76	4.26	3.94	3.71	3.54	3.41	3.30	3.21	3.07	2.93	2.78	2.70	2.62	2.54	2.45	2.35	2.26
24	7.82	5.61	4.72	4.22	3.90	3.67	3.50	3.36	3.26	3.17	3.03	2.89	2.74	2.66	2.58	2.49	2.40	2.31	2.21
25	7.77	5.57	4.68	4.18	3.85	3.63	3.46	3.32	3.22	3.13	2.99	2.85	2.70	2.62	2.54	2.45	2.36	2.27	2.17
26	7.72	5.53	4.64	4.14	3.82	3.59	3.42	3.29	3.18	3.09	2.96	2.81	2.66	2.58	2.50	2.42	2.33	2.23	2.13
27	7.68	5.49	4.60	4.11	3.78	3.56	3.39	3.26	3.15	3.06	2.93	2.78	2.63	2.55	2.47	2.38	2.29	2.20	2.10
28	7.64	5.45	4.57	4.07	3.75	3.53	3.36	3.23	3.12	3.03	2.90	2.75	2.60	2.52	2.44	2.35	2.26	2.17	2.06
29	7.60	5.42	4.54	4.04	3.73	3.50	3.33	3.20	3.09	3.00	2.87	2.73	2.57	2.49	2.41	2.33	2.23	2.14	2.03
30	7.56	5.39	4.51	4.02	3.70	3.47	3.30	3.17	3.07	2.98	2.84	2.70	2.55	2.47	2.39	2.30	2.21	2.11	2.01
40	7.31	5.18	4.31	3.83	3.51	3.29	3.12	2.99	2.89	2.80	2.66	2.52	2.37	2.29	2.20	2.11	2.02	1.92	1.80
60	7.08	4.98	4.13	3.65	3.34	3.12	2.95	2.82	2.72	2.63	2.50	2.35	2.20	2.12	2.03	1.94	1.84	1.73	1.60
120	6.85	4.79	3.95	3.48	3.17	2.96	2.79	2.66	2.56	2.47	2.34	2.19	2.03	1.95	1.86	1.76	1.66	1.53	1.38
∞	6.63	4.61	3.78	3.32	3.02	2.80	2.64	2.51	2.41	2.32	2.18	2.04	1.88	1.79	1.70	1.59	1.47	1.32	1.00

Note: v_1 is the degrees of freedom for the numerator and v_2 is the degrees of freedom for the denominator.

TABLE D
Power Values for Two-Sided *t*-Test

Level of Significance $\alpha = 0.05$

					δ				
df	1.0	2.0	3.0	4.0	5.0	6.0	7.0	8.0	9.0
1	0.07	0.13	0.19	0.25	0.31	0.36	0.42	0.47	0.52
2	0.10	0.22	0.39	0.56	0.72	0.84	0.91	0.96	0.98
3	0.11	0.29	0.53	0.75	0.90	0.97	0.99	1.00	1.00
4	0.12	0.34	0.62	0.84	0.95	0.99	1.00	1.00	1.00
5	0.13	0.37	0.67	0.89	0.98	1.00	1.00	1.00	1.00
6	0.14	0.39	0.71	0.91	0.98	1.00	1.00	1.00	1.00
7	0.14	0.41	0.73	0.93	0.99	1.00	1.00	1.00	1.00
8	0.14	0.42	0.75	0.94	0.99	1.00	1.00	1.00	1.00
9	0.15	0.43	0.76	0.94	0.99	1.00	1.00	1.00	1.00
10	0.15	0.44	0.77	0.95	0.99	1.00	1.00	1.00	1.00
11	0.15	0.45	0.78	0.95	0.99	1.00	1.00	1.00	1.00
12	0.15	0.45	0.79	0.96	1.00	1.00	1.00	1.00	1.00
13	0.15	0.46	0.79	0.96	1.00	1.00	1.00	1.00	1.00
14	0.15	0.46	0.80	0.96	1.00	1.00	1.00	1.00	1.00
15	0.16	0.46	0.80	0.96	1.00	1.00	1.00	1.00	1.00
16	0.16	0.47	0.80	0.96	1.00	1.00	1.00	1.00	1.00
17	0.16	0.47	0.81	0.96	1.00	1.00	1.00	1.00	1.00
18	0.16	0.47	0.81	0.97	1.00	1.00	1.00	1.00	1.00
19	0.16	0.48	0.81	0.97	1.00	1.00	1.00	1.00	1.00
20	0.16	0.48	0.81	0.97	1.00	1.00	1.00	1.00	1.00
21	0.16	0.48	0.82	0.97	1.00	1.00	1.00	1.00	1.00
22	0.16	0.48	0.82	0.97	1.00	1.00	1.00	1.00	1.00
23	0.16	0.48	0.82	0.97	1.00	1.00	1.00	1.00	1.00
24	0.16	0.48	0.82	0.97	1.00	1.00	1.00	1.00	1.00
25	0.16	0.49	0.82	0.97	1.00	1.00	1.00	1.00	1.00
26	0.16	0.49	0.82	0.97	1.00	1.00	1.00	1.00	1.00
27	0.16	0.49	0.82	0.97	1.00	1.00	1.00	1.00	1.00
28	0.16	0.49	0.83	0.97	1.00	1.00	1.00	1.00	1.00
29	0.16	0.49	0.83	0.97	1.00	1.00	1.00	1.00	1.00
30	0.16	0.49	0.83	0.97	1.00	1.00	1.00	1.00	1.00
40	0.16	0.50	0.83	0.97	1.00	1.00	1.00	1.00	1.00
50	0.17	0.50	0.84	0.98	1.00	1.00	1.00	1.00	1.00
60	0.17	0.50	0.84	0.98	1.00	1.00	1.00	1.00	1.00
100	0.17	0.51	0.84	0.98	1.00	1.00	1.00	1.00	1.00
120	0.17	0.51	0.85	0.98	1.00	1.00	1.00	1.00	1.00
∞	0.17	0.52	0.85	0.98	1.00	1.00	1.00	1.00	1.00

(continued)

TABLE D (continued)
Power Values for Two-Sided *t*-Test

Level of Significance $\alpha = 0.01$

δ

df	1.0	2.0	3.0	4.0	5.0	6.0	7.0	8.0	9.0
1	0.01	0.03	0.04	0.05	0.06	0.08	0.09	0.10	0.11
2	0.02	0.05	0.09	0.16	0.23	0.31	0.39	0.48	0.56
3	0.02	0.08	0.17	0.31	0.47	0.62	0.75	0.85	0.92
4	0.03	0.10	0.25	0.45	0.65	0.82	0.92	0.97	0.99
5	0.03	0.12	0.31	0.55	0.77	0.91	0.97	0.99	1.00
6	0.04	0.14	0.36	0.63	0.84	0.95	0.99	1.00	1.00
7	0.04	0.16	0.40	0.68	0.88	0.97	1.00	1.00	1.00
8	0.04	0.17	0.43	0.72	0.91	0.98	1.00	1.00	1.00
9	0.04	0.18	0.45	0.75	0.93	0.99	1.00	1.00	1.00
10	0.04	0.19	0.47	0.77	0.94	0.99	1.00	1.00	1.00
11	0.04	0.19	0.49	0.79	0.95	0.99	1.00	1.00	1.00
12	0.04	0.20	0.50	0.80	0.96	0.99	1.00	1.00	1.00
13	0.05	0.21	0.52	0.82	0.96	1.00	1.00	1.00	1.00
14	0.05	0.21	0.53	0.83	0.96	1.00	1.00	1.00	1.00
15	0.05	0.21	0.54	0.83	0.97	1.00	1.00	1.00	1.00
16	0.05	0.22	0.55	0.84	0.97	1.00	1.00	1.00	1.00
17	0.05	0.22	0.55	0.85	0.97	1.00	1.00	1.00	1.00
18	0.05	0.22	0.56	0.85	0.97	1.00	1.00	1.00	1.00
19	0.05	0.23	0.56	0.86	0.98	1.00	1.00	1.00	1.00
20	0.05	0.23	0.57	0.86	0.98	1.00	1.00	1.00	1.00
21	0.05	0.23	0.57	0.86	0.98	1.00	1.00	1.00	1.00
22	0.05	0.23	0.58	0.87	0.98	1.00	1.00	1.00	1.00
23	0.05	0.24	0.58	0.87	0.98	1.00	1.00	1.00	1.00
24	0.05	0.24	0.59	0.87	0.98	1.00	1.00	1.00	1.00
25	0.05	0.24	0.59	0.88	0.98	1.00	1.00	1.00	1.00
26	0.05	0.24	0.59	0.88	0.98	1.00	1.00	1.00	1.00
27	0.05	0.24	0.59	0.88	0.98	1.00	1.00	1.00	1.00
28	0.05	0.24	0.60	0.88	0.98	1.00	1.00	1.00	1.00
29	0.05	0.25	0.60	0.88	0.98	1.00	1.00	1.00	1.00
30	0.05	0.25	0.60	0.88	0.98	1.00	1.00	1.00	1.00
40	0.05	0.26	0.62	0.90	0.99	1.00	1.00	1.00	1.00
50	0.05	0.26	0.63	0.90	0.99	1.00	1.00	1.00	1.00
60	0.05	0.26	0.63	0.91	0.99	1.00	1.00	1.00	1.00
100	0.06	0.27	0.65	0.91	0.99	1.00	1.00	1.00	1.00
120	0.06	0.27	0.65	0.91	0.99	1.00	1.00	1.00	1.00
∞	0.06	0.28	0.66	0.92	0.99	1.00	1.00	1.00	1.00

TABLE E
Durbin–Watson Test Bounds

Level of Significance $\alpha = 0.05$

n	$p-1=1$ d_L	d_U	$p-1=2$ d_L	d_U	$p-1=3$ d_L	d_U	$p-1=4$ d_L	d_U	$p-1=5$ d_L	d_U
15	1.08	1.36	0.95	1.54	0.82	1.75	0.69	1.97	0.56	2.21
16	1.10	1.37	0.98	1.54	0.86	1.73	0.74	1.93	0.62	2.15
17	1.13	1.38	1.02	1.54	0.90	1.71	0.78	1.90	0.67	2.10
18	1.16	1.39	1.05	1.53	0.93	1.69	0.82	1.87	0.71	2.06
19	1.18	1.40	1.08	1.53	0.97	1.68	0.86	1.85	0.75	2.02
20	1.20	1.41	1.10	1.54	1.00	1.68	0.90	1.83	0.79	1.99
21	1.22	1.42	1.13	1.54	1.03	1.67	0.93	1.81	0.83	1.96
22	1.24	1.43	1.15	1.54	1.05	1.66	0.96	1.80	0.86	1.94
23	1.26	1.44	1.17	1.54	1.08	1.66	0.99	1.79	0.90	1.92
24	1.27	1.45	1.19	1.55	1.10	1.66	1.01	1.78	0.93	1.90
25	1.29	1.45	1.21	1.55	1.12	1.66	1.04	1.77	0.95	1.89
26	1.30	1.46	1.22	1.55	1.14	1.65	1.06	1.76	0.98	1.88
27	1.32	1.47	1.24	1.56	1.16	1.65	1.08	1.76	1.01	1.86
28	1.33	1.48	1.26	1.56	1.18	1.65	1.10	1.75	1.03	1.85
29	1.34	1.48	1.27	1.56	1.20	1.65	1.12	1.74	1.05	1.84
30	1.35	1.49	1.28	1.57	1.21	1.65	1.14	1.74	1.07	1.83
31	1.36	1.50	1.30	1.57	1.23	1.65	1.16	1.74	1.09	1.83
32	1.37	1.50	1.31	1.57	1.24	1.65	1.18	1.73	1.11	1.82
33	1.38	1.51	1.32	1.58	1.26	1.65	1.19	1.73	1.13	1.81
34	1.39	1.51	1.33	1.58	1.27	1.65	1.21	1.73	1.15	1.81
35	1.40	1.52	1.34	1.58	1.28	1.65	1.22	1.73	1.16	1.80
36	1.41	1.52	1.35	1.59	1.29	1.65	1.24	1.73	1.18	1.80
37	1.42	1.53	1.36	1.59	1.31	1.66	1.25	1.72	1.19	1.80
38	1.43	1.54	1.37	1.59	1.32	1.66	1.26	1.72	1.21	1.79
39	1.43	1.54	1.38	1.60	1.33	1.66	1.27	1.72	1.22	1.79
40	1.44	1.54	1.39	1.60	1.34	1.66	1.29	1.72	1.23	1.79
45	1.48	1.57	1.43	1.62	1.38	1.67	1.34	1.72	1.29	1.78
50	1.50	1.59	1.46	1.63	1.42	1.67	1.38	1.72	1.34	1.77
55	1.53	1.60	1.49	1.64	1.45	1.68	1.41	1.72	1.38	1.77
60	1.55	1.62	1.51	1.65	1.48	1.69	1.44	1.73	1.41	1.77
65	1.57	1.63	1.54	1.66	1.50	1.70	1.47	1.73	1.44	1.77
70	1.58	1.64	1.55	1.67	1.52	1.70	1.49	1.74	1.46	1.77
75	1.60	1.65	1.57	1.68	1.54	1.71	1.51	1.74	1.49	1.77
80	1.61	1.66	1.59	1.69	1.56	1.72	1.53	1.74	1.51	1.77
85	1.62	1.67	1.60	1.70	1.57	1.72	1.55	1.75	1.52	1.77
90	1.63	1.68	1.61	1.70	1.59	1.73	1.57	1.75	1.54	1.78
95	1.64	1.69	1.62	1.71	1.60	1.73	1.58	1.75	1.56	1.78
100	1.65	1.69	1.63	1.72	1.61	1.74	1.59	1.76	1.57	1.78

(*continued*)

TABLE E (continued)
Durbin–Watson Test Bounds

Level of Significance $\alpha = 0.01$

n	$p-1=1$		$p-1=2$		$p-1=3$		$p-1=4$		$p-1=5$	
	d_L	d_U	d_L	d_U	d_L	d_U	d_L	d_U	d_L	d_U
15	0.81	1.07	0.70	1.25	0.59	1.46	0.49	1.70	0.39	1.96
16	0.84	1.09	0.74	1.25	0.63	1.44	0.53	1.66	0.44	1.90
17	0.87	1.10	0.77	1.25	0.67	1.43	0.57	1.63	0.48	1.85
18	0.90	1.12	0.80	1.26	0.71	1.42	0.61	1.60	0.52	1.80
19	0.93	1.13	0.83	1.26	0.74	1.41	0.65	1.58	0.56	1.77
20	0.95	1.15	0.86	1.27	0.77	1.41	0.68	1.57	0.60	1.74
21	0.97	1.16	0.89	1.27	0.80	1.41	0.72	1.55	0.63	1.71
22	1.00	1.17	0.91	1.28	0.83	1.40	0.75	1.54	0.66	1.69
23	1.02	1.19	0.94	1.29	0.86	1.40	0.77	1.53	0.70	1.67
24	1.04	1.20	0.96	1.30	0.88	1.41	0.80	1.53	0.72	1.66
25	1.05	1.21	0.98	1.30	0.90	1.41	0.83	1.52	0.75	1.65
26	1.07	1.22	1.00	1.31	0.93	1.41	0.85	1.52	0.78	1.64
27	1.09	1.23	1.02	1.32	0.95	1.41	0.88	1.51	0.81	1.63
28	1.10	1.24	1.04	1.32	0.97	1.41	0.90	1.51	0.83	1.62
29	1.12	1.25	1.05	1.33	0.99	1.42	0.92	1.51	0.85	1.61
30	1.13	1.26	1.07	1.34	1.01	1.42	0.94	1.51	0.88	1.61
31	1.15	1.27	1.08	1.34	1.02	1.42	0.96	1.51	0.90	1.60
32	1.16	1.28	1.10	1.35	1.04	1.43	0.98	1.51	0.92	1.60
33	1.17	1.29	1.11	1.36	1.05	1.43	1.00	1.51	0.94	1.59
34	1.18	1.30	1.13	1.36	1.07	1.43	1.01	1.51	0.95	1.59
35	1.19	1.31	1.14	1.37	1.08	1.44	1.03	1.51	0.97	1.59
36	1.21	1.32	1.15	1.38	1.10	1.44	1.04	1.51	0.99	1.59
37	1.22	1.32	1.16	1.38	1.11	1.45	1.06	1.51	1.00	1.59
38	1.23	1.33	1.18	1.39	1.12	1.45	1.07	1.52	1.02	1.58
39	1.24	1.34	1.19	1.39	1.14	1.45	1.09	1.52	1.03	1.58
40	1.25	1.34	1.20	1.40	1.15	1.46	1.10	1.52	1.05	1.58
45	1.29	1.38	1.24	1.42	1.20	1.48	1.16	1.53	1.11	1.58
50	1.32	1.40	1.28	1.45	1.24	1.49	1.20	1.54	1.16	1.59
55	1.36	1.43	1.32	1.47	1.28	1.51	1.25	1.55	1.21	1.59
60	1.38	1.45	1.35	1.48	1.32	1.52	1.28	1.56	1.25	1.60
65	1.41	1.47	1.38	1.50	1.35	1.53	1.31	1.57	1.28	1.61
70	1.43	1.49	1.40	1.52	1.37	1.55	1.34	1.58	1.31	1.61
75	1.45	1.50	1.42	1.53	1.39	1.56	1.37	1.59	1.34	1.62
80	1.47	1.52	1.44	1.54	1.42	1.57	1.39	1.60	1.36	1.62
85	1.48	1.53	1.46	1.55	1.43	1.58	1.41	1.60	1.39	1.63
90	1.50	1.54	1.47	1.56	1.45	1.59	1.43	1.61	1.41	1.64
95	1.51	1.55	1.49	1.57	1.47	1.60	1.45	1.62	1.42	1.64
100	1.52	1.56	1.50	1.58	1.48	1.60	1.46	1.63	1.44	1.65

TABLE F
Bonferroni Corrected Jackknife Residual Critical Values

Level of Significance $\alpha = 0.1$

k	n = 5	10	15	20	25	50	100	200	400	800
1	6.96	3.50	3.27	3.22	3.21	3.27	3.39	3.54	3.70	3.86
2	31.82	3.71	3.33	3.25	3.23	3.28	3.39	3.54	3.70	3.86
3		4.03	3.41	3.29	3.25	3.28	3.40	3.54	3.70	3.86
4		4.60	3.51	3.33	3.27	3.29	3.40	3.54	3.70	3.86
5		5.84	3.63	3.37	3.30	3.29	3.40	3.54	3.70	3.86
6		9.92	3.81	3.43	3.33	3.30	3.40	3.54	3.70	3.86
7		63.66	4.06	3.50	3.36	3.30	3.40	3.54	3.70	3.86
8			4.46	3.58	3.39	3.31	3.40	3.54	3.70	3.86
9			5.17	3.69	3.44	3.31	3.40	3.54	3.70	3.86
10			6.74	3.83	3.49	3.32	3.40	3.54	3.70	3.86
15			7.45	3.99	3.36	3.41	3.54	3.70	3.86	
20				8.05	3.41	3.42	3.55	3.70	3.86	
40					4.50	3.47	3.55	3.70	3.86	
80						3.92	3.58	3.70	3.86	

Level of Significance $\alpha = 0.05$

k	n = 5	10	15	20	25	50	100	200	400	800
1	9.92	4.03	3.65	3.54	3.50	3.51	3.60	3.73	3.87	4.02
2	63.66	4.32	3.73	3.58	3.53	3.51	3.60	3.73	3.87	4.02
3		4.77	3.83	3.62	3.55	3.52	3.60	3.73	3.87	4.02
4		5.60	3.95	3.67	3.58	3.53	3.61	3.73	3.87	4.02
5		7.45	4.12	3.73	3.61	3.53	3.61	3.73	3.87	4.02
6		14.09	4.36	3.81	3.65	3.54	3.61	3.73	3.87	4.02
7		127.32	4.70	3.89	3.69	3.54	3.61	3.73	3.88	4.02
8			5.25	4.00	3.73	3.55	3.61	3.73	3.88	4.02
9			6.25	4.15	3.79	3.56	3.61	3.73	3.88	4.02
10			8.58	4.33	3.85	3.57	3.61	3.73	3.88	4.02
15			9.46	4.50	3.61	3.62	3.74	3.88	4.03	
20				10.21	3.67	3.63	3.74	3.88	4.03	
40					5.04	3.69	3.75	3.88	4.03	
80						4.23	3.78	3.88	4.03	

Level of Significance $\alpha = 0.01$

k	n = 5	10	15	20	25	50	100	200	400	800
1	22.33	5.41	4.55	4.29	4.17	4.03	4.06	4.15	4.27	4.40
2	318.31	5.96	4.68	4.35	4.20	4.04	4.06	4.15	4.27	4.40
3		6.87	4.85	4.42	4.24	4.05	4.06	4.15	4.27	4.40
4		8.61	5.08	4.50	4.28	4.06	4.06	4.15	4.27	4.40
5		12.92	5.37	4.60	4.33	4.07	4.07	4.15	4.27	4.40
6		31.60	5.80	4.72	4.39	4.07	4.07	4.15	4.27	4.40
7		636.62	6.43	4.86	4.45	4.08	4.07	4.15	4.27	4.40

(continued)

TABLE F (continued)
Bonferroni Corrected Jackknife Residual Critical Values

Level of Significance $\alpha = 0.1$

k	n = 5	10	15	20	25	50	100	200	400	800
8			7.50	5.05	4.53	4.09	4.07	4.15	4.27	4.40
9			9.57	5.29	4.62	4.10	4.07	4.15	4.27	4.40
10			14.82	5.62	4.72	4.12	4.08	4.15	4.27	4.40
15				16.33	5.81	4.18	4.09	4.15	4.27	4.40
20					17.60	4.28	4.10	4.16	4.27	4.40
40						6.44	4.18	4.17	4.27	4.40
80							4.97	4.21	4.28	4.40

TABLE G
Bonferroni Corrected Studentized Residual Critical Values

Level of Significance $\alpha = 0.1$

k	n = 5	10	15	20	25	50	100	200	400	800
1	1.70	2.26	2.48	2.61	2.71	2.98	3.23	3.44	3.64	3.82
2	1.41	2.21	2.46	2.60	2.70	2.98	3.22	3.44	3.64	3.82
3		2.14	2.43	2.59	2.69	2.98	3.22	3.44	3.64	3.82
4		2.05	2.40	2.57	2.69	2.98	3.22	3.44	3.64	3.82
5		1.92	2.37	2.56	2.68	2.98	3.22	3.44	3.64	3.82
6		1.71	2.32	2.54	2.66	2.97	3.22	3.44	3.64	3.82
7		1.41	2.27	2.51	2.65	2.97	3.22	3.44	3.64	3.82
8			2.19	2.49	2.64	2.97	3.22	3.44	3.64	3.82
9			2.09	2.45	2.62	2.96	3.22	3.44	3.64	3.82
10			1.94	2.41	2.60	2.96	3.22	3.44	3.64	3.82
15				1.95	2.45	2.94	3.21	3.44	3.64	3.82
20					1.96	2.92	3.21	3.44	3.64	3.82
40						2.54	3.18	3.43	3.64	3.82
80							2.96	3.41	3.63	3.82

Level of Significance $\alpha = 0.05$

k	n = 5	10	15	20	25	50	100	200	400	800
1	1.71	2.36	2.61	2.77	2.87	3.16	3.40	3.61	3.81	3.99
2	1.41	2.30	2.59	2.75	2.86	3.15	3.40	3.61	3.81	3.99
3		2.22	2.56	2.73	2.85	3.15	3.40	3.61	3.81	3.99
4		2.11	2.52	2.71	2.84	3.15	3.40	3.61	3.81	3.99
5		1.95	2.47	2.69	2.82	3.15	3.40	3.61	3.81	3.99
6		1.72	2.42	2.67	2.81	3.14	3.40	3.61	3.81	3.99
7		1.41	2.35	2.64	2.79	3.14	3.40	3.61	3.81	3.99
8			2.25	2.60	2.78	3.13	3.39	3.61	3.81	3.99
9			2.13	2.56	2.76	3.13	3.39	3.61	3.81	3.99
10			1.96	2.51	2.73	3.13	3.39	3.61	3.81	3.99
15				1.97	2.54	3.10	3.39	3.61	3.81	3.99

(continued)

TABLE G (continued)
Bonferroni Corrected Jackknife Residual Critical Values

Level of Significance $\alpha = 0.05$

k	n = 5	10	15	20	25	50	100	200	400	800
20					1.97	3.07	3.38	3.61	3.81	3.99
40						2.62	3.35	3.60	3.80	3.99
80							3.08	3.58	3.80	3.99

Level of Significance $\alpha = 0.01$

k	n = 5	10	15	20	25	50	100	200	400	800
1	1.73	2.54	2.87	3.06	3.19	3.51	3.77	3.99	4.18	4.35
2	1.41	2.45	2.83	3.03	3.17	3.51	3.77	3.99	4.18	4.35
3		2.33	2.78	3.01	3.15	3.51	3.77	3.99	4.18	4.35
4		2.18	2.72	2.98	3.14	3.50	3.77	3.99	4.18	4.35
5		1.98	2.65	2.94	3.11	3.50	3.77	3.99	4.18	4.35
6		1.73	2.57	2.91	3.09	3.49	3.77	3.99	4.18	4.35
7		1.41	2.47	2.86	3.07	3.49	3.76	3.99	4.18	4.35
8			2.35	2.81	3.04	3.48	3.76	3.98	4.18	4.35
9			2.19	2.75	3.01	3.47	3.76	3.98	4.18	4.35
10			1.99	2.68	2.97	3.47	3.76	3.98	4.17	4.35
15				1.99	2.70	3.43	3.75	3.98	4.17	4.35
20					1.99	3.38	3.74	3.98	4.17	4.35
40						2.75	3.69	3.97	4.17	4.35
80							3.31	3.94	4.17	4.34

TABLE H
Critical Values for Leverages, n = Sample Size, k = Number of Predictors

Level of Significance α = 0.10

n	k=1	2	3	4	5	6	7	8	9	10	15	20	40	80
10	0.626	0.759	0.847	0.911	0.956	0.984	0.997	1.000						
15	0.481	0.595	0.679	0.748	0.806	0.855	0.897	0.932	0.959	0.980	0.988			
20	0.394	0.491	0.565	0.627	0.682	0.731	0.775	0.815	0.851	0.883	0.918	0.992		
25	0.335	0.419	0.484	0.540	0.589	0.635	0.676	0.715	0.751	0.784	0.837	0.937		
30	0.293	0.366	0.424	0.474	0.519	0.560	0.599	0.635	0.669	0.701	0.701	0.806		
40	0.236	0.295	0.342	0.383	0.420	0.455	0.487	0.518	0.547	0.576	0.524	0.612	0.888	
60	0.172	0.214	0.248	0.279	0.306	0.332	0.356	0.380	0.402	0.424	0.418	0.491	0.737	
80	0.137	0.170	0.197	0.221	0.242	0.263	0.283	0.301	0.319	0.337	0.348	0.410	0.625	0.941
100	0.114	0.141	0.164	0.183	0.201	0.219	0.235	0.250	0.266	0.280	0.192	0.227	0.353	0.568
200	0.064	0.079	0.091	0.102	0.111	0.121	0.130	0.138	0.146	0.155	0.104	0.122	0.190	0.311
400	0.036	0.043	0.050	0.055	0.060	0.065	0.070	0.075	0.079	0.083	0.055	0.065	0.100	0.164
800	0.020	0.024	0.027	0.030	0.032	0.035	0.037	0.040	0.042	0.044				

Level of Significance α = 0.05

n	k=1	2	3	4	5	6	7	8	9	10	15	20	40	80
10	0.683	0.802	0.879	0.933	0.969	0.990	0.999	1.000						
15	0.531	0.639	0.719	0.782	0.835	0.880	0.916	0.946	0.969	0.986				
20	0.436	0.531	0.602	0.662	0.714	0.761	0.802	0.839	0.872	0.901	0.991			
25	0.372	0.454	0.518	0.573	0.621	0.665	0.705	0.742	0.776	0.807	0.931	0.994		
30	0.325	0.398	0.455	0.505	0.549	0.589	0.627	0.662	0.695	0.726	0.855	0.947		

(continued)

TABLE H (continued)
Critical Values for Leverages, n = Sample Size, k = Number of Predictors

Level of Significance α = 0.05

n	1	2	3	4	5	6	7	8	9	10	15	20	40	80
40	0.261	0.321	0.368	0.409	0.446	0.480	0.512	0.543	0.572	0.600	0.722	0.823		
60	0.190	0.233	0.268	0.298	0.326	0.352	0.376	0.400	0.422	0.444	0.543	0.630	0.898	
80	0.151	0.185	0.212	0.236	0.258	0.279	0.299	0.318	0.336	0.353	0.435	0.508	0.751	
100	0.126	0.154	0.176	0.196	0.215	0.232	0.248	0.264	0.279	0.294	0.363	0.425	0.638	0.946
200	0.070	0.085	0.098	0.108	0.119	0.128	0.137	0.146	0.154	0.162	0.201	0.236	0.362	0.570
400	0.039	0.047	0.053	0.059	0.064	0.069	0.074	0.079	0.083	0.088	0.108	0.127	0.196	0.317
800	0.021	0.025	0.029	0.032	0.034	0.037	0.039	0.042	0.044	0.046	0.057	0.067	0.103	0.168

Level of Significance α = 0.01

n	1	2	3	4	5	6	7	8	9	10	15	20	40	80
10	0.785	0.875	0.930	0.965	0.986	0.997	1.000	1.000						
15	0.629	0.724	0.792	0.844	0.887	0.921	0.948	0.969	0.984	0.994				
20	0.524	0.612	0.677	0.731	0.777	0.817	0.852	0.883	0.910	0.933	0.996			
25	0.450	0.529	0.589	0.640	0.685	0.724	0.761	0.794	0.824	0.851	0.953	0.997		
30	0.394	0.466	0.521	0.568	0.610	0.648	0.683	0.716	0.746	0.774	0.889	0.964		
40	0.318	0.377	0.424	0.464	0.501	0.534	0.565	0.595	0.622	0.649	0.763	0.855		
60	0.231	0.275	0.310	0.341	0.369	0.395	0.420	0.443	0.465	0.487	0.584	0.668	0.917	
80	0.183	0.218	0.246	0.271	0.293	0.314	0.334	0.353	0.372	0.389	0.471	0.543	0.778	
100	0.152	0.181	0.205	0.225	0.244	0.262	0.279	0.295	0.310	0.325	0.394	0.456	0.666	0.956
200	0.085	0.100	0.113	0.124	0.135	0.145	0.154	0.163	0.172	0.180	0.219	0.255	0.383	0.598
400	0.046	0.054	0.061	0.067	0.073	0.078	0.083	0.088	0.092	0.097	0.118	0.138	0.208	0.330
800	0.025	0.029	0.033	0.036	0.039	0.041	0.044	0.046	0.049	0.051	0.062	0.073	0.110	0.175

TABLE I
Lower-Tail (Too Few Runs) Cumulative Table for a Number of Runs (r) of a Sample (n_1, n_2)

$(n_1, n_2)r =$	2	3	4	5	6	7
(3, 7)	0.017	0.083				
(3, 8)	0.012	0.067				
(3, 9)	0.009	0.055				
(3, 10)	0.007	0.045				
(4, 6)	0.010	0.048				
(4, 7)	0.006	0.033				
(4, 8)	0.004	0.024				
(4, 9)	0.003	0.018	0.085			
(4, 10)	0.002	0.014	0.068			
(5, 5)	0.008	0.040				
(5, 6)	0.004	0.024				
(5, 7)	0.003	0.015	0.076			
(5, 8)	0.002	0.010	0.054			
(5, 9)	0.001	0.007	0.039			
(5, 10)	0.001	0.005	0.029	0.095		
(6, 6)	0.002	0.013	0.067			
(6, 7)	0.001	0.008	0.043			
(6, 8)	0.001	0.005	0.028	0.086		
(6, 9)	0.000	0.003	0.019	0.063		
(6, 10)	0.000	0.002	0.013	0.047		
(7, 7)	0.001	0.004	0.025	0.078		
(7, 8)	0.000	0.002	0.015	0.051		
(7, 9)	0.000	0.001	0.010	0.035		
(7, 10)	0.000	0.001	0.006	0.024	0.080	
(8.8)	0.000	0.001	0.009	0.032	0.100	
(8, 9)	0.000	0.001	0.005	0.020	0.069	
(8, 10)	0.000	0.000	0.003	0.013	0.048	
(9, 9)	0.000	0.000	0.003	0.012	0.044	
(9, 10)	0.000	0.000	0.002	0.008	0.029	0.077
(10, 10)	0.000	0.000	0.001	0.004	0.019	0.051

Note: Less than 0.10 probability values provided. If $n_1 < n_2$, simply exchange n_1 and n_2.

TABLE J
Upper-Tail (Too Many Runs) Cumulative Table for a Number of Runs (r) of a Sample (n_1, n_2)

(n_1, n_2)r =	9	10	11	12	13	14	15	16	17	18	19	20
(4, 6)	0.024											
(4, 7)	0.046											
(4, 8)	0.071											
(4, 9)	0.098											
(4, 10)												
(5, 5)	0.040	0.008										
(5, 6)	0.089	0.024	0.002									
(5, 7)		0.045	0.008									
(5, 8)		0.071	0.016									
(5, 9)		0.098	0.028									
(5, 10)			0.042									
(6, 6)		0.067	0.013	0.002								
(6, 7)			0.034	0.008	0.001							
(6, 8)			0.063	0.016	0.002							
(6, 9)			0.098	0.028	0.006							
(6, 10)				0.042	0.010							
(7, 7)			0.078	0.025	0.004	0.001						
(7, 8)				0.051	0.012	0.002	0.000					
(7, 9)				0.084	0.025	0.006	0.001					
(7, 10)					0.043	0.010	0.002					
(8, 8)				0.100	0.032	0.009	0.001	0.000				
(8, 9)					0.061	0.020	0.004	0.001	0.000			
(8, 10)					0.097	0.036	0.010	0.002	0.000			
(9, 9)						0.044	0.012	0.003	0.000	0.000		
(9, 10)						0.077	0.026	0.008	0.001	0.000	0.000	
(10, 10)							0.051	0.019	0.004	0.001	0.000	0.000

Note: Less than 0.10 probability values provided. If $n_1 < n_2$, simply exchange n_1 and n_2.

TABLE K
Cook's Distance Table: Critical Values for the Maximum of n Values of Cook's $d(i) \times (n - k - 1)$ (Bonferroni Correction Used) n Observations and k Predictors

Level of Significance $\alpha = 0.1$

k	$n = 5$	10	15	20	25	50	100	200	400	800
1	14.96	11.13	11.84	12.68	13.46	16.39	19.97	23.94	28.70	33.80
2	40.53	12.21	12.09	12.63	13.22	15.65	18.64	22.09	25.96	30.12
3		13.30	12.09	12.35	12.79	14.84	17.48	20.52	23.86	27.50
4		15.21	12.18	12.14	12.45	14.23	16.62	19.36	22.30	25.97
5		19.33	12.44	12.03	12.21	13.76	15.95	18.49	21.39	24.51
6		31.06	12.94	12.01	12.04	13.39	15.43	17.81	20.36	23.51
7		96.01	13.79	12.08	11.94	13.10	15.02	17.27	19.75	22.42
8			15.26	12.26	11.90	12.85	14.70	16.83	19.20	21.73
9			18.00	12.55	11.91	12.66	14.40	16.52	18.62	21.45
10			23.93	13.02	11.97	12.50	14.16	16.16	18.43	20.55
15				27.66	13.60	12.01	13.39	15.16	17.00	19.34
20					30.94	11.83	12.92	14.53	16.31	18.35
40						15.95	12.26	13.56	15.10	16.83
80							13.49	13.05	14.39	15.85

Level of Significance $\alpha = 0.05$

k	$n = 5$	10	15	20	25	50	100	200	400	800
1	24.97	15.24	15.55	16.37	17.18	20.41	24.31	28.83	33.88	40.15
2	82.06	16.56	15.63	16.01	16.56	19.08	22.33	26.05	30.20	33.96
3		18.16	15.50	15.49	15.85	17.93	20.72	24.14	27.57	32.06
4		21.28	15.59	15.14	15.33	17.06	19.63	22.49	25.83	29.31
5		28.40	15.94	14.95	14.96	16.41	18.70	21.39	24.42	28.24
6		50.22	16.70	14.91	14.70	15.91	17.97	20.54	23.48	26.68
7		192.90	17.99	15.00	14.55	15.50	17.49	20.00	22.35	25.67
8			20.32	15.25	14.48	15.19	17.05	19.31	22.06	24.44
9			24.78	15.69	14.49	14.92	16.69	18.85	21.34	24.29
10			34.72	16.38	14.58	14.70	16.38	18.42	20.49	23.33
15				39.98	16.94	14.03	15.36	17.16	19.39	21.75
20					44.63	13.79	14.81	16.52	18.46	20.32
40						19.50	13.92	15.22	16.83	18.76
80							15.55	14.58	15.99	17.52

Level of Significance $\alpha = 0.01$

k	$n = 5$	10	15	20	25	50	100	200	400	800
1	77.29	28.72	26.88	27.24	27.92	31.46	36.10	41.22	49.42	68.39
2	415.27	30.97	26.13	25.65	25.81	28.12	32.61	37.34	44.99	57.70
3		35.12	25.66	24.22	24.33	26.17	29.15	34.23	37.55	52.58

(continued)

TABLE K (continued)
Cook's Distance Table: Critical Values for the Maximum of n Values of Cook's $d(i) \times (n - k - 1)$ (Bonferroni Correction Used) n Observations and k Predictors

Level of Significance $\alpha = 0.01$

k	$n = 5$	10	15	20	25	50	100	200	400	800
4		44.09	25.82	23.58	23.20	24.56	27.31	31.26	35.28	40.60
5		66.83	26.66	23.20	22.49	23.39	25.84	29.44	34.14	36.91
6		150.47	28.48	23.12	22.00	22.55	24.35	28.42	31.04	36.91
7		964.09	31.80	23.34	21.71	21.79	24.19	26.87	31.04	33.55
8			37.84	23.93	21.59	21.26	23.28	25.83	29.31	33.55
9			50.10	24.93	21.64	20.76	22.23	25.62	28.21	30.50
10			80.67	26.54	21.83	20.37	22.11	24.53	28.21	30.50
15				92.09	27.02	19.16	20.22	22.40	25.64	27.73
20					102.32	18.82	19.18	21.32	23.31	25.21
40						29.95	18.04	19.32	21.17	22.91
80							20.67	18.57	20.12	22.90

TABLE L
Chi-Square Table

df	$1 - \alpha = \chi^2_{0.005}$	$\chi^2_{0.025}$	$\chi^2_{0.05}$	$\alpha = 0.10$ $\chi^2_{0.90}$	0.05 $\chi^2_{0.95}$	0.025 $\chi^2_{0.975}$	0.01 $\chi^2_{0.99}$	0.005 $\chi^2_{0.995}$
1	0.0000393	0.000982	0.00393	2.706	3.841	5.024	6.635	7.879
2	0.0100	0.0506	0.103	4.605	5.991	7.378	9.210	10.597
3	0.0717	0.216	0.352	6.251	7.815	9.348	11.345	12.838
4	0.207	0.484	0.711	7.779	9.488	11.143	13.277	14.860
5	0.412	0.831	1.145	9.236	11.070	12.832	15.086	16.750
6	0.676	1.237	1.635	10.645	12.592	14.449	16.812	18.548
7	0.989	1.690	2.167	12.017	14.067	16.013	18.475	20.278
8	1.344	2.180	2.733	13.362	15.507	17.535	20.090	21.955
9	1.735	2.700	3.325	14.684	16.919	19.023	21.666	23.589
10	2.156	3.247	3.940	15.987	18.307	20.483	23.209	25.188
11	2.603	3.816	4.575	17.275	19.675	21.920	24.725	26.757
12	3.074	4.404	5.226	18.549	21.026	23.336	26.217	28.300
13	3.565	5.009	5.892	19.812	22.362	24.736	27.688	29.819
14	4.075	5.629	6.571	21.064	23.685	26.119	29.141	31.319
15	4.601	6.262	7.261	22.307	24.996	27.488	30.578	32.801
16	5.142	6.908	7.962	23.542	26.296	28.845	32.000	34.267
17	5.697	7.564	8.672	24.769	27.587	30.191	33.409	35.718
18	6.265	8.231	9.390	25.989	28.869	31.526	34.805	37.156
19	6.844	8.907	10.117	27.204	30.144	32.852	36.191	38.582
20	7.434	9.591	10.851	28.412	31.410	34.170	37.566	39.997
21	8.034	10.283	11.591	29.615	32.671	35.479	38.932	41.401

(continued)

TABLE L (continued)
Chi-Square Table

df	$1 - \alpha = \chi^2_{0.005}$	$\chi^2_{0.025}$	$\chi^2_{0.05}$	$\alpha = 0.10$ $\chi^2_{0.90}$	0.05 $\chi^2_{0.95}$	0.025 $\chi^2_{0.975}$	0.01 $\chi^2_{0.99}$	0.005 $\chi^2_{0.995}$
22	8.643	10.982	12.338	30.813	33.924	36.781	40.289	42.796
23	9.260	11.688	13.091	32.007	35.172	38.076	41.638	44.181
24	9.886	12.401	13.848	33.196	36.415	39.364	42.980	45.558
25	10.520	13.120	14.611	34.382	37.652	40.646	44.314	46.928
26	11.160	13.844	15.379	35.563	38.885	41.923	45.642	48.290
27	11.808	14.573	16.151	36.741	40.113	43.194	46.963	49.645
28	12.461	15.308	16.928	37.916	41.337	44.461	48.278	50.993
29	13.121	16.047	17.708	39.087	42.557	45.722	49.588	52.336
30	13.787	16.791	18.493	40.256	43.773	46.979	50.892	53.672
35	17.192	20.569	22.465	46.059	49.802	53.203	57.342	60.275
40	20.707	24.433	26.509	51.805	55.758	59.342	63.691	66.766
45	24.311	28.366	30.612	57.505	61.656	65.410	69.957	73.166
50	27.991	32.357	34.764	63.167	67.505	71.420	76.154	79.490
60	35.535	40.482	43.188	74.397	79.082	83.298	88.379	91.952
70	43.275	48.758	51.739	85.527	90.531	95.023	100.425	104.215
80	51.172	57.153	60.391	96.578	101.879	106.629	112.329	116.321
90	59.196	65.647	69.126	107.565	113.145	118.136	124.116	128.299
100	67.328	74.222	77.929	118.498	124.342	129.561	135.807	140.169

TABLE M
Friedman ANOVA Table [Exact Distribution of χ^2_r for Tables with Two to Nine Sets of Three Ranks ($k = 3$; $n = 2, 3, 4, 5, 6, 7, 8, 9$)]

$n = 2$		$n = 3$		$n = 4$		$n = 5$	
χ^2_r	p	χ^2_r	p	χ^2_r	p	χ^2_r	p
0	1.000	0.000	1.000	0.0	1.000	0.0	1.000
1	0.833	0.667	0.944	0.5	0.931	0.4	0.954
3	0.500	2.000	0.528	1.5	0.653	1.2	0.691
4	0.167	2.667	0.361	2.0	0.431	1.6	0.522
		4.667	0.194	3.5	0.273	2.8	0.367
		6.000	0.028	4.5	0.125	3.6	0.182
				6.0	0.069	4.8	0.124
				6.5	0.042	5.2	0.093
				8.0	0.0046	6.4	0.039
						7.6	0.024
						8.4	0.0085
						10.0	0.00077

(continued)

TABLE M (continued)
Friedman ANOVA Table [Exact Distribution of χ_r^2 for Tables with Two to Nine Sets of Three Ranks ($k = 3; n = 2, 3, 4, 5, 6, 7, 8, 9$)]

$n = 6$		$n = 7$		$n = 8$		$n = 9$	
χ_r^2	p	χ_r^2	p	χ_r^2	p	χ_r^2	p
0.00	1.000	0.000	1.000	0.00	1.000	0.000	1.000
0.33	0.956	0.286	0.964	0.25	0.967	0.222	0.971
1.00	0.740	0.857	0.768	0.75	0.794	0.667	0.814
1.33	0.570	1.143	0.620	1.00	0.654	0.889	0.865
2.33	0.430	2.000	0.486	1.75	0.531	1.556	0.569
3.00	0.252	2.571	0.305	2.25	0.355	2.000	0.398
4.00	0.184	3.429	0.237	3.00	0.285	2.667	0.328
4.33	0.142	3.714	0.192	3.25	0.236	2.889	0.278
5.33	0.072	4.571	0.112	4.00	0.149	3.556	0.187
6.33	0.052	5.429	0.085	4.75	0.120	4.222	0.154
7.00	0.029	6.000	0.052	5.25	0.079	4.667	0.107
8.33	0.012	7.143	0.027	6.25	0.047	5.556	0.069
9.00	0.0081	7.714	0.021	6.75	0.038	6.000	0.057
9.33	0.0055	8.000	0.016	7.00	0.030	6.222	0.048
10.33	0.0017	8.857	0.0084	7.75	0.018	6.889	0.031
12.00	0.00013	10.286	0.0036	9.00	0.0099	8.000	0.019
		10.571	0.0027	9.25	0.0080	8.222	0.016
		11.143	0.0012	9.75	0.0048	8.667	0.010
		12.286	0.00032	10.75	0.0024	9.556	0.0060
		14.000	0.000021	12.00	0.0011	10.667	0.0035
				12.25	0.00086	10.889	0.0029
				13.00	0.00026	11.556	0.0013
				14.25	0.000061	12.667	0.00066
				16.00	0.0000036	13.556	0.00035
						14.000	0.00020
						14.222	0.000097
						14.889	0.000054
						16.222	0.000011
						18.000	0.0000006

$n = 2$		$n = 3$		$n = 4$			
χ_r^2	p	χ_r^2	p	χ_r^2	p	χ_r^2	p
0.0	1.000	0.2	1.000	0.0	1.000	5.7	0.141
0.6	0.958	0.6	0.958	0.3	0.992	6.0	0.105
1.2	0.834	1.0	0.910	0.6	0.928	6.3	0.094
1.8	0.792	1.8	0.727	0.9	0.900	6.6	0.077
2.4	0.625	2.2	0.608	1.2	0.800	6.9	0.068
3.0	0.542	2.6	0.524	1.5	0.754	7.2	0.054
3.6	0.458	3.4	0.446	1.8	0.677	7.5	0.052

(*continued*)

TABLE M (continued)
Friedman ANOVA Table [Exact Distribution of χ_r^2 for Tables with Two to Nine Sets of Three Ranks ($k = 3$; $n = 2, 3, 4, 5, 6, 7, 8, 9$)]

$n = 2$		$n = 3$				$n = 4$	
χ_r^2	p	χ_r^2	p	χ_r^2	p	χ_r^2	p
4.2	0.375	3.8	0.342	2.1	0.649	7.8	0.036
4.8	0.208	4.2	0.300	2.4	0.524	8.1	0.033
5.4	0.167	5.0	0.207	2.7	0.508	8.4	0.019
6.0	0.042	5.4	0.175	3.0	0.432	8.7	0.014
		5.8	0.148	3.3	0.389	9.3	0.012
		6.6	0.075	3.6	0.355	9.6	0.0069
		7.0	0.054	3.9	0.324	9.9	0.0062
		7.4	0.033	4.5	0.242	10.2	0.0027
		8.2	0.017	4.8	0.200	10.8	0.0016
		9.0	0.0017	5.1	0.190	11.1	0.00094
				5.4	0.158	12.0	0.000072

Note: p is the probability of obtaining a value of χ_r^2 as great as or greater than the corresponding value of χ_r^2.

TABLE N
Studentized Range Table

$q_{0.05}(p, f)c = f$

f	2	3	4	5	6	7	8	9	10	11	12	13	14	15	16	17	18	19	20
1	18.1	26.7	32.8	37.2	40.5	43.1	45.4	47.3	49.1	50.6	51.9	53.2	54.3	55.4	56.3	57.2	58.0	58.8	59.6
2	6.09	8.28	9.80	10.89	11.73	12.43	13.03	13.54	13.99	14.39	14.75	15.08	15.38	15.65	15.91	16.14	16.36	16.57	16.77
3	4.50	5.88	6.83	7.51	8.04	8.47	8.85	9.18	9.46	9.72	9.95	10.16	10.35	10.52	10.69	10.84	10.98	11.12	11.24
4	3.93	5.00	5.76	6.31	6.73	7.06	7.35	7.60	7.83	8.03	8.21	8.37	8.52	8.67	8.80	8.92	9.03	9.14	9.24
5	3.64	4.60	5.22	5.67	6.03	6.33	6.58	6.80	6.99	7.17	7.32	7.47	7.60	7.72	7.83	7.93	8.03	8.12	8.21
6	3.46	4.34	4.90	5.31	5.63	5.89	6.12	6.32	6.49	6.65	6.79	6.92	7.04	7.14	7.24	7.34	7.43	7.51	7.59
7	3.34	4.16	4.68	5.06	5.35	5.59	5.80	5.99	6.15	6.29	6.42	6.54	6.65	6.75	6.84	6.93	7.01	7.08	7.16
8	3.26	4.04	4.53	4.89	5.17	5.40	5.60	5.77	5.92	6.05	6.18	6.29	6.39	6.48	6.57	6.65	6.73	6.80	6.87
9	3.20	3.95	4.42	4.76	5.02	5.24	5.43	5.60	5.74	5.87	5.98	6.09	6.19	6.28	6.36	6.44	6.51	6.58	6.65
10	3.15	3.88	4.33	4.66	4.91	5.12	5.30	5.46	5.60	5.72	5.83	5.93	6.03	6.12	6.20	6.27	6.34	6.41	6.47
11	3.11	3.82	4.26	4.58	4.82	5.03	5.20	5.35	5.49	5.61	5.71	5.81	5.90	5.98	6.06	6.14	6.20	6.27	6.33
12	3.08	3.77	4.20	4.51	4.75	4.95	5.12	5.27	5.40	5.51	5.61	5.71	5.80	5.88	5.95	6.02	6.09	6.15	6.21
13	3.06	3.73	4.15	4.46	4.69	4.88	5.05	5.19	5.32	5.43	5.53	5.63	5.71	5.79	5.86	5.93	6.00	6.06	6.11
14	3.03	3.70	4.11	4.41	4.64	4.83	4.99	5.13	5.25	5.36	5.46	5.56	5.64	5.72	5.79	5.86	5.92	5.98	6.03
15	3.01	3.67	4.08	4.37	4.59	4.78	4.94	5.08	5.20	5.31	5.40	5.49	5.57	5.65	5.72	5.79	5.85	5.91	5.96
16	3.00	3.65	4.05	4.34	4.56	4.74	4.90	5.03	5.15	5.26	5.35	5.44	5.52	5.59	5.66	5.73	5.79	5.84	5.90
17	2.98	3.62	4.02	4.31	4.52	4.70	4.86	4.99	5.11	5.21	5.31	5.39	5.47	5.55	5.61	5.68	5.74	5.79	5.84
18	2.97	3.61	4.00	4.28	4.49	4.67	4.83	4.96	5.07	5.17	5.27	5.35	5.43	5.50	5.57	5.63	5.69	5.74	5.79
19	2.96	3.59	3.98	4.26	4.47	4.64	4.79	4.92	5.04	5.14	5.23	5.32	5.39	5.46	5.53	5.59	5.65	5.70	5.75
20	2.95	3.58	3.96	4.24	4.45	4.62	4.77	4.90	5.01	5.11	5.20	5.28	5.36	5.43	5.50	5.56	5.61	5.66	5.71
24	2.92	3.53	3.90	4.17	4.37	4.54	4.68	4.81	4.92	5.01	5.10	5.18	5.25	5.32	5.38	5.44	5.50	5.55	5.59
30	2.89	3.48	3.84	4.11	4.30	4.46	4.60	4.72	4.83	4.92	5.00	5.08	5.15	5.21	5.27	5.33	5.38	5.43	5.48
40	2.86	3.44	3.79	4.04	4.23	4.39	4.52	4.63	4.74	4.82	4.90	4.98	5.05	5.11	5.17	5.22	5.27	5.32	5.36
60	2.83	3.40	3.74	3.98	4.16	4.31	4.44	4.55	4.65	4.73	4.81	4.88	4.94	5.00	5.06	5.11	5.15	5.20	5.24

f																			
120	2.80	3.36	3.69	3.92	4.10	4.24	4.36	4.47	4.56	4.64	4.71	4.78	4.84	4.90	4.95	5.00	5.04	5.09	5.13
∞	2.77	3.32	3.63	3.86	4.03	4.17	4.29	4.39	4.47	4.55	4.62	4.68	4.74	4.80	4.84	4.98	4.93	4.97	5.01
1	90.0	135	164	186	202	216	227	237	246	253	260	266	272	272	282	286	290	294	298
2	14.0	19.0	22.3	24.7	26.6	282	29.5	30.7	31.7	32.6	33.4	34.1	34.8	35.4	36.0	36.5	37.0	37.5	37.9
3	8.26	10.6	12.2	13.3	14.2	15.0	15.6	16.2	16.7	17.1	17.5	17.9	182	18.5	18.8	19.1	19.3	19.5	19.8
4	6.51	8.12	9.17	9.96	10.6	11.1	11.5	11.9	12.3	12.6	12.8	13.1	13.3	13.5	13.7	13.9	14.1	14.2	14.4
5	5.70	6.97	7.80	8.42	8.91	9.32	9.67	9.97	10.24	10.48	10.70	10.89	11.08	11.24	11.40	11.55	11.68	11.81	11.93
6	5.24	6.33	7.03	7.56	7.97	8.32	8.61	8.87	9.10	9.30	9.49	9.65	9.81	9.95	10.08	10.21	10.32	10.43	10.54
7	4.95	5.92	6.54	7.01	7.37	7.68	7.94	8.17	8.37	8.55	8.71	8.86	9.00	9.12	9.24	9.35	9.46	9.55	9.65
8	4.74	5.63	6.20	6.63	6.96	7.24	7.47	7.68	7.87	8.03	8.18	8.31	8.44	8.55	8.66	8.76	8.85	8.94	9.03
9	4.60	5.43	5.96	6.35	6.66	6.91	7.13	7.32	7.49	7.65	718	7.91	8.03	8.13	8.23	8.32	8.41	8.49	8.57
10	4.48	5.27	5.77	6.14	6A3	6.67	6.87	7.05	7.21	7.36	7.48	7.60	7.71	7.81	7.91	7.99	8.07	8.15	8.22
11	4.39	5.14	5.62	5.97	625	6.48	6.67	6.84	6.99	7.13	7.25	7.36	7.46	7.56	7.65	7.73	7.81	7.88	7.95
12	4.32	5.04	5.50	5.84	6.10	6.32	6.51	6.67	6.81	6.94	7.16	7.17	7.26	7.36	7.44	7.52	7.59	7.66	7.73
13	4.26	4.96	5.40	5.73	5.98	6.19	6.37	6.53	6.67	6.79	6.90	7.01	7.10	7.19	7.27	7.34	7.42	7.48	7.55
14	4.21	4.89	5.32	5.63	5.88	6.08	6.26	6A1	6.54	6.66	6.77	6.87	696	7.05	7.12	7.20	7.27	7.33	7.39
15	4.17	4.83	5.25	5.56	5.80	5.99	6.16	6.31	6.44	6.55	6.66	6.76	6.84	6.93	7.00	7.07	7.14	7.20	7.26
16	4.13	4.78	5.19	5.49	5.72	5.92	6.08	6.22	6.35	6.46	6.56	6.66	6.74	6.82	6.90	6.97	7.03	7.09	7.15
17	4.10	414	5.14	5.43	5.66	5.85	6.01	6.15	627	6.38	6.48	6.57	6.66	6.73	6.80	6.87	6.94	7.00	7.05
18	4.07	4.70	5.09	5.38	5.60	5.79	5.94	6.08	6.20	6.31	6.41	6.50	6.58	6.65	6.72	6.79	6.85	6.91	6.96
19	4.05	4.67	5.05	5.33	5.55	5.73	5.89	6.02	6.14	6.25	6.34	6.43	6.51	6.58	6.65	6.72	6.78	6.84	6.89
20	4.02	4.64	5.02	5.29	5.51	5.69	5.84	5.97	6.09	6.19	6.29	6.37	6.45	6.52	6.59	6.65	6.71	6.76	6.82
24	3.96	4.54	4.91	5.17	5.37	5.54	5.69	5.81	5.92	6.02	6.11	6.19	626	6.33	6.39	6.45	6.51	6.56	6.61
30	3.89	4A5	4.80	5.05	5.24	5.40	5.54	5.65	5.76	5.85	5.93	6.01	6.08	6.14	620	6.26	6.31	636	6.41
40	3.82	4.37	4.70	4.93	5.11	527	5.39	5.50	5.60	5.69	5.77	5.84	5.90	5.96	6.02	6.07	6.12	6.17	6.21
60	3.76	4.28	4.60	4£2	4.99	5.13	5.25	5.36	5.45	5.53	5.60	5.67	5.73	5.79	5.84	5.89	5.93	5.98	6.02
120	3.70	4.20	4.50	4.71	4.87	5.01	5.12	5.21	5.30	5.38	5.44	5.51	5.56	5.61	5.66	5.71	5.75	5.79	5.83
∞	3.64	4.12	4.40	4.60	4.76	4.88	4.99	5.08	5.16	523	5.29	5.35	5.40	5.45	5.49	5.54	5.57	5.61	5.65

Note: f denotes degrees of freedom.

TABLE O
Fisher Z Transformation Table Values of $\frac{1}{2}\ln\frac{1+r}{1-r}$ for Given Values of r

r	0.000	0.001	0.002	0.003	0.004	0.005	0.006	0.007	0.008	0.009
0.000	0.0000	0.0010	0.0020	0.0030	0.0040	0.0050	0.0060	0.0070	0.0080	0.0090
0.010	0.0100	0.0110	0.0120	0.0130	0.0140	0.0150	0.0160	0.0170	0.0180	0.0190
0.020	0.0200	0.0210	0.0220	0.0230	0.0240	0.0250	0.0260	0.0270	0.0280	0.0290
0.030	0.0300	0.0310	0.0320	0.0330	0.0340	0.0350	0.0360	0.0370	0.0380	0.0390
0.040	0.0400	0.0410	0.0420	0.0430	0.0440	0.0450	0.0460	0.0470	0.0480	0.0490
0.050	0.0501	0.0511	0.0521	0.0531	0.0541	0.0551	0.0561	0.0571	0.0581	0.0591
0.060	0.0601	0.0611	0.0621	0.0631	0.0641	0.0651	0.0661	0.0671	0.0681	0.0691
0.070	0.0701	0.0711	0.0721	0.0731	0.0741	0.0751	0.0761	0.0771	0.0782	0.0792
0.080	0.0802	0.0812	0.0822	0.0832	0.0842	0.0852	0.0862	0.0872	0.0882	0.0892
0.090	0.0902	0.0912	0.0922	0.0933	0.0943	0.0953	0.0963	0.0973	0.0983	0.0993
0.100	0.1003	0.1013	0.1024	0.1034	0.1044	0.1054	0.1064	0.1074	0.1084	0.1094
0.110	0.1105	0.1115	0.1125	0.1135	0.1145	0.1155	0.1165	0.1175	0.1185	0.1195
0.120	0.1206	0.1216	0.1226	0.1236	0.1246	0.1257	0.1267	0.1277	0.1287	0.1297
0.130	0.1308	0.1318	0.1328	0.1338	0.1348	0.1358	0.1368	0.1379	0.1389	0.1399
0.140	0.1409	0.1419	0.1430	0.1440	0.1450	0.1460	0.1470	0.1481	0.1491	0.1501
0.150	0.1511	0.1522	0.1532	0.1542	0.1552	0.1563	0.1573	0.1583	0.1593	0.1604
0.160	0.1614	0.1624	0.1634	0.1644	0.1655	0.1665	0.1676	0.1686	0.1696	0.1706
0.170	0.1717	0.1727	0.1737	0.1748	0.1758	0.1768	0.1779	0.1789	0.1799	0.1810
0.180	0.1820	0.1830	0.1841	0.1851	0.1861	0.1872	0.1882	0.1892	0.1903	0.1913
0.190	0.1923	0.1934	0.1944	0.1954	0.1965	0.1975	0.1986	0.1996	0.2007	0.2017
0.200	0.2027	0.2038	0.2048	0.2059	0.2069	0.2079	0.2090	0.2100	0.2111	0.2121
0.210	0.2132	0.2142	0.2153	0.2163	0.2174	0.2184	0.2194	0.2205	0.2215	0.2226
0.220	0.2237	0.2247	0.2258	0.2268	0.2279	0.2289	0.2300	0.2310	0.2321	0.2331

0.230	0.2342	0.2353	0.2363	0.2374	0.2384	0.2395	0.2405	0.2416	0.2427	0.2437
0.240	0.2448	0.2458	0.2469	0.2480	0.2490	0.2501	0.2511	0.2522	0.2533	0.2543
0.250	0.2554	0.2565	0.2575	0.2586	0.2597	0.2608	0.2618	0.2629	0.2640	0.2650
0.260	0.2661	0.2672	0.2682	0.2693	0.2704	0.2715	0.2726	0.2736	0.2747	0.2758
0.270	0.2769	0.2779	0.2790	0.2801	0.2812	0.2823	0.2833	0.2844	0.2855	0.2866
0.280	0.2877	0.2888	0.2898	0.2909	0.2920	0.2931	0.2942	0.2953	0.2964	0.2975
0.290	0.2986	0.2997	0.3008	0.3019	0.3029	0.3040	0.3051	0.3062	0.3073	0.3084
0.300	0.3095	0.3106	0.3117	0.3128	0.3139	0.3150	0.3161	0.3172	0.3183	0.3195
0.310	0.3206	0.3217	0.3228	0.3239	0.3250	0.3261	0.3272	0.3283	0.3294	0.3305
0.320	0.3317	0.3328	0.3339	0.3350	0.3361	0.3372	0.3384	0.3395	0.3406	0.3417
0.330	0.3428	0.3439	0.3451	0.3462	0.3473	0.3484	0.3496	0.3507	0.3518	0.3530
0.340	0.3541	0.3552	0.3564	0.3575	0.3586	0.3597	0.3609	0.3620	0.3632	0.3643
0.350	0.3654	0.3666	0.3677	0.3689	0.3700	0.3712	0.3723	0.3734	0.3746	0.3757
0.360	0.3769	0.3780	0.3792	0.3803	0.3815	0.3826	0.3838	0.3850	0.3861	0.3873
0.370	0.3884	0.3896	0.3907	0.3919	0.3931	0.3942	0.3954	0.3966	0.3977	0.3989
0.380	0.4001	0.4012	0.4024	0.4036	0.4047	0.4059	0.4071	0.4083	0.4094	0.4106
0.390	0.4118	0.4130	0.4142	0.4153	0.4165	0.4177	0.4189	0.4201	0.4213	0.4225
0.400	0.4236	0.4248	0.4260	0.4272	0.4284	0.4296	0.4308	0.4320	0.4332	0.4344
0.410	0.4356	0.4368	0.4380	0.4392	0.4404	0.4416	0.4429	0.4441	0.4453	0.4465
0.420	0.4477	0.4489	0.4501	0.4513	0.4526	0.4538	0.4550	0.4562	0.4574	0.4587
0.430	0.4599	0.4611	0.4623	0.4636	0.4648	0.4660	0.4673	0.4685	0.4697	0.4710
0.440	0.4722	0.4735	0.4747	0.4760	0.4772	0.4784	0.4797	0.4809	0.4822	0.4835
0.450	0.4847	0.4860	0.4872	0.4885	0.4897	0.4910	0.4923	0.4935	0.4948	0.4961
0.460	0.4973	0.4986	0.4999	0.5011	0.5024	0.5037	0.5049	0.5062	0.5075	0.5088
0.470	0.5101	0.5114	0.5126	0.5139	0.5152	0.5165	0.5178	0.5191	0.5204	0.5217
0.480	0.5230	0.5243	0.5256	0.5269	0.5282	0.5295	0.5308	0.5321	0.5334	0.5347
0.490	0.5361	0.5374	0.5387	0.5400	0.5413	0.5427	0.5440	0.5453	0.5466	0.5480

(continued)

TABLE O (continued)
Fisher Z Transformation Table Values of $\frac{1}{2}\ln\frac{1+r}{1-r}$ for Given Values of r

r	0.000	0.001	0.002	0.003	0.004	0.005	0.006	0.007	0.008	0.009
0.500	0.5493	0.5506	0.5520	0.5533	0.5547	0.5560	0.5573	0.5587	0.5600	0.5614
0.510	0.5627	0.5641	0.5654	0.5668	0.5681	0.5695	0.5709	0.5722	0.5736	0.5750
0.520	0.5763	0.5777	0.5791	0.5805	0.5818	0.5832	0.5846	0.5860	0.5874	0.5888
0.530	0.5901	0.5915	0.5929	0.5943	0.5957	0.5971	0.5985	0.5999	0.6013	0.6027
0.540	0.6042	0.6056	0.6070	0.6084	0.6098	0.6112	0.6127	0.6141	0.6155	0.6170
0.550	0.6184	0.6198	0.6213	0.6227	0.6241	0.6256	0.6270	0.6285	0.6299	0.6314
0.560	0.6328	0.6343	0.6358	0.6372	0.6387	0.6401	0.6416	0.6431	0.6446	0.6460
0.570	0.6475	0.6490	0.6505	0.6520	0.6535	0.6550	0.6565	0.6579	0.6594	0.6610
0.580	0.6625	0.6640	0.6655	0.6670	0.6685	0.6700	0.6715	0.6731	0.6746	0.6761
0.590	0.6777	0.6792	0.6807	0.6823	0.6838	0.6854	0.6869	0.6885	0.6900	0.6916
0.600	0.6931	0.6947	0.6963	0.6978	0.6994	0.7010	0.7026	0.7042	0.7057	0.7073
0.610	0.7089	0.7105	0.7121	0.7137	0.7153	0.7169	0.7185	0.7201	0.7218	0.7234
0.620	0.7250	0.7266	0.7283	0.7299	0.7315	0.7332	0.7348	0.7364	0.7381	0.7398
0.630	0.7414	0.7431	0.7447	0.7464	0.7481	0.7497	0.7514	0.7531	0.7548	0.7565
0.640	0.7582	0.7599	0.7616	0.7633	0.7650	0.7667	0.7684	0.7701	0.7718	0.7736
0.650	0.7753	0.7770	0.7788	0.7805	0.7823	0.7840	0.7858	0.7875	0.7893	0.7910
0.660	0.7928	0.7946	0.7964	0.7981	0.7999	0.8017	0.8035	0.8053	0.8071	0.8089
0.670	0.8107	0.8126	0.8144	0.8162	0.8180	0.8199	0.8217	0.8236	0.8254	0.8273
0.680	0.8291	0.8310	0.8328	0.8347	0.8366	0.8385	0.8404	0.8423	0.8442	0.8461
0.690	0.8480	0.8499	0.8518	0.8537	0.8556	0.8576	0.8595	0.8614	0.8634	0.8653
0.700	0.8673	0.8693	0.8712	0.8732	0.8752	0.8772	0.8792	0.8812	0.8832	0.8852
0.710	0.8872	0.8892	0.8912	0.8933	0.8953	0.8973	0.8994	0.9014	0.9035	0.9056
0.720	0.9076	0.9097	0.9118	0.9139	9.9160	0.9181	0.9202	0.9223	0.9245	0.9266
0.730	0.9287	0.9309	0.9330	0.9352	0.9373	0.9395	0.9417	0.9439	0.9461	0.9483
0.740	0.9505	0.9527	0.9549	0.9571	0.9594	0.9616	0.9639	0.9661	0.9684	0.9707
0.750	0.9730	0.9752	0.9775	0.9799	0.9822	0.9845	0.9868	0.9892	0.9915	0.9939
0.760	0.9962	0.9986	1.0010	1.0034	1.0058	1.0082	1.0106	1.0130	1.0154	1.0179

r	.000	.001	.002	.003	.004	.005	.006	.007	.008	.009
0.770	1.0203	1.0228	1.0253	1.0277	1.0302	1.0327	1.0352	1.0378	1.0403	1.0428
0.780	1.0454	1.0479	1.0505	1.0531	1.0557	1.0583	1.0609	1.0635	1.0661	1.0688
0.790	1.0714	1.0741	1.0768	1.0795	1.0822	1.0849	1.0876	1.0903	1.0931	1.0958
0.800	1.0986	1.1014	1.1041	1.1070	1.1098	1.1127	1.1155	1.1184	1.1212	1.1241
0.810	1.1270	1.1299	1.1329	1.1358	1.1388	1.1417	1.1447	1.1477	1.1507	1.1538
0.820	1.1568	1.1599	1.1630	1.1660	1.1692	1.1723	1.1754	1.1786	1.1817	1.1849
0.830	1.1870	1.1913	1.1946	1.1979	1.2011	1.2044	1.2077	1.2111	1.2144	1.2178
0.840	1.2212	1.2246	1.2280	1.2315	1.2349	1.2384	1.2419	1.2454	1.2490	1.2526
0.850	1.2561	1.2598	1.2634	1.2670	1.2708	1.2744	1.2782	1.2819	1.2857	1.2895
0.860	1.2934	1.2972	1.3011	1.3050	1.3089	1.3129	1.3168	1.3209	1.3249	1.3290
0.870	1.3331	1.3372	1.3414	1.3456	1.3498	1.3540	1.3583	1.3626	1.3670	1.3714
0.880	1.3758	1.3802	1.3847	1.3892	1.3938	1.3984	1.4030	1.4077	1.4124	1.4171
0.890	1.4219	1.4268	1.4316	1.4366	1.4415	1.4465	1.4516	1.4566	1.4618	1.4670
0.900	1.4722	1.4775	1.4828	1.4883	1.4937	1.4992	1.5047	1.5103	1.5160	1.5217
0.910	1.5275	1.5334	1.5393	1.5453	1.5513	1.5574	1.5636	1.5698	1.5762	1.5825
0.920	1.5890	1.5956	1.6022	1.6089	1.6157	1.6226	1.6296	1.6366	1.6438	1.6510
0.930	1.6584	1.6659	1.6734	1.6811	1.6888	1.6967	1.7047	1.7129	1.7211	1.7295
0.940	1.7380	1.7467	1.7555	1.7645	1.7736	1.7828	1.7923	1.8019	1.8117	1.8216
0.950	1.8318	1.8421	1.8527	1.8635	1.8745	1.8857	1.8972	1.9090	1.9210	1.9333
0.960	1.9459	1.9588	1.9721	1.9857	1.9996	2.0140	2.0287	2.0439	2.0595	2.0756
0.970	2.0923	2.1095	2.1273	2.1457	2.1649	2.1847	2.2054	2.2269	2.2494	2.2729
0.980	2.2976	2.3223	2.3507	2.3796	2.4101	2.4426	2.4774	2.5147	2.5550	2.5988
0.990	2.6467	2.6996	2.7587	2.8257	2.9031	2.9945	3.1063	3.2504	3.4534	3.8002

r	z
0.9999	4.95172
0.99999	6.10303

Note: To obtain $\frac{1}{2}\log_e \frac{(1+r)}{(1-r)}$ when r is negative, use the negative of the value corresponding to the absolute value of r, e.g.,

$$r = 0.242, \quad \frac{1}{2}\log_e \frac{(1+0.242)}{(1-0.242r)} = -0.2469.$$

Appendix II

MATRIX ALGEBRA APPLIED TO REGRESSION

Matrix algebra is extremely useful in regression analysis when more than one x_i variable is used. Although matrix algebraic procedures are straightforward, they are extremely time-consuming. Hence, in practice, it is feasible to do by hand only the simplest models with very small sample sizes. MiniTab is used in this work.

A matrix is simply an array of numbers arranged in equal or nonequal rows and columns. For example,

$$A = \begin{bmatrix} 3 & 7 \\ 5 & 8 \end{bmatrix}, \quad b = \begin{bmatrix} 2 \\ 1 \\ 5 \\ 7 \\ 9 \end{bmatrix}, \quad c = \begin{bmatrix} 5 & 3 & 6 & 2 & 1 \end{bmatrix}, \quad D = \begin{bmatrix} 0 & 4 & 2 \\ 5 & 9 & 6 \\ 2 & 7 & 7 \\ 1 & 0 & 1 \\ 3 & 5 & 3 \end{bmatrix}.$$

The dimensions of a matrix are by row and column, or i and j. Usually, the matrix values or elements are lettered as a_{ij} for the value a and its location in the ith row and jth column. Notations for the matrix identifiers, A, B, X, and Y, are always a capital bold letter. The exception is the vector, which is usually denoted by a small bold letter, but this is not always the case in statistical applications.

For example, A given here is a 2×2 matrix (read 2 by 2, not 2 times 2), b is a 5×1 matrix, c is a 1×5 matrix, and D is a 5×3 matrix. Single-row or column matrices, such as b and c, are also known as vectors. Notation can also be written in the form, for example, $A_{r \times c}$, where r is the row and c is the column, that is, given as $A_{2 \times 2}$, $b_{5 \times 1}$, $c_{1 \times 5}$, and $D_{5 \times 3}$. In b, the value 5, by matrix notation, is at space a_{31} (see the following).

$$\mathbf{A}_{r \times c} = \begin{bmatrix} a_{11} & a_{12} & a_{13} & \cdots & a_{1c} \\ a_{21} & a_{22} & a_{23} & \cdots & a_{2c} \\ a_{31} & a_{32} & a_{33} & \cdots & a_{3c} \\ \vdots & \vdots & \vdots & \vdots & \vdots \\ a_{r1} & a_{r2} & a_{r3} & \cdots & a_{rc} \end{bmatrix}.$$

An alternative form of notation is $\mathbf{A} = \{a_{ij}\}$, for $i = 1, 2, \ldots, r$ and $j = 1, 2, \ldots,$ c. The individual elements, $\{a_{ij}\}$, are the matrix values, each referred to as an ijth element. Note that element values do not have to be whole numbers:

$$\mathbf{A}_{2 \times 3} = \begin{bmatrix} -4.15 & 0 & 6 \\ -3.2 & 2.51 & 1 \end{bmatrix}.$$

When $r = c$, the matrix is said to be square. In regression, diagonal elements in square matrices become important. Note below that the diagonal elements of $\mathbf{A}_{4 \times 4}$ are a_{11}, a_{22}, a_{33}, and a_{44}, or 1, 5, 6, and 1:

$$\mathbf{A}_{4 \times 4} = \begin{bmatrix} 1 & 5 & 6 & 7 \\ 6 & 5 & 1 & 3 \\ 0 & 5 & 6 & 1 \\ 2 & 3 & 5 & 1 \end{bmatrix}.$$

Sometimes, a matrix will have values of 0 for all its nondiagonal elements. In such cases, it is called a diagonal matrix, as depicted in the following:

$$\mathbf{B}_{4 \times 4} = \begin{bmatrix} 1 & 0 & 0 & 0 \\ 0 & 3 & 0 & 0 \\ 0 & 0 & 5 & 0 \\ 0 & 0 & 0 & 2 \end{bmatrix}.$$

Other matrix forms important in statistical analysis are "triangular-like" matrices. These are $r = c$ matrices with all the elements either above or below the diagonal 0, as illustrated in the following:

$$\mathbf{A}_{3 \times 3} = \begin{bmatrix} 1 & 0 & 0 \\ 13 & -3 & 0 \\ 2 & 5 & 6 \end{bmatrix} \quad \text{or} \quad \mathbf{B}_{3 \times 3} = \begin{bmatrix} 5 & 3 & 7 \\ 0 & 1 & 6 \\ 0 & 0 & -2 \end{bmatrix}.$$

In these matrices, elements a_{12}, a_{13}, a_{23}, b_{21}, b_{31}, and b_{32} are zeros.

A matrix consisting of only one column is a column vector

$$x = \begin{bmatrix} 5 \\ 3 \\ 1 \\ 7 \end{bmatrix}.$$

A matrix consisting of only one row is called a row vector

$$x = \begin{bmatrix} 5 & -3 & 7 & 1 \end{bmatrix}.$$

A single value matrix is termed a *Scalar*

$$x = [6] \quad y = [1].$$

MATRIX OPERATIONS

The transposition of matrix **A** is written as **A′**. It is derived by merely exchanging the **A** rows and columns: $A_{r \times c} \Rightarrow A_{c \times r} \Rightarrow A'$

$$A_{4 \times 2} = \begin{bmatrix} 2 & 5 \\ 7 & 8 \\ 9 & 6 \\ 5 & 2 \end{bmatrix} \Rightarrow A'_{2 \times 4} = \begin{bmatrix} 2 & 7 & 9 & 5 \\ 5 & 8 & 6 & 2 \end{bmatrix}.$$

The transposition of $A' = A$.

$$A' = \begin{bmatrix} 1 \\ 7 \\ 3 \end{bmatrix} \Rightarrow A = \begin{bmatrix} 1 & 7 & 3 \end{bmatrix}$$

$$A' = \begin{bmatrix} 1 & 5 & 7 & 8 \\ 9 & 2 & -3 & 6 \\ 5 & 1 & 9 & 2 \end{bmatrix} \Rightarrow A = \begin{bmatrix} 1 & 9 & 5 \\ 5 & 2 & 1 \\ 7 & -3 & 9 \\ 8 & 6 & 2 \end{bmatrix}.$$

Two matrices are considered equal if their row or column elements are equal.

$$A = \begin{bmatrix} 3 & 2 \\ 6 & 4 \end{bmatrix} \Rightarrow B = \begin{bmatrix} 3 & 2 \\ 6 & 4 \end{bmatrix}.$$

ADDITION

Matrix addition procedures require that the matrices added are of the same order, that is,

$$\text{for } \mathbf{A}_{r \times c} + \mathbf{B}_{r \times c}, \quad r_{\mathbf{A}} = r_{\mathbf{B}} \text{ and } c_{\mathbf{A}} = c_{\mathbf{B}}.$$

The corresponding elements of each matrix are added.

$$
\begin{array}{ccccc}
\mathbf{A} & + & \mathbf{B} & = & \mathbf{C}
\end{array}
$$

$$
\begin{bmatrix} a_{11} \\ a_{21} \\ a_{31} \end{bmatrix} + \begin{bmatrix} b_{11} \\ b_{21} \\ b_{31} \end{bmatrix} = \begin{bmatrix} a_{11} + b_{11} \\ a_{21} + b_{21} \\ a_{31} + b_{31} \end{bmatrix}
$$

or

$$
\begin{array}{ccccc}
\mathbf{A} & + & \mathbf{B} & = & \mathbf{C}
\end{array}
$$

$$
\begin{bmatrix} 5 & 7 & 9 & 3 \\ 2 & 1 & 8 & 9 \\ 6 & 5 & 1 & 0 \end{bmatrix} + \begin{bmatrix} 7 & 3 & 2 & -1 \\ -10 & 6 & 1 & 3 \\ 7 & 2 & 9 & 11 \end{bmatrix} = \begin{bmatrix} 5+7 & 7+3 & 9+2 & 3-1 \\ 2-10 & 1+6 & 8+1 & 9+3 \\ 6+7 & 5+2 & 1+9 & 0+11 \end{bmatrix}
$$

$$
\begin{array}{c}
\mathbf{C}
\end{array}
$$

$$
= \begin{bmatrix} 12 & 10 & 11 & 2 \\ -8 & 7 & 9 & 12 \\ 13 & 7 & 10 & 11 \end{bmatrix}.
$$

If $\mathbf{A}_r \neq \mathbf{B}_r$ or $\mathbf{A}_c \neq \mathbf{B}_c$, the matrices cannot be summed.

SUBTRACTION

The matrix subtraction process also requires row–column order equality.

$$
\begin{array}{ccccc}
\mathbf{A} & - & \mathbf{B} & = & \mathbf{C}
\end{array}
$$

$$
\begin{bmatrix} a_{11} \\ a_{21} \\ a_{31} \end{bmatrix} - \begin{bmatrix} b_{11} \\ b_{21} \\ b_{31} \end{bmatrix} = \begin{bmatrix} a_{11} - b_{11} \\ a_{21} - b_{21} \\ a_{31} - b_{31} \end{bmatrix}
$$

$$
\begin{array}{ccccc}
\mathbf{A} & - & \mathbf{B} & = & \mathbf{C}
\end{array}
$$

$$
\begin{bmatrix} 7 & 5 & 3 & 9 \\ 6 & 5 & 3 & 5 \\ 1 & 9 & -3 & 0 \end{bmatrix} - \begin{bmatrix} 2 & 1 & 5 & 9 \\ 12 & -1 & 8 & 10 \\ 8 & 9 & 5 & 0 \end{bmatrix} = \begin{bmatrix} 7-2 & 5-1 & 3-5 & 9-9 \\ 6-12 & 5+1 & 3-8 & 5-10 \\ 1-8 & 9-9 & -3-5 & 0-0 \end{bmatrix}
$$

$$
\begin{array}{c}
\mathbf{C}
\end{array}
$$

$$
= \begin{bmatrix} 5 & 4 & -2 & 0 \\ -6 & 6 & -5 & -5 \\ -7 & 0 & -8 & 0 \end{bmatrix}.
$$

MULTIPLICATION

Matrix multiplication is a little more difficult. It is done by the following steps:

Step 1: Write down both matrices. To multiply the two matrices, the values of A_c and B_r must be the same (inside values; see later). If not, multiplication cannot be performed.

$$\mathbf{A}_{r \times c} \times \mathbf{B}_{r \times c}.$$

Step 2: The product of the multiplication provides an $r \times c$-size matrix (outside values; see the following).

$$\mathbf{A}_{r \times c} \times \mathbf{B}_{r \times c}.$$

Example: $a_{3 \times 1} = \begin{bmatrix} 1 \\ 2 \\ 7 \end{bmatrix}$ $\qquad b_{1 \times 3} = \begin{bmatrix} 12 & 3 & 9 \end{bmatrix}.$

Step 1: Write down both matrices, and note if inside terms are equal.

$$a_{3 \times 1} \times b_{1 \times 3}.$$

where $1 = 1$, the matrices can be multiplied, giving $\begin{bmatrix} a_r \times b_c \end{bmatrix}_{3 \times 3}$, that is a 3 row $\times$ 3 column matrix

$$a_{3 \times 1} \times b_{1 \times 3} = \mathbf{C} = \begin{bmatrix} c_{11} & c_{12} & c_{13} \\ c_{21} & c_{22} & c_{23} \\ c_{31} & c_{32} & c_{33} \end{bmatrix},$$

where $c_{11} = a$ (row 1)$\times b$ (column 1), $c_{12} = a$ (row 1)$\times b$ (column 2), and so on.

$$
\begin{array}{ccccc}
a_{3 \times 1} & \times & b_{1 \times 3} & = & c_{3 \times 3}
\end{array}
$$

$$\begin{bmatrix} 1 \\ 2 \\ 7 \end{bmatrix} \times \begin{bmatrix} 12 & 3 & 9 \end{bmatrix} = \begin{bmatrix} 1 \times 12 = 12 & 1 \times 3 = 3 & 1 \times 9 = 9 \\ 2 \times 12 = 24 & 2 \times 3 = 6 & 2 \times 9 = 18 \\ 7 \times 12 = 84 & 7 \times 3 = 21 & 7 \times 9 = 63 \end{bmatrix}.$$

Let us look at another example.

$$\mathbf{A}_{3 \times 3} = \begin{bmatrix} 3 & 2 & 5 \\ 6 & 7 & 9 \\ 8 & 2 & 1 \end{bmatrix} \quad \mathbf{B}_{3 \times 4} = \begin{bmatrix} 5 & -1 & 8 & 0 \\ 2 & 0 & 5 & 2 \\ 3 & 1 & 7 & 5 \end{bmatrix}.$$

Let us multiply.

Step 1: Write out the matrix order.

$$\mathbf{A}_{3\times3} \times \mathbf{B}_{3\times4}.$$

The inside dimensions are the same, so we can multiply.

Step 2: Write out the product matrix (outside terms).

$$\mathbf{A}_{3\times3} \times \mathbf{B}_{3\times4} = \mathbf{C}_{3\times4}.$$

$$\mathbf{C}_{3\times4} = \begin{bmatrix} c_{11} & c_{12} & c_{13} & c_{14} \\ c_{21} & c_{22} & c_{23} & c_{24} \\ c_{31} & c_{32} & c_{33} & c_{34} \end{bmatrix}.$$

The c_{11} element is the sum of the products for the entire row 1 of **A** multiplied by the entire column 1 of **B**.

$$\mathbf{A} = \begin{bmatrix} 3 & 2 & 5 \\ 6 & 7 & 9 \\ 8 & 2 & 1 \end{bmatrix} \times \mathbf{B} = \begin{bmatrix} 5 & -1 & 8 & 0 \\ 2 & 0 & 5 & 2 \\ 3 & 1 & 7 & 5 \end{bmatrix} = \mathbf{C}$$

$$= \begin{bmatrix} c_{11} = 3 \times 5 + 2 \times 2 + 5 \times 3 = 34 \\ \\ \\ \end{bmatrix}.$$

Let us work the entire problem by the following demonstration:

$c_{11} = 34$

$c_{12} = \mathbf{A}$ row $1\times\mathbf{B}$ column $2 = 3\times-1 + 2\times0 + 5\times1 = 2$

$c_{13} = \mathbf{A}$ row $1\times\mathbf{B}$ column $3 = 3\times8 + 2\times5 + 5\times7 = 69$

$c_{14} = \mathbf{A}$ row $1\times\mathbf{B}$ column $4 = 3\times0 + 2\times2 + 5\times5 = 29$

$c_{21} = \mathbf{A}$ row $2\times\mathbf{B}$ column $1 = 6\times5 + 7\times2 + 9\times3 = 71$

$c_{22} = \mathbf{A}$ row $2\times\mathbf{B}$ column $2 = 6\times-1 + 7\times0 + 9\times1 = 3$

$c_{23} = \mathbf{A}$ row $2\times\mathbf{B}$ column $3 = 6\times8 + 7\times5 + 9\times7 = 146$

$c_{24} = \mathbf{A}$ row $2\times\mathbf{B}$ column $4 = 6\times0 + 7\times2 + 9\times5 = 59$

$c_{31} = \mathbf{A}$ row $3\times\mathbf{B}$ column $1 = 8\times5 + 2\times2 + 1\times3 = 47$

$c_{32} = \mathbf{A}$ row $3\times\mathbf{B}$ column $2 = 8\times-1 + 2\times0 + 1\times1 = -7$

$c_{33} = \mathbf{A}$ row $3\times\mathbf{B}$ column $3 = 8\times8 + 2\times5 + 1\times7 = 81$

$c_{34} = \mathbf{A}$ row $3\times\mathbf{B}$ column $4 = 8\times0 + 2\times2 + 1\times5 = 9$

$$\mathbf{C}_{3\times4}\begin{bmatrix} c_{11} & c_{12} & c_{13} & c_{14} \\ c_{21} & c_{22} & c_{23} & c_{24} \\ c_{31} & c_{32} & c_{33} & c_{34} \end{bmatrix} = \begin{bmatrix} 34 & 2 & 69 & 29 \\ 71 & 3 & 146 & 59 \\ 47 & -7 & 81 & 9 \end{bmatrix}.$$

Needless to say, the job is far easier using a computer. To perform this same process interactively using MiniTab software, one merely inputs the $r \times c$ size and matrix data to create M1.

MTB > read 3 by 3 in M1

DATA > 3 2 5

DATA > 6 7 9   } = A

DATA > 8 2 1

3 rows read.

MTB > read 3 by 4 in M2

DATA > 5 − 1 8 0

DATA > 2 0 5 2   } = B

DATA > 3 1 7 5

3 rows read.

MTB > print M1

Data Display

Matrix M1 = A

3 2 5

6 7 9

8 2 1

MTB > print M2

Data Display

Matrix M2 = B

5−1 8 0

2 0 5 2

3 1 7 5

MTB > mult m1 by m2 put in m3 (A $\times$ B = C)

MTB> print m3

Data Display

Matrix M3

$$\mathbf{C} = \begin{bmatrix} 34 & 2 & 69 & 29 \\ 71 & 3 & 146 & 59 \\ 47 & -7 & 81 & 9 \end{bmatrix}$$

You can see that matrix algebra is far easier using a computer.

INVERSE OF MATRIX

In algebra, the inverse of a number is its reciprocal, $x^{-1} = 1/x$. In matrix algebra, the inverse is conceptually the same, but the conversion usually requires a great deal of computation, except for the very simplest of matrices. If a solution exists, then $\mathbf{A} \times \mathbf{A}^{-1} = \mathbf{I}$. $\mathbf{I}$ is a very useful matrix named as an identity matrix, where the diagonal elements are 1 and the nondiagonal elements are 0.

$$\text{For example,} \quad \mathbf{I} = \begin{bmatrix} 1 & 0 & 0 \\ 0 & 1 & 0 \\ 0 & 0 & 1 \end{bmatrix} \quad \text{or} \quad \mathbf{I} = \begin{bmatrix} 1 & 0 & 0 & 0 & \cdots & 0 \\ 0 & 1 & 0 & 0 & \cdots & 0 \\ 0 & 0 & 1 & 0 & \cdots & 0 \\ 0 & 0 & 0 & 1 & \cdots & 0 \\ \vdots & \vdots & \vdots & \vdots & \vdots & \vdots \\ 0 & 0 & 0 & 0 & \cdots & 1 \end{bmatrix}.$$

The inverse computation is much time-consuming to perform by hand, so its calculation is done by a computer program.

Let us now look at matrices as they relate to regression analyses.

$\mathbf{Y}_{r \times 1} = $ vector of the observed y_i values

$$\mathbf{Y}_{r \times 1} = \begin{bmatrix} y_1 \\ y_2 \\ y_3 \\ \vdots \\ y_n \end{bmatrix}$$

$$\mathbf{Y}'_{r \times 1} = \begin{bmatrix} y_1 & y_2 & y_3 & \cdots & y_n \end{bmatrix}.$$

The x_i values are placed in an **X** matrix. For example, in simple linear regression,

$$\hat{y} = b_0 + b_1 x.$$

The **X** matrix is

$$\mathbf{X}_{r \times c} = \begin{matrix} x_0 & x_1 \\ \begin{bmatrix} 1 & x_1 \\ 1 & x_2 \\ 1 & x_3 \\ \vdots & \vdots \\ n & x_n \end{bmatrix} \end{matrix}.$$

For any regression equation of k parameters, $(b_1, b_2, \ldots, b_k)$, there are $k + 1$ columns and n rows.

The first column contains all ones, which are dummy variables, where $x_0 = 1$

$$\mathbf{X}' = \begin{matrix} x_0 \\ x_1 \end{matrix} \begin{bmatrix} 1 & 1 & \cdots & n \\ x_1 & x_2 & \cdots & x_n \end{bmatrix}.$$

Sometimes, it is necessary to compute $\sum y_i^2$. From a matrix standpoint, the operation is

$$\mathbf{y}'\mathbf{y} = [y_1, y_2, \ldots, y_n] \begin{bmatrix} y_1 \\ y_2 \\ \vdots \\ y_n \end{bmatrix} = a_{1 \times 1} \text{matrix}, \quad \text{which is } \sum_{i=1}^{n} y_i^2.$$

In simple linear regression, the matrix $\mathbf{X}'\mathbf{X}$ produces several useful calculations

$$\mathbf{X}'\mathbf{X} = \begin{bmatrix} 1 & 1 & \cdots & 1 \\ x_1 & x_2 & \cdots & x_n \end{bmatrix} \begin{bmatrix} 1 & x_1 \\ 1 & x_2 \\ \vdots & \vdots \\ 1 & x_n \end{bmatrix} = \begin{bmatrix} n & \sum x_i \\ \sum x_i & \sum x_i^2 \end{bmatrix}.$$

In addition, $\mathbf{X'Y}$ produces

$$\mathbf{X'Y} = \begin{bmatrix} 1 & 1 & \cdots & 1 \\ x_1 & x_2 & \cdots & x_n \end{bmatrix} \begin{bmatrix} y_1 \\ y_2 \\ \vdots \\ y_n \end{bmatrix} = \begin{bmatrix} \sum y_i \\ \sum x_i y_i \end{bmatrix}.$$

This makes the elementary calculations of n, $\sum x_i$, $\sum y_i$, $\sum x_i y_i$, and so on, unnecessary.

Let us look further into simple linear regression through matrix algebra: $\hat{y}_i = b_0 + b_1 x_1 + e_i$ is given in matrix terms as $\mathbf{Y} = \mathbf{Xb} + e$, where

$$\begin{matrix} \mathbf{Y} & & \mathbf{X} & & & e \end{matrix}$$
$$\begin{bmatrix} y_1 \\ y_2 \\ \vdots \\ y_n \end{bmatrix} = \begin{bmatrix} 1 & x_1 \\ 1 & x_2 \\ \vdots & \vdots \\ 1 & x_n \end{bmatrix} \begin{bmatrix} b \\ b_0 \\ b_1 \end{bmatrix} + \begin{bmatrix} e_1 \\ e_2 \\ \vdots \\ e_n \end{bmatrix}.$$

Multiplying $\mathbf{Xb}$, that is, $\mathbf{X} \times b$, one gets $\hat{y}$

$$\mathbf{Xb} = \begin{bmatrix} b_0 + b_1 x_1 \\ b_0 + b_2 x_2 \\ \vdots \\ b_0 + b_1 x_n \end{bmatrix} = \hat{\mathbf{Y}} \quad \text{and} \quad \mathbf{Xb} + e = \begin{bmatrix} b_0 + b_1 x_1 + e_1 \\ b_0 + b_1 x_2 + e_3 \\ \vdots \\ b_0 + b_1 x_n + e_n \end{bmatrix} = \mathbf{Y}.$$

$$\mathbf{Y} = E[\mathbf{Y}] = \mathbf{Xb}.$$

The researcher does not know what the error values are, except that they sum to 0, $E[e] = 0$.

Also,

$$\boldsymbol{\sigma}_\varepsilon^2 = \begin{bmatrix} \sigma^2 & 0 & 0 & 0 \\ 0 & \sigma^2 & 0 & 0 \\ \vdots & \vdots & \vdots & \vdots \\ 0 & 0 & 0 & \sigma^2 \end{bmatrix}$$

or

$$\sigma^2 \mathbf{I} = \sigma_{(E)}^2.$$

The normal matrix equation for all regression work is $\mathbf{Y} = \mathbf{X}b + e$, and the least-square calculation by matrix algebra is $b = (\mathbf{X'X})^{-1} \mathbf{X'Y}$.

Let us do a regression using a simple linear model.

For $\hat{y} = b_0 + b_1 x_1$, we compute $b = (\mathbf{X'X})^{-1} \mathbf{X'Y}$,

where

y	x
9	1
8	1
10	1
10	2
12	2
11	2
15	3
14	3
13	3
17	4
18	4
19	4

For an interactive system, such as MiniTab, the data are keyed in as

```
MTB > read 12 1 m1        Reads a 12×1 matrix labeled
                          M1. This is the Y vector.

DATA > 9
DATA > 8
DATA > 10
DATA > 10
DATA > 12
DATA > 11
DATA > 15
DATA > 14
DATA > 13
DATA > 17
DATA > 18
DATA > 19
```

The result of M1 is displayed as

$$Y = \begin{bmatrix} 9 \\ 8 \\ 10 \\ 10 \\ 12 \\ 11 \\ 15 \\ 14 \\ 13 \\ 17 \\ 18 \\ 19 \end{bmatrix}.$$

For **X**, we key in x_0 and x_1.

MTB > read 12 2 m2	Reads a 12 × 2 matrix labeled
DATA > 1 1	M2
DATA > 1 1	
DATA > 1 1	
DATA > 1 2	
DATA > 1 2	
DATA > 1 2	
DATA > 1 3	
DATA > 1 3	
DATA > 1 3	
DATA > 1 4	
DATA > 1 4	
DATA > 1 4	

The result of M2 is displayed as

$$X = \begin{bmatrix} 1 & 1 \\ 1 & 1 \\ 1 & 1 \\ 1 & 2 \\ 1 & 2 \\ 1 & 2 \\ 1 & 3 \\ 1 & 3 \\ 1 & 3 \\ 1 & 4 \\ 1 & 4 \\ 1 & 4 \end{bmatrix}.$$

The transposition of **X** is M3:

$$\mathbf{X}' = \begin{bmatrix} 1 & 1 & 1 & 1 & 1 & 1 & 1 & 1 & 1 & 1 & 1 & 1 \\ 1 & 1 & 1 & 2 & 2 & 2 & 3 & 3 & 3 & 4 & 4 & 4 \end{bmatrix}.$$

Next, we multiply—that is, $\mathbf{X}'\mathbf{X}$—and put the product into M4.

$\mathbf{X}'_{2\times12} \times \mathbf{X}_{12\times2}$, hence, the resultant product will be a 2×2 matrix.

The MiniTab command is

MTB > mult m3 m2, m4

$$\mathbf{X}'\mathbf{X} = \begin{bmatrix} 12 & 30 \\ 30 & 90 \end{bmatrix}.$$

Recall

$$\mathbf{X}'\mathbf{X} = \begin{bmatrix} n & \sum x_i \\ \sum x_i & \sum x_i^2 \end{bmatrix} = \begin{bmatrix} 12 & 30 \\ 30 & 90 \end{bmatrix},$$

which is very useful for other computations by hand.
Next, we find the inverse of $(\mathbf{X}'\mathbf{X})^{-1}$.
The MiniTab command is
MTB > inverse m4, m5

$$(\mathbf{X}'\mathbf{X})^{-1} = \begin{bmatrix} 0.500000 & -0.166667 \\ -0.166667 & 0.066667 \end{bmatrix}.$$

The inverse is multiplied by $\mathbf{X}'$:

$$(\mathbf{X}'\mathbf{X})^{-1}_{2\times2} \quad \mathbf{X}'_{2\times12}$$

MTB > mult m5, m3, m6

$$\mathbf{X}' = \begin{bmatrix} 0.333333 & 0.333333 & 0.333333 & 0.166667 & 0.166667 & 0.166667 & 0.000000 & -0.00000 & -0.000000 & -0.166667 & -0.166667 & -0.166667 \\ -0.100000 & -0.100000 & -0.100000 & -0.033333 & -0.033333 & -0.033333 & 0.033333 & 0.033333 & 0.033333 & 0.100000 & 0.100000 & 0.100000 \end{bmatrix}.$$

Finally, we multiply by **Y**, $(\mathbf{X}'\mathbf{X})^{-1}\mathbf{X}'\mathbf{Y}$
    MTB > mult m5 by m1, m7, which gives us

$$b = \begin{bmatrix} 5.5 \\ 3.0 \end{bmatrix}, \quad \text{that is,} \quad \begin{cases} b_0 = 5.5, \\ b_1 = 3.0. \end{cases}$$

Therefore, the final regression equation is
$\hat{y} = 5.5 + 3.0x$ or, in matrix form, $\hat{Y} = Xb$.
The key strokes are
MTB > mult m2 by m7, m8

$$\hat{Y} = \begin{bmatrix} 8.5 \\ 8.5 \\ 8.5 \\ 11.5 \\ 11.5 \\ 11.5 \\ 14.5 \\ 14.5 \\ 14.5 \\ 17.5 \\ 17.5 \\ 17.5 \end{bmatrix}.$$

This vector consists of the predicted $\hat{y}_i$ values to determine the error $Y - \hat{Y} = e$.
Subtract M8 from M1, M9 for matrix M9:

$$e = Y - \hat{Y} = \begin{bmatrix} 0.50000 \\ -0.50000 \\ 1.50000 \\ -1.50000 \\ 0.50000 \\ -0.50000 \\ 0.50000 \\ -0.50000 \\ -1.50000 \\ -0.50000 \\ 0.50000 \\ 1.50000 \end{bmatrix}.$$

Now, for larger sets of data, one does not want to key the data into a matrix, but rather, would read it from a text file. Finally, in statistics, use of the Hat Matrix is valuable, particularly in diagnostics such as discovering outlier values by the Studentized and jackknife tests. The diagonal is used in these tests.

$$\mathbf{H}_{n \times n} = \mathbf{X}(\mathbf{X'X})^{-1}\mathbf{X'}.$$

The regression can also be determined by

$$\widehat{\mathbf{Y}} = \mathbf{HY}.$$

Several other matrix operations we use are as follows:

$$SS_T = \mathbf{Y'Y} - \left(\frac{1}{n}\right)\mathbf{Y'JY}$$

$$SS_E = \mathbf{Y'Y} - \boldsymbol{b'}\mathbf{X'Y}$$

$$SS_R = \boldsymbol{b'}\mathbf{X'Y} - \left(\frac{1}{n}\right)\mathbf{Y'JY},$$

where $\mathbf{J}$ is the matrix of $\begin{bmatrix} 1 & 1 & 1 & 1 \\ 1 & 1 & 1 & 1 \end{bmatrix}$ and is an $n \times n$ size.

The variance matrix is the diagonal of

$$s^2\boldsymbol{b} = MS_E(\mathbf{X'X})^{-1}$$

$$s^2\boldsymbol{b} = \begin{bmatrix} s_{b_0}^2 & & & \\ & s_{b_1}^2 & & \\ & & \ddots & \\ & & & s_{b_k}^2 \end{bmatrix}.$$

References

Aitkin, M.A. (1974). "Simultaneous inference and the choice of variable subsets." *Technometrics*, 16, 221–227.

Assagioli, R. 1973. *The Act of Will*. New York: Viking Press.

Belsley, D.A., Kuh, E., and Welsch, R.F. 1980. *Regression Diagnostics: Identifying influential data sources of collinearity*. New York: John Wiley & Sons.

Box, G.E.P., Hunter, J.S., and Hunter, W.G. 2005. *Statistics for Experimenters: Design, Innovation, and Discovery*, 2nd edn. Hoboken, NJ: John Wiley & Sons, Inc.

Draper, N.R. and Smith, H. 1998. *Applied Regression Analysis*, 3rd edn. New York, NY: John Wiley & Sons.

Green, R.H. 1979. *Sampling Designs and Statistical Methods for Environmental Biologists*. New York: John Wiley & Sons.

Hoaglin, D.C. and Welsch, R.E. 1978. The hat matrix in regression and ANOVA. *Am. Stat.*, 32, 17–22.

Hoerl, A.E. and Kennard, R.W. 1976. Ridge regression: iterative estimation of the biasing parameter. *Commun. Stat.*, 5, 77–88.

Hoerl, A.E., Kennard, R.W., and Baldwin, K.F. 1975. Ridge regression: some simulations. *Commun. Stat.*, 4, 105–123.

Kleinbaum, D.G., Kupper, L.L., Muller, K.E., and Nizam, Azhar. 1998. *Applied Regression Analysis and Other Multivariable Methods*, 3rd edn. Pacific Grove, CA: Duxbury Press.

Kutner, M.H., Nachtsheim, C.J., Neter, J., and Li, W. 2005. *Applied Linear Statistical Models*, 5th edn. New York: McGraw-Hill.

Lapin, L. 1977. *Statistics: Meaning and Method*. New York: Harcourt Brace Jovanovich, Inc.

Maslow, A.H. 1971. *The Farther Reaches of Human Nature*. New York: Viking.

Montgomery, D.C., Peck, E.A., and Vining, G.G. 2001. *Introduction to Linear Regression Analysis*, 3rd edn. New York, NY: John Wiley & Sons.

Neter, J. and Wasserman, W. 1983. *Applied Linear Statistical Models*. Homewood, IL: Irwin.

Neter, J., Wasserman, W., and Kutner, M.H. 1983. *Applied Linear Regression Models*. Homewood, IL: Irwin.

Paulson, D.S. 2003. *Applied Statistical Designs for the Researcher*. New York: Marcel Dekker, Inc.

Polkinghorne, D. 1983. *Methodology For The Human Sciences*. Albany, NY: State University of New York Press.

Riffenburg, R.H. 2006. *Statistics in Medicine*, 2nd edn. Boston: Elsevier.

Salsburg, D.S. 1992. *The use of Restricted Significance Tests in Clinical Trials*. New York: Springer-Verlag.

Searle, R. 1995. *The Construction of Social Reality*. New York: Free Press.

Sears, D.O., Peplau, L.A., and Taylor, S.E. 1991. *Social Psychology,* 7th edn. New York: McGraw-Hill.

Sokal, R.R and Rohlf, F.J. (1994). *Biometry. The principles and practice of statistics in biological research,* 3rd ed. San Francisco, CA: W.H. Freeman and Company.

Tukey, J.W. 1971. *Exploratory Data Analysis.* Reading, MA: Addison-Wesley.

Varela, F. and Shear, J. 1999. *The view from within.* Lawrence, KS: Imprint Academic Press.

Index